MICROALBUMINURIA
BIOCHEMISTRY, EPIDEMIOLOGY
AND CLINICAL PRACTICE

Microalbuminuria, the abnormal urinary excretion of albumin, is recognised as an important independent marker of both renal and cardiovascular disease, particularly in diabetes mellitus. This volume is the only comprehensive and up-to-date review of the relevance of microalbuminuria to health and disease. It covers the pathophysiology and epidemiology of microalbuminuria, methodology of laboratory assessment, as well as a discussion of the non-specific nature of microalbuminuria in less well-recognised clinical situations. This is the first book to deal in detail with the treatment of microalbuminuria in diabetic and non-diabetic subjects.

It will provide an essential source of reference and a guide to clinical practice for diabetologists, endocrinologists, cardiologists, renal physicians and clinical biochemists.

DR PETER WINOCOUR trained in diabetes and endocrinology in Manchester and Newcastle and has published numerous articles on dyslipidaemia, hypertension and nephropathy, particularly in diabetes mellitus. Born in Glasgow on 2nd December 1956, he trained at the University of Glasgow and has served as a committee member of the British Hyperlipidaemia Association. His MD thesis was on the subject of metabolic control and complications in insulin-dependent diabetes mellitus. He is Consultant Physician at the Queen Elizabeth II Hospital, Welwyn Garden City, and Honorary Senior Lecturer at the Royal Free Hospital School of Medicine, London.

DR SALLY MARSHALL graduated with first class honours in biochemistry from the University of Glasgow in 1975, and with MB ChB in 1978. Her MD, for a thesis on microalbuminuria in diabetes, was awarded in 1990. She has published numerous articles on diabetes, particularly on several aspects of diabetic nephropathy. She has served as a committee member of the European Diabetic Nephropathy Study Group and is currently Chairman of the Professional Advisory Committee of the British Diabetic Association. She is Reader in Diabetes in the University of Newcastle upon Tyne, and Honorary Consultant Physician in the Royal Victoria Infirmary NHS Trust.

MICROALBUMINURIA

Biochemistry, epidemiology and clinical practice

PETER H. WINOCOUR

Consultant Physician, Queen Elizabeth II Hospital, Welwyn Garden City,
Honorary Senior Lecturer, Royal Free Hospital School of Medicine

and

SALLY M. MARSHALL

Reader in Diabetes Medicine, Department of Medicine, University of Newcastle upon Tyne,
Honorary Consultant Physician, Royal Victoria Infirmary, Newcastle upon Tyne

Foreword by
K. G. M. M. ALBERTI

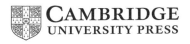

CAMBRIDGE
UNIVERSITY PRESS

PUBLISHED BY THE PRESS SYNDICATE OF THE UNIVERSITY OF CAMBRIDGE
The Pitt Building, Trumpington Street, Cambridge CB2 1RP, United Kingdom

CAMBRIDGE UNIVERSITY PRESS
The Edinburgh Building, Cambridge CB2 2RU, UK http://www.cup.cam.ac.uk
40 West 20th Street, New York, NY 10011-4211, USA http://www.cup.org
10 Stamford Road, Oakleigh, Melbourne 3166, Australia

First published 1998

Printed in the United Kingdom at the University Press, Cambridge

Typeset in Times 11/14pt by Keyword plc, Wallington, Surrey

A catalogue record for this book is available from the British Library

ISBN 0 521 45703 3 paperback

Contents

v

Preface

The interest in, and importance of, microalbuminuria is reflected in the exponential increase in the number of publications on the topic over the last few years. We recognised at commissioning of this book in 1993 that we were chasing a rapidly moving target. In persevering with this flood of literature our objective was to temper the enthusiastic discussion of microalbuminuria as a one-dimensional risk factor in diabetes and to broaden the discussion into other areas of general medicine. At the same time, we have tried to put the difficulties surrounding the measurement of microalbuminuria and the treatment of microalbuminuria in diabetes into an appropriate clinical context. We were also encouraged by the knowledge that such a book covering the broadest aspects of microalbuminuria had not previously been written.

Our interest in the subject has been stimulated over the last 15 years by our initially separately developed interests in Manchester and Newcastle, and subsequently by the opportunity to work together in George Alberti's powerhouse in the Department of Medicine, University of Newcastle upon Tyne from 1993 to 1997. The unplanned geographical splitting and conversion for one of us, from a University teaching post to a full-time National Health Service position, has added a touch of excitement regarding communication and ensuring that the manuscript is up to date. Modern technology has not totally alleviated these difficulties.

In addition to our undoubted gratitude to George Alberti, we would like to thank our many other colleagues and mentors who have provided stimulation and moral support over the last 15 years: Professor David Anderson, Dr Harold Cohen, Professor Paul Durrington, the late Dr John Ireland, Dr Rudy Bilous, Dr Jean Mcleod, Dr Carlo Catalano, Dr Steve Jones, Dr Martin Rutter, Dr Deepak Bhatnagar, Dr Laura Baines, Mrs Catherine White, Mrs Pat Shearing, Professor Philip Home, Professor Robert Wilkinson, Dr Trevor Thomas, and Professor Roy Taylor.

Finally we must acknowledge the patient and expert support from the staff of Cambridge University Press for bearing with us in times of chaos and confusion.

The book is dedicated to our families and friends who have borne the brunt of our frustrations in the preparation of this manuscript.

Peter H. Winocour
Welwyn Garden City
Sally M. Marshall
Newcastle upon Tyne

Foreword

The appearance of small amounts of albumin in the urine, which were less than those detected by conventional methods at the time but higher than normal, was first noted by Professor Keen and colleagues in the 1960s. Little further was done for 15 years until groups in London and Denmark started to look in more detail at urine protein excretion in people with diabetes. This intermediate grade of proteinuria between dip-stick detectable and normal was referred to as microalbuminuria – a totally inaccurate name but one that has stuck! Since then a vast amount of work has accumulated and many publications on the subject have appeared. Of particular interest is the fact that these small amounts of protein in the urine are associated not just with more rapid progression to end stage renal failure but with subsequent cardiovascular disease mortality and morbidity. Initially, studies focused on type 1 diabetes, but now there is much literature on type 2 as well, and increasing awareness of the relevance of microalbuminuria in non-diabetic renal and vascular disease.

For many physicians the amount of literature on microalbuminuria is overwhelming and hence tends not to be read. The present book by Drs Winocour and Marshall provides a succinct account of what we know about microalbuminuria, not just in relation to renal function but with regard to the broader aspects of diabetes. The book fills a large gap in the diabetes and renal literature. Importantly, the relevance of microalbuminuria in non-diabetic hypertension and other medical conditions is also examined. The book will, I hope, be of benefit to many people working in diabetes who would like to be updated but do not have time to hunt through voluminous tomes in dusty libraries or scan the Internet. It should be of particular interest to those working on complications in diabetes, but will also appeal to students and generalists alike interested in glomerular and cardiovascular disease.

K.G.M.M. Alberti
President,
Royal College of Physicians, London

1

Renal structure and physiology

The kidney is an organ with endocrine properties, and the capacity to synthesise and catabolise proteins. However, its fundamental role is to remove fluid and potentially toxic substances by the production of urine as an ultrafiltrate of plasma, and to maintain homeostasis of body protein. These latter functions are the task of the nephron, a microscopic unit comprising the glomerulus, Bowman's capsule, proximal and distal convoluted tubules, and the collecting ducts (Fig. 1.1). The various components of the nephron interact with the systemic circulation, thereby influencing renal handling of plasma proteins. Before discussing this in detail, the structure of the nephron components will be summarised briefly.

The glomerulus is a capillary network composed of a thin layer of endothelial cells, a central region of mesangial cells with surrounding mesangial matrix material, visceral epithelial cells with associated basement membrane, and the parietal epithelial cells of Bowman's capsule with its basement membrane. Bowman's (urinary) space lies between these two epithelial layers, and afferent and efferent arterioles control the capillary blood flow (Fig. 1.1). Glomeruli are innervated by autonomic nerves, and neural control may be particularly important in the larger juxtamedullary glomeruli, close to which is the site of renin secretion.

Molecules in the glomerular ultrafiltrate may traverse the filtration barrier from blood into the urinary space. The barrier has three major components (Fig. 1.2):

1. **Capillary endothelial cells:** These are perforated by fenestrae up to 100 nm in diameter, close to which is an extensive network of filaments and microtubules. They have a negative surface charge due to the presence of podocalcyn, a polyanionic glycoprotein. The structure and function of endothelial cells will be discussed in more detail in Chapter 5.

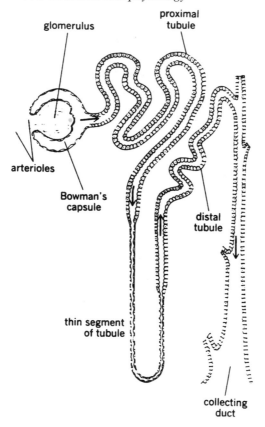

Fig. 1.1 The basic structure of a nephron.

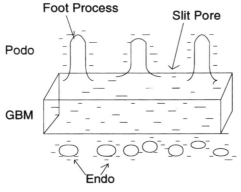

Fig. 1.2 The components of the glomerular filtration barrier. Podo: podocyte or epithelial cell. GBM: glomerular basement membrane. Endo: capillary endothelial cell.

2. **Glomerular basement membrane:** These also possess a fixed negative charge, the anionic sites consisting of glycosaminoglycans (GAGs) associated with procollagen-like molecules.
3. **Visceral epithelial cells:** These are also known as podocytes, and are the largest cells in the glomerulus. They possess long cytoplasmic trabeculae which divide into 'foot processes' and come into close contact with the glomerular basement membrane. The 'slit pores' are the gaps between adjacent foot processes. As with the other barrier components, the surface of the podocyte foot processes is negatively charged, due to the presence of sialic acid. Podocytes are responsible in part for the synthesis and maintenance of basement membrane components such as collagen, prostaglandins and GAG.

The glomerular mesangial cells, adjacent to the endothelium, are in fact specialised pericytes which possess smooth muscle cell and phagocytic properties. Their main function is to provide structural support for capillary loops, but contractile properties in response to vasoactive agents confer the ability to reduce glomerular filtration. The surrounding matrix is composed of sulphated GAG, fibronectin, and laminin. The cells of the proximal convoluted tubule contain membrane bound organelles (lysosomes) adjacent to the lumen, which are involved in endocytotic protein reabsorption. The subsequent tubular components are more fundamentally involved with electrolyte handling and urinary concentration and acidification, although distal tubular feedback in response to rate of urine flow and solute (particularly chloride) entry appears to then exert control over intrarenal (i.e. glomerular) haemodynamics, a process known as autoregulation.

Mechanisms of urinary protein excretion (Table 1.1)

Under physiological conditions, normal urine contains no more than one-millionth of the 12 600 g of protein filtered daily by the glomeruli. This reflects the efficiency of the glomerulus as a sieve, and the reabsorptive capacity of the tubular cells (Fig. 1.3). Perhaps no more than 60 % of urinary protein excretion is normally derived from the glomerular ultrafiltrate of plasma, the remainder produced by the kidney and the lower urinary tract. Glomerular and, to a lesser extent tubular protein handling are the most important determinants of abnormal patterns of protein excretion.

The initial glomerular ultrafiltrate is the net balance of the transcapillary hydraulic pressure and intravascular colloid osmotic pressure, respectively reflecting efferent arteriolar flow rate and pressure, and plasma protein concentration. As mentioned earlier, renal vascular flow is influenced by neural

Table 1.1. *Factors determining the constituents of excreted urinary protein*

Glomerular protein filtration
1. Renal plasma flow
2. Oncotic pressure
3. Protein size
4. Protein charge
5. Protein configuration
6. Glomerular basement membrane integrity and charge

Tubular protein handling
1. Tubular reabsorptive capacity
2. Competition from other proteins and solutes
3. Tubular secretion
4. Tubular catabolism
5. Tubulo-glomerular feedback

Renal tract protein excretion
1. Distal tubular secretion

Lower genito-urinary tract protein secretion and extravasation

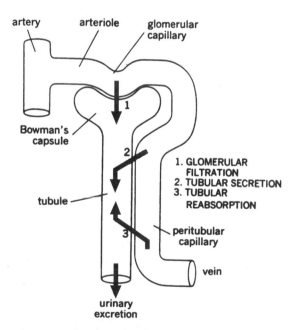

Fig. 1.3. The three basic components of normal urine production.

factors, tubulo-glomerular feedback, and also hormones and vasoactive substances (Table 1.2). Although renal blood flow usually reflects systemic blood flow and is a major determinant of glomerular filtration, it is attenuated by adrenergic neural activity. Furthermore, considerable variation in intrarenal haemodynamics is known to take place in response to local vasoconstrictive influences, such as angiotensin II and vasodilatory prostaglandins. Individual characteristics of plasma proteins (plasma concentration, size, charge, configuration and rigidity) and the integrity of the glomerular filtration barrier also determine the composition of the ultrafiltrate. Most circulating proteins have net negative charges, particularly those of the molecular weight of albumin or lower, and there is electrostatic repulsion between the protein molecules and the filtration barrier, since both are polyanionic. Molecules with neutral electrical charge such as IgG are less influenced by the polyanionic nature of the barrier, whereas molecules with a net positive charge more easily interact with the barrier[1]. Thus small uncharged molecules such as beta$_2$- microglobulin, retinol-binding protein and alpha$_1$-microglobulin (up to 30 kdaltons (kd)) pass freely into the urinary space in addition to water and electrolytes, whereas the passage of negatively charged molecules of intermediate size, such as albumin (67 kd), is normally impeded at the endothelial surface of the glomerular basement membrane.

Both diffusion and filtration (bulk flow) contribute to transglomerular protein passage. The selectivity index is based on the fractional excretion of two molecules of different size and charge, such as albumin and IgG. It can be used to confirm that the restrictive properties of the glomerular barrier remain intact. Factors such as non-enzymatic glycation (*vide infra*) may alter the charge of proteins and of the filtration barrier, thereby modifying this process[2]. Molecular heterogeneity of individual proteins may also alter glomerular handling in healthy subjects. For example, there is evidence that excessive binding of non-esterified fatty acids to albumin leads to distinctive changes in conformation, size, charge and ligand reactivity, with subsequent increased excretion and different chromatographic patterns of albuminuria[3]. This selectivity is lost in disease, when albumin with a low fatty acid content is excreted in greater amounts.

Thereafter, filtered proteins are normally reabsorbed by cells of the proximal convoluted tubule. This is achieved by pinocytosis, an energy-dependent process with high capacity but low affinity. As in the glomerulus, tubular cells selectively reabsorb proteins. The mechanism is not fully understood, although charge–charge interactions appear to influence the concentration of luminal proteins stored in endocytotic vesicles at the apex of tubular epithelial cells. Specific receptor-mediated uptake has not yet been demon-

Table 1.2. *Hormonal and vasoactive factors which modify renal blood flow*

Vasodilators	Vasoconstrictors
Prostaglandin E_1 and E_2	Angiotensin II
Serotonin (5HT)	Adrenaline
Acetylcholine	Insulin-like growth factor 1
Cyclic AMP	Epidermal growth factor
Endothelial-derived relaxing factor (nitric oxide)	Leukotrienes
Growth hormone	Endothelin
Atrial natriuretic peptide	Vasopressin
Bradykinin	
Insulin	
Insulin-like growth factor I (pharmacological effect)	
Glucagon	

strated, but it does appear that proteins may compete for uptake, with increased filtration of either low or high molecular weight proteins leading to increased urinary excretion of other proteins[4,5]. Tubular protein uptake may also be modified by urinary flow rates, and impeded by solute components such as glucose, amino acids, ketone bodies and toxic proteins such as immunoglobulin light chains. Following reabsorption, partial intracellular hydrolysis to amino acids, and then secretion into the circulation takes place. Under certain conditions, transtubular transport of intact protein may occur. Fractional reabsorption of low molecular weight proteins in healthy individuals has been estimated at 99.97 %, whereas that of albumin varies between 92 and 99 %.

Direct tubular secretion of proteins also contributes to urinary protein excretion. The Tamm Horsfall mucoprotein is a large (23 000 kd) acidic glycoprotein derived from the epithelial surface membranes of the thick ascending loop of Henle and the early distal convoluted tubule. It is the major constituent of urinary casts, and has recently been shown to be identical in sequence to uromodulin, suggesting a common role in inactivation of lymphokines such as interleukin (IL-1) and tumour necrosis factor.

Secretory IgA normally accounts for < 3 % of urinary protein. It is secreted from tubular epithelial cells to help maintain a sterile urine. Urokinase is one of several urinary enzymes of intermediate size (31 and 55 kd) which appear in normal urine. It probably acts as an antifibrinolytic agent and may help in cast removal. Tubular secretion of enzymes such as n-acetyl-glucosaminosidase (NAG) may have functional importance, and excretion of high concentrations may reveal tubular damage. Lesser amounts of urinary proteins and glycoproteins are also derived from seminal, prostatic, urethral and vaginal secretion, but ejaculation does not appear to influence the albumin excretion rate[6].

Structure and function of albumin and other plasma proteins excreted in normal urine (Table 1.3)

Albumin is the most abundant plasma protein (usual concentration 36–50 g/l). It is derived from the liver, and synthetic rates are highly responsive to any change in requirements consequent upon loss of circulating albumin. It has a relatively long half-life of 2–3 weeks. Its main functions are to maintain colloid osmotic pressure within the intravascular compartment, and as a transporter of ions, water insoluble substances such as lipids and non-esterified fatty acids, hormones and drugs. Catabolism of albumin takes place predominantly in the liver and kidney.

Retinol-binding protein (RBP) is an α-globulin, which is synthesised in the liver, and circulates in the blood bound to prealbumin. The size of the circulating complex prevents filtration through the glomerulus. The affinity for prealbumin lessens following delivery of retinol to the target epithelial tissues, when RBP then undergoes complete glomerular filtration and catabolism in the proximal renal tubules. In normal subjects serum levels of RBP are over one thousand times higher than in urine[7].

β_2-microglobulin is a cationic low molecular weight protein, which is thought to be produced by normal white blood cells, and may be related to the human leucocyte antigen (HLA) complex. It is freely filtered by the glomerulus, but is not ideal as a marker of tubular function, as it is unstable in urine, particularly at low pH.

α_1-microglobulin is a glycoprotein synthesised in the liver, which appears to be stable in acidic urine. It may bind to IgA and influence immune function[8]. IgG is one of the group of immunoglobulins synthesised by plasma cells and which function as antibodies. They are synthesised from two heavy and two light polypeptide chains. They form particularly in response to soluble antigens such as bacterial toxins. Components of IgG such as kappa or gamma light chains may also circulate and are freely filtered by the glomerulus. Some 96 % of IgG is either neutral or cationic in charge, which is in marked contrast to IgG4, the anionic subclass which is preferentially excreted in normoalbuminuric subjects[9].

Transferrin is the major iron-binding protein present in plasma. It transports iron from the sites of absorption and red cell breakdown, to the developing red cells in bone marrow. The binding sites of transferrin are normally

Table 1.3. *Size, charge, and renal excretion of plasma proteins in normal subjects*

Name	Molecular weight (Daltons)	Charge	Normal 24 h excretion (μg/min; range)
Albumin	67 000	—	0.100–15.000
Retinol-binding protein	21 000	0	0.016–0.173
β_2-microglobulin	11 815	0	0.021–0.257
IgG	160 000	0	1.340–1.700
Transferrin	90 000	0	0.090–0.326
α_1-microglobulin	30 000	0	0.902–6.250
α_1-acid glycoprotein	44 000	0	0.125–0.469
α_1 antitrypsin	45 000	0	0.130–0.391
Caeruloplasmin	160 000	—	0.032–0.042
Haptoglobin	85 000	—	0.000–0.290
G_c-globulin	50 000	0	0.011–0.033
Haemopexin	80 000	—	0.099–0.199
β_2-glycoprotein	40 000	0	0.150–0.338

Charge: 0 neutral;—anionic

about 30 % saturated. It has a slightly larger molecular weight than albumin, but is of greater molecular charge, favouring tubular reabsorption over albumin.

Physiological determinants of proteinuria

Although a large number of plasma protein constituents of normal urine have been identified (Table 1.3), the majority of proteins are not derived from blood but, like Tamm Horsfall protein, are secreted from the kidney or from the lower genito-urinary tract. Urinary excretion of albumin and lower molecular weight proteins is enhanced by any factors which increase the load filtered by the glomerulus, either by saturating tubular reabsorptive capacity, or simply as a result of increased tubular volume and flow rate. Thus, increased proteinuria in normal subjects would result from any situation of increased renal blood flow and glomerular filtration rates and/or increased intraglomerular pressure and permeability. This is most clearly seen during extracellular volume expansion with saline, but even simple oral water loading appears to increase acutely the urinary excretion of albumin [10–12]. The effect of water loading on excretion of retinol-binding protein and other lower molecular weight proteins is less marked.

Urinary albumin excretion also increases during the assumption and maintenance of an upright posture, regardless of the time, although particularly by day, suggesting additional diurnal variation. The actual magnitude of postural variation varies considerably between individuals, and within-individual day-to-day variation of up to 80 % is recognised. The mechanism is presumed to be glomerular, the consequence of an increased filtration fraction due to respective increases and reductions in systemic blood pressure and renal blood flow. This is supported by the observation that normally renal blood flow will increase and systemic and renal vascular resistance will fall whilst recumbent. This is not the case if there is autonomic dysfunction. Upright posture does not appear to increase excretion of retinol-binding protein, strengthening the view that tubular proteinuria is not normally influenced by postural changes in blood flow and vascular resistance. Exercise-induced increase in albumin excretion is well recognised[13], and is the likely consequence of increases in renal blood flow, systemic and intraglomerular pressure and filtration fraction.

Although it has been argued that albuminuria after exercise predominantly reflects a failure of proximal tubular reabsorption, excretion of lower molecular weight proteins may not necessarily increase during exercise[13]. This suggests either an alternative mechanism for the increased albuminuria, or could be compatible with the concept of selective tubular reabsorption of smaller molecular weight proteins, in preference to albumin. Oral glucose loading in healthy individuals also acutely increases albuminuria although not low molecular weight proteinuria[14]. Tubular protein–protein interaction is again the likeliest explanation for this phenomenon, although acute increases in renal blood flow may also be implicated, in part as a response to physiological hyperinsulinaemia. By contrast, acute and chronic dietary protein loads appear to increase both albuminuria and low molecular weight proteinuria, primarily as a result of the increased glomerular filtration and urine flow rate which is a homeostatic response to the increased nitrogenous load[10,15].

Pregnancy is another physiological state of increased urinary protein excretion[16,17]. Urinary albumin excretion appears to increase some threefold in the third trimester, and similar changes in other proteins, including retinol binding protein and transferrin, have been recorded. The mechanism is likely to be complex, and not simply the result of increased renal blood flow and intraglomerular pressure, but may also be due to increased protein synthesis, selective filtration and tubular reabsorption, and altered capillary permeability, reflecting physiological changes in neuro-endocrine balance.

References

1. Christensen EI, Rennke HG, Carone FA. Renal tubular uptake of protein: effect of molecular charge. *Am J Physiol* 1983; **244**:F436–F441.
2. Cavallo-Perin P, Chiambretti A, Calefato V, Tomalino M, Cecchini G, Gruden G, Pagano G. Urinary excretion of glycated albumin in insulin-dependent diabetic patients with micro- and macroalbuminuria. *Clin Nephrol* 1992; **38**:9–13.
3. Hayashi Y, Morikawa A, Makino M. Heterogeneity of urinary albumin from diabetic patients. *Clin Chim Acta* 1990; **190**:93–104.
4. Bernard A, Viau C, Ouled A, Lauwerys R. Competition between low- and high- molecular weight proteins for tubular uptake. *Nephron* 1987; **45**:115–118.
5. Nguyen-Simonnet H, Vincent C, Revillard JP. Competition between albumin and beta-2-microglobulin for renal tubular uptake: brush border and/or lysosomes? *Nephron* 1988; **48**:159–160.
6. Hirsch IB, Farkas-Hirsch R, Herbst JS, Skyler JS. The effect of ejaculation on albumin excretion rate. *J Diabet Compl* 1992; **6**:163–165.
7. Tomlinson PA, Dalton RN, Turner C, Chantler C. Measurement of ß$_2$-microglobulin, retinol-binding protein, alpha$_1$-microglobulin and urine protein I in healthy children using enzyme-linked immunosorbent assay. *Clin Chim Acta* 1990; **192**:99–106.
8. Yu H, Yanagisawa Y, Forbes MA, Cooper EH, Crockson RA, MacLennan ICM. Alpha-1-microglobulin: an indicator protein for renal tubular function. *J Clin Pathol* 1983; **36**:253–259.
9. Pietravalle P, Morano S, Cristina G, Grazia de Rossi M, Mariani G, Cotroneo P, *et al*. Charge selectivity of proteinuria in type 1 diabetes explored by Ig subclass clearance. *Diabetes* 1991; **40**:1685–1690.
10. Amore A, Coppo R, Rocattello D, Martina G, Rollino C, Basolo B *et al*. Single kidney function: effect of acute protein and water loading on micro-albuminuria. *Am J Med* 1988; **84**:711–715.
11. First MR, Sloan DE, Pesce AJ, Pollak VE. Albumin excretion by the kidney: The effect of volume expansion. *J Lab Clin Med* 1977; **89**:25–29.
12. Viberti GC, Mogensen CE, Keen H, Jacobsen FK, Jarrett RJ, Christensen CK. Urinary excretion of albumin in normal man: the effect of water loading. *Scand J Clin Lab Invest* 1982; **42**:147–151.
13. Watts GF, Williams I, Morris RW, Mandalia S, Shaw KM, Polak A. An acceptable exercise to study microalbuminuria in type 1 diabetes. *Diabet Med* 1989; **6**:787–792.
14. Hegedus L, Christiansen NJ, Mogensen CE, Gundersen HJG. Oral glucose increases urinary albumin excretion in normal subjects but not in insulin-dependent diabetics. *Scand J Clin Lab Invest* 1980; **40**:479–480.
15. Shestakova MV, Mukhin NA, Dedov II, Titov VN, Warshavsky VA. Protein-loading test, urinary albumin excretion and renal morphology in diagnosis of subclinical diabetic nephropathy. *J Intern Med* 1992; **231**:213–217.
16. Lopez-Espinoza I, Dhar H, Humphreys S, Redman WG. Urinary albumin excretion in pregnancy. *Br J Obstet Gynaecol* 1986; **93**:176–181.
17. Wright A, Steele P, Bennett JR, Watts G, Polak A. The urinary excretion of albumin in normal pregnancy. *Br J Obstet Gynaecol* 1987; **94**:408–412.

2

Measurement and expression of microalbuminuria

Introduction

Until the 1960s, quantitative methods of measuring low concentrations of albumin were laborious as they depended on the separation of protein by electrophoresis after concentration of the urine. In 1963, Keen and Chlouverakis[1] described an immunoassay which was specific for albumin, required only small volumes of urine, was accurate and sensitive and was capable of dealing with large numbers of samples. This trail-blazing paper was not only the forerunner of many methodological developments, but also the starting point of much exciting research which has eventually established the significance of small amounts of albumin in the urine. Such increases in albuminuria which are undetectable by conventional dip-stick testing but greater than the normal excretion have been called microalbuminuria.

Laboratory measurement of microalbuminuria

General considerations

As discussed above, the assay must be specific for albumin, and hence have an immunological basis. It must be precise, sensitive and practicable. Currently the techniques commonly used are radioimmunoassay (RIA), single radial immunodiffusion (RID), immunoturbidimetry (IT), laser immuno-nephelometry (IN), and enzyme-linked immunosorbent assays (ELISA) (Table 2.1). There are many variations of each method and little has been published on comparisons of different techniques.

Radioimmunoassay

Most currently used RIA methods are variations of the original assay[1], human albumin being labelled with ^{125}I[2,3]. Most are 'saturation assays',

11

Table 2.1. *Methods for measurement of microalbuminuria*

Laboratory methods	Side-room tests
Radioimmunoassay	Side agglutination tests
Single radial immunodiffusion	Sensitive dip-stick tests
Immunoturbidimetry	'Tablet' tests
Laser immunonephelometry	
Enzyme-linked immunosorbent assay	

performed in liquid phase with an excess of antigen being added[2], although solid-phase assays have been described[4]. Separation of bound and free albumin may be by precipitation with polyethylene glycol[2,5] or a second antibody[1,6]. Several commercially produced RIA kits are available. The sensitivity of an albumin RIA is generally < 1 mg/l.

Radial immunodiffusion

In this technique, the antigen–antibody reaction takes place in an antibody-containing well. The antigen travels through the gel to reach equilibrium, at which point antigen–antibody complexes precipitate when antibody is present in excess. The complexes are then stained and the diameter of the antigen–antibody ring measured manually[2]. The technique is obviously labour intensive and laborious, and the sensitivity generally less than that of RIA, being around 2.5 mg/l.

Immunoturbidimetry

This is a kinetic assay whereby the rate of formation of antigen–antibody complex in solution and in the presence of antibody excess is measured by changes in absorbence of transmitted light at 340 nm. Sensitivity is around 2–4 mg/l[2,7,8]. Samples should be tested initially by conventional dip-stick tests for proteinuria, as proteinuria in excess of 200 mg/l may cause antigen excess and the 'hook' or 'prozone' phenomenon, leading to a falsely low result.

Laser immunonephelometry

Laser immunonephelometry quantifies light scattering caused by antigen–antibody complexes precipitated in a liquid phase. Several methods have been described[9,10]. Sensitivity is generally less than RIA[11], but accuracy and precision are similar.

Enzyme-linked immunosorbent assay

An early publication on this technique described a 'three-site' assay, with the first anti-human albumin antibody being immobilised on a solid phase. After added antigen has bound to this first antibody, the second antibody, goat anti-human albumin, is added. A third anti-goat antibody conjugated to an enzyme label is then added[12]. Subsequent publications have detailed a simplified 'two-site' immunoassay, whereby bound complexes are detected and quantified by addition of a second antibody conjugated to an enzyme label[2,13–15]. Other 'competitive' variations of this technique, in which standard or sample are added at the same time as the second antibody, have been described[16–18]. Most conjugates contain horse-radish peroxidase which, on addition of *o*-phenylenediamine and hydrogen peroxide, generates a quantifiable colour reaction. The sensitivity is generally around 6 µg/l, lower than other immunoassay systems[2].

Other immunological methods

A solid phase fluorescent immunoassay has been described, in which the primary albumin antibody is coupled to an immunobead matrix[19] and the second antibody conjugated with fluorescein isothiocyanate. Although no direct comparisons have been made, this method does seem to have sensitivity and precision on a par with radioimmunoassay techniques and the standard curve is linear over a wide range of albumin concentrations. In a variation of this technique, the assay is carried out in the liquid phase, separation being achieved by addition of a second antibody[20]. The authors of this report suggested that the fluorescein-labelled albumin could be replaced by ^{125}I-albumin without altering the assay characteristics significantly.

Solomon and colleagues[21] have described an immunological assay utilising the ability of oxirane-bearing polymethyl-methacrylate beads to bind anti-human albumin antibodies. The assay properties appear satisfactory, apart from the rather limited linear range of the standard curve (1–25 mg/l).

Comparison of immunological methods

Comparison of immunological methods is limited. Most have used radio-immunoassay as the reference technique because it is the longest established and has been used in many of the longitudinal studies demonstrating the significance of microalbuminuria in diabetes. All types of assay generally have satisfactory performance criteria when studied individually, although it is important to realise that different techniques, and indeed similar methods run in different laboratories, will report differing absolute values. There is general agreement that RIA is the most precise technique with acceptable sensitivity[2,22,23], although one study reported better precision with a nephelometry method[24].

Watts and colleagues[2] found that there were no systematic differences between RIA and RID, but that immunoturbidimetry gave consistently lower values than RIA, the mean difference being 1.8 mg/l. The differences between the methods increased with increasing albumin concentration. In contrast, some other immunoturbidimetric methods appear to give higher albumin concentrations than RIA[23,24], whilst others yield similar results[8,25]. With the ELISA technique, some authors report results similar to those from RIA[13] whilst others report a consistent underestimate with ELISA of around 9.7 mg/l[2]. In a somewhat superficial comparison of commercially available RIA, RID, immunoturbidimetry and nephelometry methods, the correlation of the methods with the radioimmunoassay were excellent ($r > 0.97$)[26]. However, although no further statistical comparison was undertaken, the correlation graphs provided in the paper suggest that the relationships between assays were not unity. Marre and colleagues[9] found an excellent agreement between RIA and laser nephelometry.

Radioimmunoassay necessitates the use of radioisotopes with limited shelf-life, has high capital costs but low running costs and requires sample batching for greatest efficiency. Immunoturbidimetry probably has the highest running costs, but fastest turn-around time. Radial immunodiffusion requires a high degree of technical skill and is time consuming. ELISA methods also have high capital costs. The final choice of methodology will rest more on the individual laboratory's expertise and currently available equipment, and the demand for the service, rather than on perceived advantages of one particular assay type.

Non-immunological methods

Because of the complexities of the immunological methods, other techniques of detecting low concentrations of 'albumin' in the urine have been sought. These, however measure total protein rather than albumin. A colourimetric method using pyrogallol red–molybdate has been described, based on the shift in the absorption spectrum of the pyrogallol red–molybdate complex when protein is bound[27]. The method has a range of 10–1000 mg/l and is simple and easy to perform. A comparison of a modification of this method[28], with a nephelometric assay specific for albumin showed that all samples with a urinary protein concentration greater than 60 mg/l by the pyrogallol red method had an albumin concentration > 30 mg/l. The authors suggested a role for the pyrogallol red test as a screening test for microalbuminuria. However, it should be remembered that the proportion of albumin to total protein in the urine varies enormously with the severity of diabetic nephropathy, thus limiting the usefulness of this type of test.

Side-room tests for microalbuminuria

A number of side-room tests have been developed for the detection of microalbuminuria (Table 2.1). With one exception, they are immunologically based and therefore specific for albumin. All are semi-quantitative at best, so potentially useful for screening purposes rather than strict quantification of microalbuminuria. They depend on a variety of principles, described below.

Slide agglutination tests

In the original description of this method, anti-human albumin antibody is immobilised on latex beads[29]. When antigen and then the same antibody in liquid phase are added, visible agglutination appears. Proportions of the reagents are adjusted so that agglutination occurs in the microalbuminuric range of albumin concentrations. The test is easy to perform, requiring only the application to a latex agglutination plate of drops of three reagents in the correct sequence, followed by gentle rocking of the plate for 5 min. A simplified modification of this method has been compared with RIA[30]. Agglutination was detected in all samples with albumin concentration > 30 mg/l, although there were a considerable number of false positive results in samples with albumin concentration < 30 mg/l. Some attempt was made to quantitate the reaction by grading the degree of agglutination by means of an analogue scale, but although there was very good agreement between ten observers, each point on the scale represented a wide range of albumin concentrations. It should be noted that because of the prozone phenomenon, no agglutination was seen in samples with albumin concentration > 400 mg/l, thus emphasising the need for prior testing of all specimens by conventional protein dip-stick.

Commercial versions of this method have been developed and tested. In an initial version (Albuscreen, Cambridge Life Sciences, Cambridge, UK) the proportions of reagents were adjusted so that agglutination occurred at an albumin concentration of approximately 25 mg/l. This gave low sensitivity in detecting an albumin:creatinine ratio > 2.5 mg/mmol in a random urine sample[31]. A revised version, the Albusure kit (Cambridge Life Sciences, Cambridge, UK) appears to have acceptable sensitivity and specificity as a screening tool with good reproducibility[23,32]. However, the wide spectrum of albumin concentrations represented by each point on the analogue scale renders the test only semi-quantitative.

Sensitive and specific dip-stick tests

Conventional dip-stick tests detect total protein rather than albumin and are neither sufficiently sensitive nor reproducible enough to detect micro-albuminuria[23,32,33]. A sensitive dip-stick test specific for urinary albumin has been developed using complex dry chemistry (Micral-Test, Boehringer Mannheim, Mannheim, Germany). In the original version of this strip, urinary albumin was bound to a soluble conjugate of albumin antibodies and ß-galactosidase. Unbound conjugate is removed in a separate zone containing immobilised albumin, so that only bound albumin–antibody-β-galactosidase reaches a third zone where a colourimetric reaction takes place. The intensity of the developed colour is compared to a scale of five colour blocks denoting albumin concentrations of 0, 10, 20, 50 and 100 mg/l. Difficulties with this test include the five minute reaction time, making multiple tests in a busy out-patient clinic inconvenient. Evaluations of this version suggested that the test-strip had sufficient sensitivity and specificity to be used as a screening test for microalbuminuria but was at best only semi-quantitative[26,34–39]. One large study in general practice suggested that sensitivity and specificity only reached acceptable levels if multiple repeat tests were performed[40].

A revised version of Micral-Test, Micral-Test II (Boehringer Mannheim, Germany) has been marketed. In this version, the absorbed urine enters a zone containing a soluble antibody–gold conjugate which specifically binds to albumin. Excess conjugate is retained in a separation zone containing immobilised human albumin, so that only the albumin–gold complex reaches the detection zone. The colour product (white to red) is directly related to the albumin content of the urine. The reaction time is one minute and colour bands represent albumin concentrations of 0, 20, 50 and 100 mg/l. Initial evaluation reports suggest that this is a useful screening tool, with the advantage that the reaction colour is stable for 60 min[41].

Other side-room tests

The third commercially available side-room test is a tablet test based on the 'protein-error of indicators' principle (Microbumintest, Ames, Stoke Poges, UK). At a constant buffered pH, the intensity of colour developed depends on the amount of albumin in a volume of urine dropped onto the tablet.

Bromophenol blue is used as the indicator and the test is obviously not specific for albumin. The colour developed is compared to the manufacturer's chart, with blocks indicating negative, one plus (approximately > 40 mg/l) or two plusses. One study has shown this test to have a sensitivity of 100 % and specificity of 83 % in detecting urine albumin concentration > 20 mg/l[26]. However, the high false positive rate resulted in a positive predictive value of 36 %. In addition, there was poor agreement between different observers. Other workers have confirmed the low specificity and positive predictive value of Microbumintest[42–44]. As with the other side-room tests, this test is not suitable for quantitative analysis.

Comparison of semi-quantitative tests

Few direct comparisons of the different side-room tests have been made. Watts and colleagues[45] found that Microbumintest was as sensitive but less specific than an in-house latex agglutination test in identifying urine albumin concentrations greater than 15 mg/l. Other workers suggested that the sensitivity of Microbumintest and a commercial latex agglutination test (Albufast, Amplifon Divisione Biomedica, Milan, Italy) were similar in their ability to identify urine albumin concentrations of > 20 and > 30 mg/l, but that the specificity of Albufast was lower. However, both tests had such low specificities that the authors questioned their usefulness[24]. In a direct comparison of Microbumintest and Micral-Test I, Bashyam and colleagues[46] found that both tests had unacceptably high false positive and false negative rates and could not recommend either as a screening test. However, whilst it was particularly true that Microbumintest recorded false negative results over a wide range of albumin concentrations, Micral-Test I recorded most false negatives in the concentration range 20–30 mg/l and gave no false positive results.

It thus seems that the side-room tests for microalbuminuria are useful as initial screening tests only, if formal laboratory testing is not readily available. In addition, they are only semi-quantitative, and hence are not suitable for monitoring changes in albumin excretion in response to intervention or with time in research studies. Thus for study purposes, laboratory confirmation of a positive screening test should be made, and monitoring the response to intervention should also be by laboratory testing. For clinical use, laboratory-based testing is also to be preferred. It has been suggested that multiple screening measurements should be made, perhaps on three consecutive days, in the hope that the false positive and negative test rates would be reduced.

Sample handling

An aliquot of urine for screening purposes can be collected without preservative. Some authors suggest that for timed collections, a preservative such as borate or sodium azide should be added, although this is probably not necessary. Urinary tract infection should be excluded before testing, either by formal culture of a mid-stream urine sample or by dip-stick testing for nitrite and blood. All samples should be tested initially by conventional dip-stick to exclude those in the proteinuric range.

Methods describing the measurement of albumin excretion rate suggest that samples should be stored at 4, –20 or –70 °C before assay, and that the sample should be vortexed, centrifuged or filtered before assay. Several workers have demonstrated that the albumin concentration in urine kept at 4 °C is stable for 7–14 days[47–49]. Some[47,50–52] but not all authors[16,48,49,53] have found falsely low albumin concentrations after storage of the urine at –20 °C. Erman and colleagues[47] suggested that freezing may induce a conformational change in urine proteins, resulting in partial precipitation. In a small number of samples from healthy individuals with low albumin concentrations, an effect of temperature of storage on the apparent rate of degradation of albumin was observed[22]. Storage at –20 °C resulted in a rate of decline which was marginally significantly different from zero ($p = 0.089$), whereas after storage at –40 °C no change was seen. Different methods of sample treatment (vortexing, centrifugation or filtering) before or after freezing and thawing, had no influence on the albumin concentration. However, the small number of samples and their low albumin concentration makes the broader application of these results difficult. In a larger study using urine samples with a wide range of albumin concentrations, no effect of storage at –20 and –40 °C for up to six months was found[49] and thawing and refreezing up to six times in a six-week period also did not alter the measured albumin concentration. In a relatively large study of children and adolescents with diabetes, storage of urine at –20 °C resulted in a significant effect on the measured albumin concentration[54]. The effect appeared to be related to the initial urine albumin concentration rather than the length of storage time, and was inconsistent in that in some samples the concentration apparently increased and in some it decreased.

Currently it seems sensible to store urine samples at 4 °C if they are to be assayed within 14 days, or at –40 °C if prolonged storage is required.

Variability in albumin excretion

Diurnal variation

Many factors, physiological and pathological, influence the albumin excretion rate (AER). There is a marked diurnal variation, day-time excretion being approximately 30 % higher than overnight albumin excretion in non-diabetic adults[55] and children[56,57] and in diabetic patients with both insulin-dependent diabetes mellitus (IDDM)[58-60] and non-insulin-dependent diabetes mellitus (NIDDM)[60]. Thus, overnight albumin excretion rates are lower than 24-hour rates in non-diabetic and diabetic subjects[59-61].

Several studies have suggested that the difference between day and night excretion rates is greater in diabetic than non-diabetic subjects, and is particularly high in those IDDM patients with an elevated albumin excretion rate[60,61]. This may be due to increased glomerular permeability to albumin in response to exercise in IDDM patients[62]. Indeed, it has been suggested that the albumin excretion response to a standard exercise test may be useful as a provocation test to identify diabetic patients at risk of developing diabetic nephropathy[63-66]. Feldt-Rasmussen and coworkers[65] studied non-diabetic control subjects and IDDM patients with normal 24 h albumin excretion or microalbuminuria (Fig. 2.1). During exercise the AER increased significantly in all three groups, the relative increase being higher in the diabetic subjects with microalbuminuria. Renal haemodynamic changes were qualitatively similar in all three groups, but the filtration fraction during exercise increased to a similar extent in the two diabetic groups, suggesting that the elevated transcapillary pressure gradient *per se* occurring during exercise is not sufficient to cause an increase in albumin excretion. A functional glomerular lesion, manifest as increased albumin excretion at rest, must also be present. However, one recent study has demonstrated that diabetic children and adolescents with normal overnight or 24-h urinary albumin excretion who have an abnormal response to an exercise test are not at increased risk of developing diabetic nephropathy in the future[67]. Sixty six patients, mean age 15 years and duration of diabetes nine years, were studied at baseline and after a mean of 6.2 years follow-up, using a standardised exercise test. At baseline, pre- and post-exercise albumin excretion rates were similar in the diabetic patients and matched non-diabetic control children, with a similar rise in AER with exercise. Eight out of 66 diabetic children had developed microalbuminuria at follow-up (AER > 20 μg/min). Baseline resting and post-exercise AER, delta AER with exercise, blood pressure, HbA_1, and age and duration of diabetes, were similar in the patients who became microalbuminuric and those who remained normoalbuminuric.

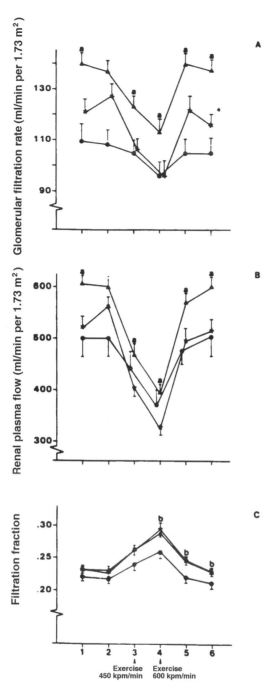

Fig. 2.1 Glomerular filtration rate (A), renal plasma flow (B) and filtration
fraction (C) before, during and after physical exercise in young
IDDM patients and non-diabetic control subjects (mean ± SEM).
Twenty-minute periods are marked on the horizontal axis. ● non-
diabetic subjects; ▲ diabetic patients with albumin excretion < 15
μg/min: group 1; ◆ diabetic patients with albumin excretion > 15
μg/min: group 2. [a] $p < 0.05$, group 1 versus group 2; [b] $p < 0.05$, non-
diabetic subjects versus groups 1 and 2. Reproduced from reference
65 with permission.

In addition to the effects of exercise, this difference in day- and night-time albumin excretion may also be due at least in part to the effects of attaining the upright posture, blood pressure changes[68] and dietary intake[69].

Day-to-day variation

Coefficients of variation for overnight albumin excretion rates are as high as 30–60 % for non-diabetic and IDDM patients with and without microalbuminuria[9,70,71]. Some studies have suggested that the variance in overnight and day-time excretion rates was similar in non-diabetic and diabetic subjects[9,55] whilst other workers have suggested that the variation is greater in diabetic subjects and is higher in day-time than overnight collections[4]. Significant day-to-day variation in overnight[57,72] and day-time[72] albumin excretion is also seen in non-diabetic children. Price and colleagues[72] found no difference in the variability of day and night collections, although variation in diabetic children was greater in both samples than in non-diabetic subjects.

Despite this apparently large variation, misclassification of subjects as normal or abnormal occurs most often when the measured parameters are in the borderline range[71] so that most patients are correctly classified on the basis of one or two collections[73]. Nonetheless, it remains important to base classification on several measurements. In research studies looking at change of albumin excretion with time or in response to intervention, it is now standard practice for three urine collections to be made at each time point. In clinical practice, trends with time on repeated testing, in addition to individual values, are important.

A complex analysis of the changes in AER over 12 months in 13 microalbuminuric, normotensive and metabolically stable IDDM or NIDDM patients has been reported[74]. Subjects were initially classified as microalbuminuric on the basis of at least two out of three 24-h urine collections. Thereafter, one collection was made each month. In only three patients was a significant trend in AER observed. In the remaining ten patients, the variability in AER from month to month was so high as to obscure any statistically significant trend. Because of this high within-person variability, only patients with an initial AER 53–76 µg/min had a high probability ($\geq$ 95 %) of having microalbuminuria on subsequent testing, the probability rising to 99 % if initial AER was $\geq$ 99 µg/min. The authors concluded that the variability in AER limits its potential as a serial marker of renal function. However, it may be that in this group of normotensive patients, AER would not be expected to change much in one year, and that a much longer time-course must be examined.

Which measurement?

Timed urine collections, either 24 h, overnight or short day-time, are regarded as the gold standard. There is no information to suggest that any one of these has superior predictive powers. Although one study found a good correlation ($r = 0.905$) between AER in an overnight and a 30 min, recumbent, fasting sample, practical difficulties limit the usefulness of such a short day-time collection[75]. However, there is general agreement that it is impractical to screen large numbers of subjects for microalbuminuria using timed collections. Alternatives which have been advocated include measurement of the albumin concentration or the albumin:creatinine ratio in either an early morning or a spot day-time urine sample.

Comparison of timed and untimed urine collections

As detailed in Table 2.2, most but not all of the studies examining the predictive power of microalbuminuria in diabetes mellitus have used timed urine collections, either 24-h, overnight or short day-time samples collected with the person resting for some time. This is particularly true for those studies examining renal risk in patients with IDDM. Timed collections are inconvenient and cumbersome for patient and laboratory staff, and open to inaccuracies of incomplete collection. These factors, plus the necessity of testing large numbers of patients with diabetes annually for microalbuminuria, have prompted the search for a more convenient screening test. The commonest strategies have measured either the albumin concentration or albumin:creatinine ratio in an aliquot of a first morning urine sample (EMU) or a day-time random urine sample. Most workers have found a highly significant correlation between the albumin concentration or albumin:creatinine ratio in an early morning or random urine sample and the overnight or 24-h albumin excretion rate[6,44,76–78]. On the basis of sensitivity, specificity and positive and negative predictive values, the workers have gone on to derive the albumin concentration or albumin:creatinine ratio which is predictive of microalbuminuria in the timed urine collection. Unfortunately, it is virtually impossible to compare these works directly because of differences in the definitions of microalbuminuria used, different laboratory methods and different tests being compared. The relevant work is summarised in Tables 2.3 and 2.4. Comparison is further hindered by the fact that the sensitivity and specificity of a test will vary with the prevalence of the abnormality being screened for. In some of the studies quoted in Tables 2.3 and 2.4, the populations are truly unselected, whilst in others some selection bias has

Table 2.2. *Predictive power of microalbuminuria in diabetic patients*

Reference	Urine collection	Albumin assay	Reference range	Discriminant AER
Insulin dependent diabetic patients				
Viberti[111]	Overnight	RIA	< 12 µg/min	30 µg/min
Parving[112]	24 h	RID	< 40 mg/24 h	40 mg/24 h
Mogensen[113]	Day-time	RIA	< 7.5 µg/min	15 µg/min
Mathiesen[114]	24 h	RID	< 20 µg/min	70 µg/min
Non-insulin-dependent diabetic patients				
Jarrett[92]	Overnight	RIA	?	> 10.0 µg/min
Mogensen[93]	EMU	RIA	?	> 15.0 mg/l
MacLeod[94]	Overnight	RIA	< 10.5 µg/min	> 10.5 µg/min
Schmitz[95]	EMU	RIA	?	15.0 µg/min
Beatty[96]	Random	RIA	?	> 35 mg/l
Gall[115]	24 h	RIA	?	> 30 mg/24 h
Neil[116]	Random	RIA	?	> 40 mg/l
Mattock[117]	Overnight	RIA	?	> 20 µg/min

EMU: early morning urine sample; RIA: radioimmunoassay
RID: radial immunodiffusion; ?: reference range not given

undoubtedly occurred, so the prevalence of microalbuminuria is not comparable between studies.

In one study, both an AER in an overnight urine collection and an albumin:creatinine ratio in a random urine sample were measured in 54 diabetic patients[79]. A ratio > 3.0 identified all patients with AER > 30 µg/min (sensitivity 100 % and specificity 92 %). In addition, a ratio < 1.0 was always associated with AER < 10.0 µg/min (specificity 100 % and sensitivity 50 %). The authors then went on to test the usefulness of the albumin:creatinine ratio < 1.0 to identify patients with normal albumin excretion in a prospective study. Overnight AER and random albumin:creatinine ratio were measured 144 times in 133 diabetic patients, 30 of whom had AER > 30 µg/min. Again, a ratio < 1.0 identified all patients with AER < 10.0 µg/min (sensitivity 80 %, specificity 100 %) whilst a ratio > 3.0 had sensitivity and specificity of 90 % in identifying patients with AER > 30 µg/min.

The major concern against a random urine sample is the variable effect of exercise and posture on albumin excretion, whilst the major advantage is ease of collection and therefore improved compliance. Problems with simple measurement of albumin concentration are that it makes no allowance for urine flow rate or concentration. In diabetic patients, particularly those with

Table 2.3. *Use of albumin concentration and albumin:creatinine ratio in untimed random urine samples to predict micro-albuminuria*

Reference	Timed collection	Laboratory assay	Definition of microalbuminuria	Cut-off	Sensitivity (%)	Specificity (%)
Nathan[6]	24 h	RIA	> 12 mg/24 h	1.5 mg/mmol	95	97
Nathan[6]	24 h	RIA	> 22 mg/24 h	2.3 mg/mmol	94	96
Nathan[6]	24 h	RIA	> 44 mg/24 h	3.4 mg/mmol	100	100
Schwab[44]	24 h	RIA	> 30 μg/min	20 mg/l	89	85
Gatling[77]	Overnight	ELISA	> 30 μg/min	3.0 mg/mmol	80	81
Gatling[118]	Overnight	ELISA	> 30 μg/min	25 mg/l	56	81
Watts[119]	Overnight	RIA	> 30 μg/min	15 mg/l	96	80
Watts[119]	Overnight	RIA	> 30 μg/min	2.9 mg/mmol	100	88
Watts[119]	Overnight	RIA	> 30 μg/min	26 mg/l	100	85
Watts[119]	Overnight	RIA	> 30 μg/min	8 mg/mmol	100	96

RIA: radioimmunoassay
ELISA: enzyme-linked immunosorbent assay

Table 2.4. *Use of albumin concentration and albumin:creatinine ratio in early morning urine samples to predict micro-albuminuria*

Reference	Timed collection	Laboratory assay	Definition of microalbuminuria	Cut-off	Sensitivity (%)	Specificity (%)
Kouri[80]	Overnight	Nephelometry	> 15 µg/min	10 mg/l	91	77
Kouri[80]	Overnight	Nephelometry	> 15 µg/min	20 mg/l	70	97
Gatling[77]	Overnight	ELISA	> 30 µg/min	20 mg/l	82	96
Gatling[77]	Overnight	ELISA	> 30 µg/min	3.5 mg/mmol	88	99
Gatling[77]	Overnight	ELISA	> 30 µg/min	2.0 mg/mmol	96	100
Cowell[78]	24 h	RIA	> 20 mg/24 h	20 mg/l	100	57
Gatling[118]	Overnight	ELISA	> 30 µg/min	20 mg/l	86	97
Gatling[118]	Overnight	ELISA	> 30 µg/min	3.5 mg/mmol	100	95
Hutchison[76]	Overnight	RIA	> 30 µg/min	3.0 mg/mmol	97	94
Hutchison[76]	Overnight	RIA	> 30 µg/min	17 mg/l	97	91
Schwab[44]	24 h	RIA	> 30 µg/min	20 mg/l	70	93
Marshall[120]	Overnight	RIA	> 30 µg/min	20 mg/l	91	74
Cohen[71]	Overnight	RIA	> 30 µg/min	2.5 mg/mmol	100	100
Marshall[120]	Overnight	RIA	> 30 µg/min	3.5 mg/mmol	98	69
Marshall[120]	Overnight	RIA	> 30 µg/min	4.5 mg/mmol	96	80

RIA: radioimmunoassay; ELISA: enzyme-linked immunosorbent assay.

glycosuria, urine volumes are liable to be high, and hence albumin concentrations low[80]. Thus, in screening for microalbuminuria, a low albumin concentration cut-off is set to avoid false negative results, with the consequence that the false positive rate is high. However, attempts to correct for differences in urine flow rate by calculating the albumin:creatinine ratio introduce further expense and sources of error and, as shown in Tables 2.3 and 2.4, may not convincingly reduce the false positive rate.

The variability of both the albumin concentration and the albumin:creatinine ratio has been stressed in one study[81]. Multiple first morning urine samples were collected from 1391 diabetic patients over two years. The mean coefficient of variation was similar for both measurements, being around 58–82 %, and bore no relation to the albumin concentration. This work emphasises the limitations of the usefulness of untimed samples to screening only and confirms the need for confirmation and follow-up of microalbuminuria by timed collections.

One recent paper has re-emphasised the forgotten fact that the creatinine excretion rate is higher by approximately a factor of two in men compared with women, because of higher muscle mass[82]. Thus, if the albumin:creatinine ratio is used to screen for microalbuminuria, different cut-offs should be applied for males and females. In the above study, figures of 2.5 mg/mmol for men and 4.5 mg/mmol for women were suggested as giving high specificity and sensitivity of identifying those patients with an overnight AER > 30 µg/min. However, recruitment of patients at high risk of microalbuminuria may have biased the results in favour of high sensitivity and specificity. In the UK, the Saint Vincent guidelines suggest a cut-off of 3.5 mg/mmol for women[83] and in non-diabetic subjects aged > 60 years a ratio of 3.0 mg/mmol has been recommended[84].

In a different approach to the problem one group of workers have measured in duplicate albumin concentration, albumin:creatinine ratio and albumin excretion rate in multiple serial samples (24 h, first morning urine and random urine) for non-diabetic and diabetic subjects[85]. In all cases, the analytical coefficient of variation was < 5 %, and contributed < 1 % to the overall total variance. The albumin concentration in the first morning urine had the lowest intra-individual and inter-individual variance, around 35–40 % and this parameter was recommended as the most satisfactory screening test. The authors further recommended a cut-off of 30 mg/l on the grounds that no healthy person would ever exceed this level and thus that anyone screening above this had undoubted disease – that is, that there would be no false positive results.

The limitations of the use of sensitivity, specificity and predictive value in assessing a screening test, and of regression of one set of results against another, have been stressed by Cundy and colleagues[86]. In an alternative approach, they have calculated an estimated albumin excretion rate derived from a random albumin:creatinine ratio using a modified version of the Cockroft and Gault equation[87] as described by Ginsberg and coworkers[88] to calculate 24-h creatinine excretion. They conclude that as the day-to-day variation of actual 24-h albumin excretion rate is as large as the imprecision of the derived 24-h excretion rate, the calculated rate is an acceptable method for monitoring albumin excretion.

From the above discussions, it should be obvious that albumin concentration, albumin:creatinine ratio or albumin excretion rate collected under different conditions and measured by different methods are not directly comparable. Albumin excretion rates measured in 24-h urine collections will be higher than rates derived from overnight collections, and albumin concentrations and albumin:creatinine ratios in day-time samples higher than concentrations and ratios in early morning urine samples. Given the widely differing methodology currently used, it is vitally important that direct comparisons are made only for comparable results.

Which parameter is measured and how results are expressed probably is best determined at the moment by the purpose of the testing. For research studies, timed collections, either 24 h or overnight, are necessary to allow comparison with other work and for good precision. In clinical practice, screening can be done on the basis of albumin concentration or albumin: creatinine ratio in an early morning urine sample. If the major concern is renal risk, confirmation and response to intervention should use a measure which makes some allowance for urine flow rate, either albumin:creatinine ratio or timed collection. For cardiovascular risk in NIDDM patients, confirmation and follow-up can be limited to either albumin concentration or to albumin:creatinine ratio; timed collections do not appear to be necessary (Table 2.2).

Cut-off points, reference ranges and predictive values

Comparatively few large studies have published reference ranges for albumin excretion (Table 2.5). It is obvious that, in adults, the reference range varies with the urine collection and laboratory assay used, perhaps more than with other biological variables. Thus it is important for each laboratory to establish their own reference range under standard conditions. In addition, such wide inter-laboratory variation makes comparison of results between

Table 2.5. *Published reference ranges for albumin excretion rates in non-diabetic subjects*

Reference	Adult/child	Number studied	Laboratory assay	Urine collection	Reference range
Tomaselli[61]	Adult	35	RIA	24 h	4.1 ± 0.8 µg/min
Tomaselli[61]	Adult	35	RIA	Overnight	2.8 ± 0.5 µg/min
Watts[55]	Adult	127	RIA	Overnight	3.2 (1.2–8.6) µg/min
Weigmann[60]	Adult	20	RIA	24 h	2.7 ± 0.6 µg/min
Marshall[120]	Adult	106	RIA	Overnight	1.7–10.5 µg/min
Marshall[102]	Child	64	RIA	Overnight	0.4–9.0 µg/min
Davies[56]	Child (M)	183	ELISA	24 h	$6.64 \times \div /1.98$ mg/24 h/1.73 m^2
Davies[56]	Child (F)	191	ELISA	24 h	$8.30 \times \div /2.21$ mg/24 h/1.73 m^2
Davies[56]	Child (M)	183	ELISA	Overnight	$2.77 \times \div /1.89$ µg/min/1.73 m^2
Davies[56]	Child (F)	191	ELISA	Overnight	$2.98 \times \div /1.84$ µg/min/1.73 m^2

RIA: radioimmunoassay.
ELISA: enzyme-linked immunosorbent assay.
Reference ranges are expressed as: mean $\pm$ SD, median (range), range, or geometric mean $\times \div$ tolerance factor.

centres very difficult and necessitates the use of one central assay in multi-centre studies.

The importance of microalbuminuria lies in its predictive value, as will be discussed in detail in subsequent chapters, of identifying diabetic patients at risk of, or with early diabetic nephropathy, and subjects at risk of premature death from large vessel disease. The original papers summarising the predictive power of microalbuminuria in diabetes are summarised in Table 2.2. Several important facts emerge. Firstly, for IDDM patients, the risk of nephropathy has been determined on the basis of timed albumin excretion rates, either overnight, 24 h or short-term, measured by a variety of laboratory assays. The discriminant cut-off above which the risk increases is different in each report and, in addition, in all but one case this cut-off is well above the upper limit quoted for the non-diabetic reference range. In order to clarify this rather confusing situation, a consensus definition of microalbuminuria above which the IDDM patient is at risk of nephropathy has been agreed[89] as 20–200 μg/min in any timed urine collection. Obviously, this is a somewhat arbitrary definition, but it at least has the virtue of allowing some standardisation. Whilst the lower limit of 20 μg/min may at first sight appear not to be justified, there is accumulating evidence that IDDM patients with an albumin excretion rate above the strict upper limit of normal but below 20 μg/min progress on to true microalbuminuria and presumably eventually to proteinuria[90,91] (Fig. 2.2). Thus in IDDM, a definition of microalbuminuria in a timed collection of 20–200 μg/min seems appropriate at the moment, but with the caveat that patients with excretion rates of 10–20 μg/min may also be at risk of progression.

It is noteworthy that, although the consensus document made proposals specifically for IDDM patients, this definition of microalbuminuria (20–200 μg/min) has also been applied in NIDDM. The two initial studies detailing the predictive power of microalbuminuria in NIDDM used timed overnight excretion rates[92] or albumin concentrations in early morning urine samples[93]. In the first study, excess early mortality was seen at an AER > 10.0 μg/min and in the second at an albumin concentration > 15.0 mg/l. Recent work has shown that the excess mortality seen when AER > 10.5 μg/min is due to cardiovascular disease[94]. Other studies have also confirmed that a simple measure of urinary albumin concentration is predictive of premature cardiovascular death in NIDDM[95,96]. Thus in NIDDM, timed urine collections are not necessary to assess cardiovascular risk, use of an albumin concentration being sufficient.

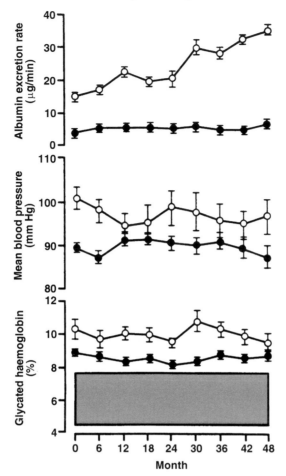

Fig. 2.2. Albumin excretion rate, mean arterial blood pressure and glycated haemoglobin concentration in insulin-dependent diabetic patients who progress to microalbuminuria (○) and in those who remain normoalbuminuric (●) throughout a four-year study period. The shaded area represents the non-diabetic normal range for glycated haemoglobin concentration. Results are expressed as mean (SD) and geometric mean (SD) for albumin excretion rate. Reproduced from reference 91 with permission.

Screening for microalbuminuria

From the above, it is obvious that any method to test for microalbuminuria has disadvantages[76,97]. Given all of these caveats, we have taken a pragmatic, practical approach to screening, which is outlined in Fig. 2.3. It is important only to test in the absence of other intercurrent illnesses which may falsely elevate albumin excretion, for example fever, urinary tract infec-

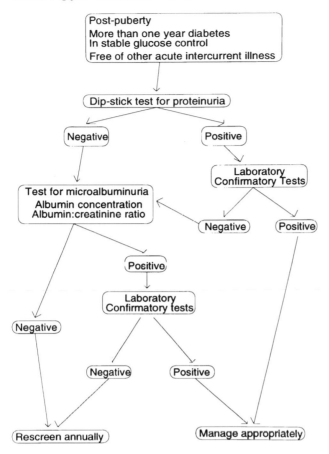

Fig. 2.3 A suggested scheme for screening for microalbuminuria in diabetes. Modified from reference 121 with permission.

tion and cardiac failure. In diabetes, the person should be in stable diabetic control as acute hyperglycaemia may temporarily elevate albumin excretion[98,99]. Also, the ketone body acetoacetate is detected in creatinine assays based on the chromogenic Jaffe reaction, but not in enzymatic-based assays[100].

Adult IDDM patients should be tested annually beginning after one year's duration of diabetes, as the prevalence of microalbuminuria may be high even at such a short duration[101]. Microalbuminuria is very rare before puberty[102,103], so that screening is only recommended from 12 years of age. NIDDM patients should be tested from diagnosis, as patients may have persistent microalbuminuria at presentation[104,105].

It is obviously pointless to perform a test for microalbuminuria if a conventional dip-stick test for protein is more than 1 plus-positive. As with other biological variables with high day-to-day variation, multiple testing should be performed before a label of microalbuminuria is given.

One of the prerequisites of screening for any abnormal state is that the natural history of the condition can be modified. There is good evidence that the risk of end-stage renal disease can be reduced in both IDDM and NIDDM patients but no studies have reported on cardiovascular outcome. Screening therefore to identify diabetic patients at risk of renal disease seems appropriate. Given the strength of the association of microalbuminuria and premature cardiovascular mortality in NIDDM, identification of NIDDM patients with microalbuminuria should lead to intensification of efforts to alter modifiable cardiovascular risk factors. In the non-diabetic population, screening for microalbuminuria is currently controversial, although it may have a role in the clinical assessment of hypertension [106].

Cost-effectiveness of screening

Several studies have attempted to estimate the cost–benefit ratio of screening for microalbuminuria in IDDM patients, followed by treatment with angiotensin-converting enzyme inhibitors. Two reported a favourable benefit[107,108] whilst the third found that screening was not cost effective[109]. This discrepancy probably relates to the uncertain estimates about the efficiency of screening and the precise magnitude of the effectiveness of intervention assumed in the studies.

Two groups have suggested that it is more cost effective to screen all samples first by sensitive dip-stick method, limiting laboratory analysis to those samples which screen positive[110,111].

Overall approach to screening

A suggested plan for screening for microalbuminuria, taking into account all of the above factors, is given in Fig. 2.3.

References

1. Keen H, Chlouverakis C. An immunoassay method for urinary albumin at low concentration. *Lancet* 1963; **ii**:913–914.
2. Watts GF, Bennett JE, Rowe DJ, Morris RW, Gatling W, Shaw KM, Polak A. Assessments of immunochemical methods for determining low concentrations of albumin in the urine. *Clin Chem* 1986; **32**:1544–1548.
3. Hutchison AS, O'Reilly DStJ, MacCuish AC. Albumin excretion rate, albumin concentration and albumin/creatinine ratio compared for screening diabetics for slight albuminuria. *Clin Chem* 1986; **34**:2019–2021.

4. Chachati A, von Frenckell R, Foidart-Willems J, Godon JP, Lefebvre PJ. Variability of albumin excretion in insulin-dependent diabetics. *Diabet Med* 1987; **4**:441–445.

5. Christensen C, Orskov C. Rapid screening PEG radioimmunoassay for quantification of pathological microalbuminuria. *Diabet Nephropath* 1984; **3**:92–97.

6. Nathan DM, Rosenbaum C, Protasowicki D. Single-void urine samples can be used to estimate quantitative microalbuminuria. *Diabetes Care* 1987; **10**:414–418.

7. McCormick CP, Shihabi ZK, Konen JC. Microtransferrinuria and microalbuminuria: enhanced immunoassay. *Ann Clin Lab Sci* 1989; **19**:444–451.

8. Lloyd DR, Hindle EJ, Marples J, Gatt JA. Urinary albumin measurement by immunoturbidimetry. *Ann Clin Biochem* 1987; **24**:209–210.

9. Marre M, Claudel JP, Ciret P, Luis N, Suarez L, Passa Ph. Laser immunonephelometry for routine quantification of urinary albumin excretion. *Clin Chem* 1987; **33**:209–213.

10. Giampietro O, Lucchetti A, Cruschelli L, Miccoli R, di Palma L, Navalesi R. Measurement of urinary albumin excretion (UAE) in diabetic patients: immunonephelometry versus radioimmunoassay. *J Nucl Med All Sci* 1989; **33**:252–257.

11. Giampietro O, Clerico A. Microalbuminuria in diabetes: which method to employ, which sample to collect. *J Nucl Med All Sci* 1990; **34**:111–120.

12. Fielding BA, Price DA, Houlton CA. Enzyme immunoassay for urinary albumin. *Clin Chem* 1983; **29**:355–357.

13. Mohammed A, Wilkin T, Leatherdale B, Davies R. A microenzyme-linked immunosorbent assay for urinary albumin, and its comparison with radioimmunoassay. *J Immunol Methods* 1984; **74**:17–22.

14. Whitfield WE, Spierto FW. Modified ELISA for the measurement of urinary albumin. *Clin Chem* 1986; **32**:561.

15. McBain AM, Brown IRF. An improved enzyme-immunoassay method suitable for screening to detect microalbuminuria. *Ann Clin Biochem* 1987; **24**:207–208.

16. Torffvit O, Wieslander J. A simplified enzyme-linked immunosorbent assay for urinary albumin. *Scand J Lab Invest* 1986; **46**:545–548.

17. Chesham J, Anderton SW, Kingdon CFM. Rapid, competitive enzyme immunoassay for albumin in urine. *Clin Chem* 1986; **32**:669–671.

18. Magnotti RA, Stephens GW, Rogers RK, Pesce AJ. Microplate measurements of urinary albumin and creatinine. *Clin Chem* 1989; **35**:1371–1375.

19. Chavers BM, Simonson J, Michael AF. A solid phase fluorescent immunoassay for the measurement of human urinary albumin. *Kidney Int* 1984; **25**:576–578.

20. Silver A, Dawney A, Landon J, Cattell WR. Immunoassays for low concentrations of albumin in the urine. *Clin Chem* 1986; **32**:1303–1306.

21. Solomon B, Fleminger G, Schwartz F, Doolman R, Sela B-A. Microalbuminuria immunoassay based on antibodies covalently conjugated to Eupergit C-coated beads. *Diabetes Care* 1992; **15**:1451–1454.

22. MacNeil ML, Mueller PW, Caudill SP, Steinberg KK. Considerations when measuring urinary albumin: precision, substances that may interfere, and conditions for sample storage. *Clin Chem* 1991; **37**:2120–2123.

23. Sawicki PT, Heinemann L, Berger M. Comparison of methods for determination of microalbuminuria in diabetic patients. *Diabet Med* 1989; **6**:412–415.

24. Giampietro O, Penno G, Clerico A, Cruschelli L, Lucchetti A, Nannipieri M *et al*. Which method for quantifying 'microalbuminuria' in diabetes? *Acta Diabetol* 1992; **28**:238–245.
25. Bakker AJ. Immunoturbidimetry of urinary albumin: prevention of adsorption of albumin influence of other urinary constituents. *Clin Chem* 1988; **34**:82–86.
26. Tiu SC, Lee SS, Cheng MW. Comparison of six commercial techniques in the measurement of microalbuminuria in diabetic patients. *Diabetes Care* 1993; **16**:616–620.
27. Watanabe N, Kamei S, Ohkubo A, Yamanaka M, Ohsawa S, Makino K, Tokuda K. Urinary protein as measured with a pyrogallol red–molybdate complex, manually and in a Hitachi 726 automated analyser. *Clin Chem* 1986; **32**:1551–1554.
28. Phillipou G, James SK, Seaborn CJ, Phillips PJ. Screening for microalbuminuria by use of a rapid, low-cost colorimetric assay. *Clin Chem* 1989; **35**:456–458.
29. Viberti GC, Vergani D. Detection of potentially reversible diabetic albuminuria. A three-drop agglutination test for urinary albumin at low concentration. *Diabetes* 1982; **31**:973–975.
30. Hodgson BW, Watts GF. A simple side-room test to screen for microalbuminuria in diabetes mellitus. *Ann Clin Biochem* 1987; **24**:581–584.
31. Spooner RJ, Weir RJ, Frier BM. Detection of microalbuminuria in diabetic patients using a simple latex agglutination test. *Clin Chim Acta* 1987; **166**: 247– 253.
32. Coonrod BA, Ellis D, Becker DJ, Dorman JS, Drash AL, Kuller LH, Orchard TJ. Assessment of Albusure and its usefulness in identifying IDDM subjects at increased risk for developing clinical diabetic nephropathy. *Diabetes Care* 1989; **12**:389–393.
33. Gatling W, Knight C, Hill RD. Testing for urinary protein: comparison of Albustix and laboratory albumin measurement. *Practical Diabetes* 1985; **2:** 38–41.
34. Marshall SM, Shearing PA, Alberti KGMM. Assessment of a new test strip for detection of microalbuminuria. *Clin Chem* 1992; **38**:588–591.
35. Bangstad H-J, Try K, Dahl-Jorgensen K, Hanssen KF. New semiquantitative dipstick test for microalbuminuria. *Diabetes Care* 1991; **14**:1094–1097.
36. Hermans MP, Selvais P, van Ypersele de Strihou M, Ketelslegers J-M. Detection of low-range diabetic microalbuminuria: Micral test revisited. *Diabet Med* 1994; **11**:715–716 (letter).
37. Gilbert RE, Akdeniz A, Jerums G. Semi-quantitative determination of microalbuminuria by urinary dipstick. *Aust NZ J Med* 1992; **22**;334–337.
38. Jury DR, Mikkelsen DJ, Glen D, Dunn PJ. Assessment of Micral Test microalbuminuria test strip in the laboratory and in diabetic outpatients. *Ann Clin Biochem* 1992; **29**:96–100.
39. Hasslacher C. Clinical significance of microalbuminuria and evaluation of the Micral-Test. *Clin Biochem* 1993; **26**:283–287.
40. de Grauw WJC, van de Lisdonk EH, van den Hoogen HJM, van Gerwent WHEM, van den Bosch WJHM, Willems JL, van Weel C. Screening for microalbuminuria in Type 2 diabetic patients: the evaluation of a dipstick in general practice. *Diabet Med* 1995; **12**:657–663.
41. Poulsen PL, Mogensen CE. Evaluation of a new semiquantative stix for microalbuminuria. *Diabetes Care* 1995; **18**:732–733.

42. Renard E, de Boisvilliers F, Monnier L, Orsetti A. Evaluation d'un test de depistage rapide de la microalbuminurie en diabetologie. *Diabete et Metab* 1990; **16**:260–263.

43. Tai J, Tze WJ. Evaluation of Micro-Bumintest reagent tablets for screening of microalbuminuria. *Diabetes Res Clin Prac* 1990; **9**:137–142.

44. Schwab SJ, Dunn FL, Feinglos MN. Screening for microalbuminuria. A comparison of single sample methods of collection and techniques of albumin assay. *Diabetes Care* 1992; **15**:1581–1584.

45. Watts GF, Hodgson B, Morris RW, Shaw KM, Polak A. Side-room tests to screen for microalbumunuria in diabetes mellitus. *Diabet Med* 1988; **3**:298–303.

46. Bashyam MM, O'Sullivan NJ, Baker HH, Duggan PF, Mitchell TH. Microalbuminuria in NIDDM. *Diabetes Care* 1993; **4**:634–635.

47. Erman A, Rabinov M, Rosenfeld J. Albumin determination in frozen urines – underestimated results. *Clin Chim Acta* 1988; **174**:255–262.

48. Silver A, Dawnay A, Landon J. Specimen preparation for assay of albumin in urine. *Clin Chem* 1987; **33**:199–200 (letter).

49. Collins ACG, Sethi M, MacDonald FA, Brown D, Viberti GC. Storage temperature and differing methods of sample preparation in the measurement of urinary albumin. *Diabetologia* 1993; **36**:993–997.

50. Townsend JC. Effect of storage temperature on the precipitation of albumin from urine. *Clin Chem* 1986; **32**:1372–1378.

51. Elving LD, Bakkeren JAJM, Jansen MJH, de Kat Angelino CM, de Nobel E, van Munster PJJ. Screening for microalbuminuria in patients with diabetes mellitus: frozen storage of urine samples decreases their albumin content. *Clin Chem* 1989; **35**:308–310.

52. Osberg I, Chase P, Garg SK, DeAndrea A, Harris S, Hamilton R, Marshall G. Effects of storage time and temperature on measurement of small concentrations of albumin in the urine. *Clin Chem* 1990; **36**:1428–1430.

53. Giampietro O, Crushelli I, Penno G, Navalesi R, Clerico A. More effects of storage time and temperature on measurement of small concentrations of albumin in urine. *Clin Chem* 1991; **37**:591–592 (letter).

54. Shield JPH, Hunt LP, Morgan JE, Pennock CA. Are frozen urine samples acceptable for estimating albumin excretion in research? *Diabet Med* 1995; **12**:713–716.

55. Watts GF, Morris RW, Khan K, Polak A. Urinary albumin excretion in healthy adult subjects: reference values and some factors affecting their interpretation. *Clin Chim Acta* 1988; **172**:191–198.

56. Davies AG, Postlethwaite RJ, Price DA, Burn JL, Houlton CA. Urinary albumin excretion in school children. *Arch Dis Child* 1984; **59**:625–630.

57. Rowe DJF, Bagga H, Betts PB. Normal variations in rate of albumin excretion and albumin to creatinine ratios in overnight and daytime urine collections in non-diabetic children. *Br Med J* 1985; **291**:693–694.

58. Davies AG, Price DA, Postlethwaite RJ, Addison GM, Burn JL, Fielding BA. Renal function in diabetes mellitus. *Arch Dis Child* 1985; **60**:299–304.

59. Eshoj O, Feldt-Rasmussen B, Larsen ML, Mogensen EF. Comparison of overnight, morning and 24-hour urine collections in the assessment of diabetic microalbuminuria. *Diabet Med* 1987; **4**:531–533.

60. Weigmann TB, Chonko AM, Barnard MJ, MacDougall ML, Folscroft J, Stephenson J *et al*. Comparison of albumin excretion rate obtained with different times of collection. *Diabetes Care* 1990; **13**:864–871.

61. Tomaselli L, Trischitti V, Vinci C, Frittitta L, Squatrito S, Vigneri R. Evaluation of albumin excretion rate in overnight versus 24-h urine. *Diabetes Care* 1989; **12**:585–587.
62. Viberti GC, Jarrett RJ, McCartney M, Keen H. Increased glomerular permeability to albumin induced by exercise in diabetic subjects. *Diabetologia* 1978; **14**:293–300.
63. Mogensen CE, Vittinghus E. Urinary albumin excetion during exercise in juvenile diabetes. *Scand J Clin Lab Invest* 1975; **35**:295–300.
64. Poortmans J, Dorchy H, Toussaint D. Urinary excretion of total proteins, albumin and β_2-microglobulin during rest and exercise in adolescents with and without retinopathy. *Diabetes Care* 1982; **5**:617–623.
65. Feldt-Rasmussen B, Baker L, Deckert T. Exercise as a provocative test in early renal disease in type 1 (insulin-dependent) diabetes: albuminuric, systemic and renal haemodynamic responses. *Diabetologia* 1985; **28**:389–396.
66. Watts GF, Williams I, Morris RW, Mandalia S, Shaw KM, Polak A. An acceptable exercise test to study microalbuminuria in Type 1 diabetes. *Diabet Med* 1989; **6**:787–792.
67. Bognetti E, Meschi F, Pattarini A, Zoja A, Chiumello G. Post-exercise albuminuria does not predict microalbuminuria in Type 1 diabetic patients. *Diabet Med* 1994; **11**:850–855.
68. Mogensen CE, Chistensen CK. Blood pressure changes and renal function in incipient and overt diabetic nephropathy. *Hypertension* 1985; **7** (suppl 2): 64–73.
69. Wiseman MJ, Hunt R, Goodwin A, Gross JL, Keen H, Viberti GC. Dietary composition and renal function in healthy subjects. *Nephron* 1987; **46**:37–42.
70. Feldt-Rasmussen B, Mathiesen ER. Variability of urinary excretion in incipient diabetic nephropathy. *Diabet Nephropath* 1984; **3**:101–103.
71. Cohen DL, Close CF, Viberti GC. Variability of overnight urinary albumin excretion in insulin-dependent diabetic and normal subjects. *Diabet Med* 1987; **4**:437–440.
72. Price DA, Fielding BA, Davies AG, Postlethwaite RJ. Short-term variability of urinary albumin excretion in normal and diabetic children. *Diabet Nephropath* 1985; **4**:169–171.
73. MacLeod JM, Marshall SM. Urinary albumin excretion: timed collections advisable. *Br Med J* 1993; **306**:1271–1272 (letter).
74. Phillipou G, Phillips P. Variability of urinary albumin excretion in patients with microalbuminuria. *Diabetes Care* 1994; **17**:425–427.
75. Giampietro O, Miccoli R, Clerico A, Crushelli I, Penno G, Navalesi R. Urinary albumin excretion in normal subjects and in diabetic patients measured by a radioimmunoassay: methodological and clinical aspects. *Clin Biochem* 1988; **21**:63–68.
76. Hutchison AS, Paterson KR. Collecting urine for microalbumin assay. *Diabet Med* 1988; **5**:527–532.
77. Gatling W, Knight C, Mullee MA, Hill RD. Microalbuminuria in diabetes: a population study of the prevalence and an assessment of three screening tests. *Diabet Med* 1988; **5**:343–347.
78. Cowell CT, Rogers S, Silink M. First morning urinary albumin concentration is a good predictor of 24-hour urinary albumin excretion in children with Type 1 (insulin-dependent) diabetes. *Diabetologia* 1986; **29**:97–99.

79. Coutarel P, Grimaldi A, Bosquet F, Bureau G, Thervet F. Which method of urine collection and expression of results for albuminuria when screening for incipient diabetic nephropathy? *Diabetes Care* 1988; **11**:371–372.

80. Kouri TT, Viikari JSA, Mattila KS, Irjala KMA. Microalbuminuria. Invalidity of simple concentration-based screening tests for early nephropathy due to urinary volumes of diabetic patients. *Diabetes Care* 1991; **14**:591–593.

81. Johnston J, Paterson KR, O'Reilly DStJ. Estimating urinary albumin excretion rate of diabetic patients in clinical practice. *Br Med J* 1993; **306**:493–494.

82. Connell SJ, Hollis S, Tieszen KL, McMurray JR, Dornan TL. Gender and the clinical usefulness of the albumin:creatinine ratio. *Diabet Med* 1994; **11**:32–36.

83. Viberti GC, Marshall SM, Beech R, Brown V, Derben P, Higson N, *et al.* Saint Vincent and improving diabetes care. Report of the Renal Subgroup. *Diabet Med* 1996; **13** (suppl 4):S6–S12.

84. James MA, Fotherby MD, Potter JF. Screening tests for microalbuminuria in non-diabetic elderly subjects and their relation to blood pressure. *Clin Sci* 1995; **88**:185–190.

85. Howey JEA, Browning MCK, Fraser CG. Selecting the optimum specimen for assessing slight albuminuria, and a strategy for clinical investigation: novel use of data on biological variation. *Clin Chem* 1987; **33**:2034–2038.

86. Cundy TF, Nixon D, Berkahn L, Baker J. Measuring the albumin excretion rate: agreement between methods and biological variability. *Diabet Med* 1992; **9**:138–143.

87. Cockroft DW, Gault MH. Prediction of creatinine clearance from serum creatinine. *Nephron* 1976 **16** 31–41.

88. Ginsberg JM, Chang BS, Matatese RA, Garella S. Use of single voided urine samples to estimate quantitative proteinuria. *N Engl J Med* 1983; **309**:1543–1546.

89. Mogensen CE, Chachati A, Christensen CK, Close CF, Deckert T, Hommel E. *et al*. Microalbuminuria: an early marker of renal involvement in diabetes. *Uremia Invest* 1985; **9**:85–95.

90. Mathiesen ER, Ronn B, Jensen T, Storm B, Deckert T. Relationship between blood pressure and urinary albumin excretion in development of microalbuminuria. *Diabetes* 1990; **39**:245–249.

91. Microalbuminuria Collaborative Study Group UK. Risk factors for development of microalbuminuria in insulin dependent diabetic patients: a cohort study. *Br Med J* 1993; **306**:1235–1239.

92. Jarrett RJ, Viberti GC, Argyropoulos A, Hill RD, Mahmud U, Murrells TJ. Microalbuminuria predicts mortality in non-insulin-dependent diabetes. *Diabet Med* 1984; **1**:17–20.

93. Mogensen CE. Microalbuminuria predicts clinical proteinuria and early mortality in maturity-onset diabetes. *N Engl J Med* 1984; **310**:356–360.

94. MacLeod JM, Lutale J, Marshall SM. Albumin excretion and vascular deaths in NIDDM. *Diabetologia* 1995; **38**:610–616.

95. Schmitz A, Vaeth M. Microalbuminuria: a major risk factor in non-insulin-dependent diabetes. A 10-year follow-up study of 503 patients. *Diabet Med* 1988; **5**:126–134.

96. Beatty OL, Ritchie CM, Bell PM, Hadden DR, Kennedy L, Atkinson AB. Microalbuminuria as identified by a spot morning urine specimen in non-insulin-treated diabetes: an eight-year follow-up. *Diabet Med* 1995; **12**: 261–266.

97. Marshall SM. Screening for microalbuminuria: Which measurement? *Diabet Med* 1991; **8**:706–711.
98. Mogensen CE. Urinary albumin excretion in early and long-term juvenile diabetes. *Scand J Clin Lab Invest* 1971; **28**:183–193.
99. Parving HH, Noer I, Deckert T, Evrin PE, Nielsen SL, Lyngsoe J, *et al*. The effect of metabolic regulation on microvascular permeability to small and large molecules in short-term juvenile diabetics. *Diabetologia* 1976; **12**: 161–166.
100. Watts GF, Pillay D. Effect of ketones and glucose on the estimation of urinary creatinine: implications for microalbuminuria screening. *Diabet Med* 1990; **7**:263–265.
101. Stephenson J, Fuller JH on behalf of the EURODIAB IDDM Complications Study Group. Microvascular and acute complications in IDDM patients: the EURODIAB IDDM Complications Study. *Diabetologia* 1994; **37**:278–285.
102. Marshall SM, Hackett A, Court S, Parkin M, Alberti KGMM. Albumin excretion in children and adolescents with diabetes. *Diabetes Res* 1986; **3**:345–348.
103. Mathiesen ER, Saurbrey N, Hommel E, Parving HH. Prevalence of microalbuminuria in children with Type 1 (insulin-dependent) diabetes mellitus. *Diabetologia* 1986; **29**:640–643.
104. Schmitz A, Hansen HH, Christensen T. Kidney function in newly diagnosed Type 2 (non-insulin-dependent) diabetic patients, before and during treatment. *Diabetologia* 1989; **32**:434–439.
105. Patrick AW, Leslie PJ, Clarke BF, Frier BM. The natural history and associations of microalbuminuria in Type 2 diabetes during the first year after diagnosis. *Diabet Med* 1990; **7**:902–908.
106. Winocour PH. Microalbuminuria. *Br Med J* 1992; **304**:1196–1197.
107. Borch-Johnsen K, Wenzell H, Viberti GC, Mogensen CE. Is screening and intervention for microalbuminuria worthwhile in patients with insulin-dependent diabetes? *Br Med J* 1993; **306**:1722–1723.
108. Siegel JE, Krolewski AS, Warram JH, Weinstein MC. Cost-effectiveness of screening and early treatment of nephropathy in patients with insulin dependent diabetes melitus. *J Am Soc Nephrol* 1992; **3**:S111–S119.
109. Kiberd BA, Jindal KK. Screening to prevent renal failure in insulin dependent diabetic patients: an economic evaluation. *Br Med J* 1995; **311**:1595–1599.
110. Le Floch JP, Charles MA, Philippon C, Perlemuter L. Cost-effectiveness of screening for microalbuminuria using immunochemical dipstick tests or laboratory assays in diabetic patients. *Diabet Med* 1994; **11**:349–356.
111. Viberti GC, Hill RD, Jarrett RJ, Argyropoulos A, Mahmud U, Keen H. Microalbuminuria as a predictor of clinical nephropathy in insulin-dependent diabetes mellitus. *Lancet* 1982; **i**:1430–1432.
112. Parving H-H, Oxenboll B, Svendsen PAa, Sandahl Christiansen J, Andersen AR. Early detection of patients at risk of developing diabetic nephropathy. A longitudinal study of urinary albumin excretion. *Acta Endocrinol (Copenh)* 1982; **100**:550–555.
113. Mogensen CE, Christensen CK. Predicting diabetic nephropathy in insulin-dependent patients. *N Engl J Med* 1984; **311**:89–93.
114. Mathiesen ER, Oxenboll B, Johansen K, Svendsen PAa, Deckert T. Incipient nephropathy in Type 1 (insulin dependent) diabetes. *Diabetologia* 1984; **26**:406–410.

115. Gall MA, Borch-Johnsen K, Hougaard P, Nielsen FS, Parving HH. Albuminuria and poor glycaemic control predict mortality in NIDDM. *Diabetes* 1995; **44**:1303–1309.
116. Neil A, Hawkins M, Potok M, Thorogood M, Cohen D, Mann J. A prospective, population-based study of microalbuminuria as a predictor of mortality in NIDDM. *Diabetes Care* 1993; **16**:994–1003.
117. Mattock MW, Morrish NJ, Viberti GC, Keen H, Fitzgerald AP, Jackson G. Prospective study of microalbuminuria as predictor of mortality in NIDDM. *Diabetes* 1992; **41**:736–741.
118. Gatling W, Knight C, Hill RD. Screening for early diabetic nephropathy: which sample to detect microalbuminuria? *Diabet Med* 1985; **2**:451–455.
119. Watts GF, Shaw KM, Polak A. The use of random urine samples to screen for microalbuminuria in the diabetic clinic. *Practical Diabetes* 1986; **3**:86–88.
120. Marshall SM, Alberti KGMM. Comparison of the prevalence and associated features of abnormal albumin excretion in insulin-dependent and non-insulin-dependent diabetes. *Q J Med* 1989; **261**:61–71.
121. Marshall SM. Strategies for monitoring diabetic nephropathy. *Current Med* 1996; **13**:67–72.

3

Epidemiology and determinants of microalbuminuria in health

The definition of microalbuminuria

The epidemiology of microalbuminuria is not straightforward. At present, large studies are few and far between, there is no standardisation of sample collection conditions and the expression of microalbuminuria, and the precise definition of 'normality' is not yet established[1,2]. Whereas it may be acceptable in standard laboratory practice to produce a clinically useful reference range, this is not the case for microalbuminuria. A more appropriate approach is to examine the distribution of microalbuminuria in a representative community sample which is not subject to selection bias. Whilst there are several early reports of microalbuminuria in ostensibly healthy populations[3–8], only the Copenhagen City Heart Study[9] has carefully defined their study population as a true random sample of a well defined population denominator. Even then it may not necessarily be correct to define 'abnormality' in these studies as values outside the 95th percentile. A useful parallel is blood pressure and lipid distribution, where even carefully defined population-based ranges may be misleading. The importance of all these three parameters is not necessarily the absolute distribution of the data, but the attributable risk for a clinical end point at various levels. Present clinical practice has taken account of this in assessment of blood pressure and lipids, and it is now necessary to consider the impact of age, gender and ethnic origin on expression of abnormality, which in turn is based upon prospective studies which have defined the relative and absolute risk of various end points. These are primarily cardiovascular (CVD), but there may be considerable variation in the role of the different factors in determining, for example coronary heart disease (CHD) as opposed to cerebrovascular disease. Furthermore, the importance of risk factors for CVD morbidity may not equate with those for mortality.

The situation with regard to microalbuminuria is even more complicated in that the majority of studies attributing a prognostic value to microalbuminuria have been carried out in small numbers of diabetic subjects where the end points have included diabetic nephropathy (i.e. persistent Albustix positive proteinuria with or without reduced filtration function), CVD mortality, and overall mortality[10–13]. The consensus definition based on earlier work suggested that microalbuminuria could be defined as overnight albumin excretion rates of 20–200 µg/min[14,15], but this is artificial and too conservative. By expressing microalbuminuria as an 'all or none' phenomenon, there is a danger that the epidemiological and pathophysiological importance of lesser and greater degrees of albuminuria will be misunderstood. It is also the case that these cut off points may be quite inappropriate for non-diabetic populations. It may be better to think of a graded risk for microalbuminuria, beyond a threshold where there is an appreciable attributable risk. This has been borne out by more recent reports that overnight albumin excretion rates > 10 µg/min are predictive of mortality in NIDDM, as well as in the elderly non-diabetic population[16,17]. Such a cut off may prove to be more appropriate, particularly since this is often the 95th percentile of many laboratory-based reference ranges. The difficulty in establishing analagous cut off points for albumin concentrations or albumin:creatinine ratios in random or timed samples has not yet been overcome. Thus according to the definition of microalbuminuria, the prevalence may vary from 2.2 % (albumin concentration > 20 mg/l *and* albumin:creatinine ratio > 3.5 mg/mmol) to 6.3 % (albumin concentration > 20 mg/l only) in the same population[6] (Tables 3.1 and 3.2).

Features associated with microalbuminuria

Notwithstanding such reservations, several studies have examined the distribution and determinants of albuminuria (Table 3.1). The largest of these was carried out by Metcalf and coworkers in Auckland, New Zealand, and will be discussed in some detail.

Metcalf and colleagues carried out a health screening survey of a local workforce of 5670 individuals, aged 40–78 years[5,18,19]. Gender-specific reference ranges were established for urinary albumin concentrations and albumin:creatinine ratios in a subgroup of 3597 people, after excluding subjects with Albustix-positive proteinuria, diabetes mellitus and current hypertension using WHO criteria, bacteriuria, obesity (body mass index $\geq 30 \text{ kg/m}^2$), or fasting serum triglycerides ≥ 2.5 mmol/l. The 95th and 97.5th centiles for urine albumin concentration were respectively 19 mg/l and 28 (men) or 29

Table 3.1 *Prevalence and expression of microalbuminuria in normoglycaemic adults, Europid and non-Europid*

Study	Sample size (M:F)	Age (mean (range))	Ethnic grouping	Type of urine collection and expression of albuminuria	Reference range	Prevalence of microalbuminuria (%)
European						
Gould[4]	959 (423:536)	> 50 (40–75)	100% Europid	Timed EMU/ Overnight AER	AER (> 20 µg/ min)	5.8
Watts[7]	127 (59:68)	33 (8–63)	Europid	Timed day		
				Conc. (mg/l)	0.9–29.6	5
				AER (µg/min)	1.0–9.1	5
				A:C Ratio	0.1–2.3	5
				Timed overnight		
				Conc. (mg/l)	0.9–16.2	5
				AER (µg/min)	1.2–8.6	5
				A:C Ratio	0.1–1.0	5
Gosling[3]	199 (99:100)	40 (20–60)	? Europid	Timed 24 h AER (µg/min)	0.2–14.0	5
Damsgaard[17]	279 (119:160)	67 (60–74)	Europid	Day 1 h timed AER (> 15 µg/min)	0–16.6 (M) 0–14.3 (F)	30 25

Reference	n (M:F)	Age	Ethnicity	Method	Reference range/cut-off	Prevalence (%)
Jensen[9]	1011 (487:524)	>50 (30–70)	Europids	Timed overnight AER (> 15 µg/min)	0–11	5
Metcalf[19]	3597 (2622:975)	49[b] (40–78)	88.6% Europid + Maori/Asian + Polynesian	EMU Conc. (mg/l) A:C Ratio	0–19 0–1.43 (M)	5 5
Winocour[6]	447 (209:238)	47 (25–70)	98% Europid	EMU Conc. (>20 mg/l) A:C Ratio (>3.5)		6.3 2.2
Non-Europid Haffner[20]	316 (117:199)	50 (25–64)	Mexican Americans	EMU Conc. (>30 mg/l)		13
Collins[22]	702 (310:392)	38 (20–65+)	Polynesians	EMU Conc. (>30 mg/l)	20	9
Woo[8]	1333 (795:538)	38 (20–56)	Chinese	EMU A:C Ratio[a]	0–1.3 (M) 0–2.1 (F)	10 10

Prevalence expressed as percentage outside reference range, or stated cut-off points.
[a]Greater than 90th centile. [b] Median.
Conc: albumin concentration. AER: albumin excretion rate, A:C Ratio: urine albumin:creatinine ratio, EMU: random untimed or early morning urine.

Table 3.2 *Prevalence and expression of microalbuminuria in normoglycaemic children*

Study	Sample size (M:F)	Age (mean (range))	Ethnic grouping	Type of urine collection and expression of albuminuria	Reference range	Prevalence of microalbuminuria (%)
Davies[23]	374 (183:191)	9 (4–16)	Europid	Timed day AER (μg/min/1.73 m^2)	1.1–28.6 (M)	5
					1.3–45.2 (F)	5
				Timed night AER (μg/min/1.73 m^2)	0.8–9.9 (M)	5
					0.9–10.1 (F)	5
Kodama[34]	1090 (582:508)	8 (6–11)	Japanese	EMU Conc. (mg/l)	0–18	5

Prevalence expressed as percentage outside reference range, or stated cut-off points.
Conc: albumin concentration
AER: albumin excretion rate
EMU: random untimed or early morning urine

(women) mg/l. For albumin:creatinine ratios the respective 95th and 97.5th centiles were 1.43 (men) or 1.80 (women), and 2.3 (men) or 2.8 (women) mg/mmol. Albumin concentrations fell with age in men and women, although the albumin:creatinine ratios only fell in women. In sterile Albustix-negative urine (5425 subjects), the degree of albuminuria showed log linear relationships with diastolic blood pressure ($p = 0.0001$, significant change in slope > 78.6 mmHg), and with body mass index ($p = 0.0001$, significant change in slope > 25.9 kg/m^2 in men, and > 28.4 kg/m^2 in women). Log linear relationships with no clear cut off were recorded with serum triglycerides, cholesterol, and systolic blood pressure (all $p = 0.0001$), and a negative linear relationship was noted with HDL cholesterol ($p = 0.0461$, significant change in slope < 1.4 mmol/l). These associations were retained after exclusion of the 183 subjects with diabetes.

Multiple regression analysis revealed that 12.4 % of the variability in albuminuria concentration could be accounted for by the independent influences of age (inverse association), gender, body mass index, diastolic blood pressure and serum triglycerides. Information on alcohol and tobacco consumption increased the prediction of variability to 14.5 %[5], and on dietary intake of fat and fibre to 13.9%. Further study of the same cohort suggested that dietary cholesterol intake > 226 mg/day and dietary fibre intake ≤ 26 g/day independently influenced albuminuria. There appeared to be no independent influence of dietary protein, salt, or altered polyunsaturated:saturated fat ratios[5]. There was also a suggestion that alcohol intake > 32 g/day influenced microalbuminuria independently of age, gender and ethnicity, although not of triglyceridaemia. Smoking was associated with a marginal yet significant univariate increase in albuminuria (5.4 versus 4.6 mg/l), with a linear association apparent on consumption of > 10 cigarettes/day[5].

Influence of ethnic variation

Before discussing the comparability of this study and other reports, it is worth scrutinising the study sample of Metcalf and colleagues. The key point of the study was to ensure that there was adequate representation of employees who were Maori and Pacific Islanders, in addition to Europids. Thus, some 20 % of the entire study population were not European, although the selected group on whom the reference range was based comprised only 10 % non-Europids. The importance of the ethnic background lies in the realisation that microalbuminuria and a host of other metabolic derangements are more prevalent amongst Westernised ethnic minority groups. This is particularly apparent in non-insulin dependent diabetes (see later), where microalbuminuria appears more prevalent in both indiginous and migrant non-Europid ethnic groups, but is also apparent in the absence of diabetes. These same ethnic groups have an increased incidence of obesity, hypertension, dyslipidaemia and non-insulin dependent diabetes, factors directly associated with microalbuminuria, and perhaps the sequelae of primary insulin insensitivity. The significant proportion (20 %) of non-Europids in Metcalf's study had a disproportionate influence on the pattern of microalbuminuria and its relationship with biological variables, which was independent of the greater prevalence of glucose intolerance in these ethnic groups[18]. Other studies in non-diabetic Mexican Americans[20], Australian Aborigines[21], Nauruan Pacific Islanders[22] and Hong Kong Chinese[8] would support this view.

Influence of other demographic factors

In the study of Woo and colleagues[8], the urinary albumin:creatinine ratio was related to blood pressure and measures of insulinaemia and glycaemia in both men and women, and to triglyceridaemia and anthropometric estimates in women. However following multivariate analyses which took account of blood pressure, fasting blood glucose in men, and fasting serum insulin in women also independently contributed to microalbuminuria, but only whilst hypertensive subjects were included in the sample.

The Copenhagen City Heart Study[9] examined an age-stratified representative geographically defined population. The main findings were that on average albuminuria remained constant with age, although men over 60 accounted for the higher albumin excretion rates in males in comparison to females. The prevalence of microalbuminuria (15–150 µg/min) was 3 %, although the 95th centile for this population was 11 µg/min.

Greater urine albumin concentrations in men have also been recorded in almost 1000 Europids in north London[4]. This could be expected from the gender-specific differences in the other variables which appear to exert an influence on microalbuminuria. The anomalous finding of a greater prevalence of microalbuminuria in non-diabetic Nauruan women[22] probably reflects the overwhelming influence of obesity and its preponderance in these women. The contrasting higher albumin:creatinine ratios in women in Auckland[19] has also been recorded in smaller studies in Newcastle upon Tyne[6] and in schoolchildren in Greater Manchester, England[23], and is in a sense an artefact reflecting less muscle bulk and hence lower creatinine excretion amongst females.

The influence of age on albuminuria is more perplexing. Jensen found that increased albumin excretion rates were confined to men more than 60 years old[9], whereas Metcalf and colleagues[19] found that albuminuria concentrations fell in men and women (as did albumin:creatinine ratios in women), and suggested this reflected the parallel age-related decline in glomerular filtration rate, although they then went on to make the interesting (and unsubstantiated) comment that 'age and sex effects were undetectable when laboratory rounding of results and analytical variation were taken into account'. Contrasting unexplained age-related reductions in albumin excretion rates in women and increases in men were noted by Gould and coworkers[4], whereas in our own study a direct correlation between age and albuminuria in men and women was noted[6], and a similar observation was made by Collins and colleagues in Nauruans[22]. Others have found no relationship with age[9]. The age spectrum varied quite a bit in the different studies, and it would appear that a direct relationship with increasing age is more likely where the age spread is not necessarily greater (i.e. 25–65, as opposed to 40–78 years), but where a major proportion is under 40 years of age. This would be compatible with the view that ageing exerts an indirect influence due to an increasing incidence of adverse age-related biological factors, and that this operates above a threshold at roughly 40 years of age.

Influence of metabolic and physiological factors

Blood pressure, body mass index, serum lipids, glucose and insulin are biological factors which are independently associated with albuminuria, and there are sound physiological bases for these relationships. Metcalf and coworkers suggested that they could account for 12.4 % of variability in albuminuria concentrations[19], whilst Gould and colleagues[4] suggested that age, height, systolic blood pressure and blood glucose two hours after a 75 g oral glucose load accounted for 8.4 % of the variability in albumin excretion rates in men. We suggested that as much as 37 % of the variabilty in albumin: creatinine ratios could be accounted for by age, gender, systolic blood pressure and estimated insulin resistance[6].

The correlation between blood pressure and albuminuria is the most consistent observation in the various studies, although there has been a suggestion that, as with insulin resistance and hypertension, the strength of this relationship might vary between ethnic groups, and may be most evident in Europids and Hong Kong Chinese. Metcalf and colleagues[19] used multiple regression and suggested that diastolic blood pressure exerted the major influence, whereas systolic blood pressure appeared more important in other studies[4,6]. An important observation was made by Gosling and Beevers[3], who only found an association with mean blood pressure beyond a threshold of 140 (systolic)/90 (diastolic) mmHg. The concept of an effect of blood pressure beyond a threshold is supported by Metcalf and collaborators[19], where a significant increase in the slope of the regression line between diastolic blood pressure and urine albumin concentration was noted when the 95th centile exceeded 82 mmHg. The relative influence of systolic and diastolic blood pressure reflects the different patterns and prevalence of hypertension in the different population studies. The likeliest mechanism is a chronic increase in capillary hydraulic pressure, in conjunction with altered glomerular permeability. It has been suggested that this could even operate in normotensive first degree relatives of those with essential hypertension, thus explaining microalbuminuria in such subjects, and reflecting the possibilty of genetic modulation of renal albumin handling[24].

The variable importance of body mass index in the several studies may be the consequence of sample, population and ethnic differences in the prevalence of obesity, and perhaps more importantly in variable patterns of regional fat distribution. The clearest direct association between body mass and albuminuria was in the reports of Metcalf and colleagues[19] and Collins and coworkers[22], where obesity (BMI > 30) was a feature of 20 % and 60 % of the respective study populations. By contrast, when obesity was present in less than 10 % of subjects, no such relationship was noted. The suggestion by Gould and colleagues[4] that reduced height was an independent associate of microalbuminuria in men is compatible with increased body mass and centrally distributed fat, but unfortunately no information was provided on the weight of their subjects. A direct physiological mechanism for such an association is speculative. Gould raised the possibility that altered intrauterine growth could be the common basis for short stature, obesity, and altered renal structure and function. An alternative, and to our mind more likely scenario, is that central obesity and additional adverse factors frequently cluster within individuals. The co-existence of cardiovascular disease, hypertension, dyslipidaemia (reduced HDL cholesterol and raised serum triglycerides), hyperuricaemia, hypofibrinolysis, and hyperinsulinaemia in association with normoglycaemia or hyperglycaemia, are increasingly recognised accompaniments of central obesity. There is currently intense interest as to whether hyperinsulinaemia and/or insulin insensitivity could be the prime mover in this constellation of metabolic and vascular abnormalities. As most if not all of these factors have been related to microalbuminuria in the population studies, it may be statistically difficult to demonstrate an independent role for one particular factor.

Fasting or post-glucose load hyperinsulinaemia and insulin insensitivity were independently related to a variable degree with microalbuminuria in Nauruan men but not women[22], in women but not men in Hong Kong Chinese[8] and in smaller studies in English Europids and Mexican Americans[6,20]. In the absence of diabetes, fasting or post oral glucose load plasma glucose values are even less consistently related to albuminuria. This is likely to be a reflection of the fact that under these circumstances plasma glucose operates as a surrogate for serum insulin, but other possibilities include a transitory impact of either glucose or insulin on albumin excretion. Acute increases in blood glucose produce a short-lived increase in albumin excretion, partly through an osmotic diuretic effect, and perhaps also through interference with tubular reabsorption[25-27]. In addition, however, the serum insulin response to glucose loading will itself increase renal blood flow and glomerular filtration of albumin. Insulin may also increase vascular permeability acutely[28]. It is not known whether such processes could operate chronically to augment albuminuria. The associated hyperuricaemia could, however, be the consequence of altered insulin action on renal tubules, and this in turn may affect renal handling of albumin.

The association between albuminuria and triglycerides and HDL cholesterol has been seen to a greater or lesser degree in several studies[6,19,20]. The role of lipids in microalbuminuria will be discussed in more detail later, but the association is of course not necessarily causal, and these cross-sectional studies could just as easily be demonstrating that dyslipidaemia may be the sequelae of microalbuminuria. The likelihood that altered lipid concentrations do not normally modify renal handling of albumin is supported by the lack of microalbuminuria amongst subjects with primary hyperlipidaemia (hypercholesterolaemia and hypertriglyceridaemia)[29].

Influence of lifestyle factors

The independent role of lifestyle in determining microalbuminuria is also probably of marginal importance. The suggestion by Metcalf and colleagues[5] that alcohol may influence albuminuria was not apparent after correction for triglycerides which often rise with chronic alcohol intake, and probably not relevant after taking account of alcohol-induced blood pressure changes. Other reports have found no suggestion that alcohol was related to albuminuria. There is no straightforward mechanism whereby alcohol could alter albumin excretion. Likewise, although smoking may well be important in the progression of microalbuminuria in established cases (particularly in diabetes), the suggestion that smoking induces renal hypoxia and urinary albumin loss appears to be at best of marginal importance. Metcalf and collea-gues[5] suggested that this was significant in those who smoked more than 10 cigarettes a day, but others have not found smoking to be more common amongst microalbuminuric subjects.

The suggestion that dietary cholesterol and fibre intake could indepen-dently influence albuminuria[5] remains unsubstantiated and difficult to explain in physiological terms. Neither dietary salt or protein intake nor the polyunsaturated:saturated fat ratio appear to be significant determinants of microalbuminuria, yet it is known that albumin excretion rates are lower in strict vegans than in omnivores[30]. Although glomerular filtration may change acutely following large animal protein loads[31], varying amounts of protein intake between individuals does not appear to be an important deter-minant of albuminuria.

Exercise is a similar example, in that whilst acute exercise clearly increases albuminuria, regular exercise is not a correlate of albuminuria in popula-tions. The role of regular exercise in albumin excretion cannot be straightfor-ward because of the impact of physical fitness on metabolic and haemodynamic factors which themselves may regulate albumin excretion.

There is virtually no current information on the role of haemostatic and fibrinolytic factors in microalbuminuria in non-diabetic subjects, although we found significant alteration of fibrinogen concentrations accompanying microalbuminuria[6]. There has been a recent intriguing suggestion that indus-trial environmental factors might also play a role in the development of microalbuminuria. Hotz and colleagues[32] examined the role of glycosoami-noglycans in workers exposed to industrial solvents and found that those hypertensive individuals exposed to greatest amounts had significantly higher levels of microalbuminuria. More recently, this finding has been attributed to alterations in the circadian rhythms with shift work rather than to prolonged exposure to nephrotoxic chemicals[33].

Summary

Microalbuminuria in the normal population is probably most precisely defined as overnight albumin excretion rates > 10 µg/min, which are likely to be more prevalent amongst males. In practical terms this might best equate to albumin:creatinine ratios > 1.43 mg/mmol in men, and 1.80 mg/mmol in women. The clearest determinant is blood pressure, but other factors closely related to blood pressure such as insulin insensitivity may also be implicated. The impact of age is probably in the main due to the greater likelihood of these factors interacting.

References

1. Marshall SM. Screening for microalbuminuria: which measurement? *Diabet Med* 1991; **8**:706–711.
2. Hutchison AS, Paterson KR. Collecting urine for microalbumin assay. *Diabet Med* 1988; **5**:527–532.
3. Gosling P, Beevers DG. Urinary albumin excretion and blood pressure in the general population. *Clin Sci* 1989; **76**:39–42.
4. Gould MM, Mohamed-Ali V, Goubet SA, Yudkin JS, Haines AP. Microalbuminuria: associations with height and sex in non-diabetic subjects. *Br Med J* 1993; **306**:240–306.
5. Metcalf PA, Baker JR, Scragg RKR, Dryson E, Scott AR, Wild CJ. Albuminuria in people at least 40 years old: effect of alcohol consumption, regular exercise, and cigarette smoking. *Clin Chem* 1993; **39**:1793–1797.
6. Winocour PH, Harland JOE, Millar JP, Laker MF, Alberti KGMM. Microalbuminuria and associated risk factors in the community. *Atherosclerosis* 1992; **93**:71–81.
7. Watts GF, Morris RW, Khan K, Polak A. Urinary albumin excretion in healthy adult subjects: reference values and some factors affecting their interpretation. *Clin Chim Acta* 1988; **172**:191–198.
8. Woo J, Cockram CS, Swaminathan R, Lau E, Chan A, Cheung R. Microalbuminuria and other cardiovascular risk factors in non-diabetic subjects. *Int J Cardiol* 1992; **37**:345-350.
9. Jensen JS, Feldt-Rasmussen B, Borch-Johnsen K, Jensen G and the Copenhagen City Heart Study Group. Urinary albumin excretion in a population based sample of 1011 middle aged non-diabetic subjects. *Scand J Clin Lab Invest* 1993; **53**:867–872.
10. Jarrett RJ, Viberti GC, Argyropoulos A, Hill RD, Mahmud U, Murrells TJ. Microalbuminuria predicts mortality in non-insulin-dependent diabetes. *Diabet Med* 1984; **1**:17–20.
11. Messent JWC, Elliot TG, Hill RD, Jarrett RJ, Keen H, Viberti GC. Prognostic significance of microalbuminuria in insulin-dependent diabetes mellitus: twenty- three year follow-up study. *Kidney Int* 1992; **41**:836-839.
12. Mogensen CE. Microalbuminuria predicts clinical proteinuria and early mortality in maturity-onset diabetes. *N Engl J Med* 1984; **310**:356–360.
13. Viberti GC, Hill RD, Jarrett RJ, Argyropoulos A, Mahmud U, Keen H. Microalbuminuria as a predictor of clinical nephropathy in insulin-dependent diabetes mellitus. *Lancet* 1982; **i**:1430–1432.
14. Mogensen CE, Chachati A, Christensen CK, Close CF, Deckert T, Hommel E, *et al*. Microalbuminuria: an early marker of renal involvement in diabetes. *Uremia Invest* 1985–86; **9**:85–95.
15. Microalbuminuria Collaborative Study Group. Microalbuminuria in type 1 diabetic patients. Prevalence and clinical characteristics. *Diabetes Care* 1992; **15**:495–501.
16. MacLeod JM, Lutale J, Marshall SM. Albumin excretion and vascular deaths in NIDDM. *Diabetologia* 1995; **38**:610–616.
17. Damsgaard EM, Fröland A, Jörgensen OD, Mogensen CE. Microalbuminuria as a predictor of increased mortality in elderly people . *Br Med J* 1990; **300**: 297–300.

18. Metcalf PA, Baker JR, Scragg RKR, Dryson E, Scott AJ, Wild CJ. Microalbuminuria in a middle-aged workforce: effect of hyperglycaemia and ethnicity. *Diabetes Care* 1993; **16**: 1485-1493.

19. Metcalf P, Baker J, Scott A, Wild C, Scragg R, Dryson E. Albuminuria in people at least 40 years old: effect of obesity, hypertension, and hyperlipidaemia. *Clin Chem* 1992; **38**:1802–1808.

20. Haffner SM, Stern MP, Gruber MKK, Hazuda HP, Mitchell BD, Patterson JK. Microalbuminuria. Potential marker for increased cardiovascular risk factors in nondiabetic subjects? *Arteriosclerosis* 1990; **10**:727–731.

21. Guest CS, Ratnaike S, Larkins RG. Albuminuria in Aborigines and Europids of South-Eastern Australia. *Med J Austr* 1993; **159**:335–338.

22. Collins VR, Dowse GK, Finch CF, Zimmet PZ, Linnane AW. Prevalence and risk factors for micro- and macroalbuminuria in diabetic subjects and entire population of Nauru. *Diabetes* 1989; **38**:1602–1610.

23. Davies AG, Postlethwaite RJ, Price DA, Berne JL, Houlton CA, Fielding BA. Urinary albumin excretion in children. *Arch Dis Child* 1984; **59**:625–630.

24. Fauvel JP, Hadj-Aissa A, Laville M, Fadat G, Labeeuw M, Zech P, Pozet N. Microalbuminuria in normotensives with genetic risk of hypertension. *Nephron* 1991; **57**: 375–376.

25. First MR, Patel VB, Pesce AJ, Bramlage RJ, Pollak VE. Albumin excretion by the kidney. The effects of osmotic diuresis. *Nephron* 1978; **20**:171–175.

26. Hegedus L, Christiansen NJ, Mogensen CE, Gundersen HJG. Oral glucose increases urinary albumin excretion in normal subjects but not in insulin-dependent diabetics. *Scand J Clin Lab Invest* 1980; **40**:479–480.

27. Jarrett RJ, Verma NP, Keen H. Urinary albumin excretion in normal and diabetic subjects. *Clin Chim Acta* 1976; **71**:55–59.

28. Nestler JE, Barlascini CO, Tetrault GA, Fratkin MJ, Clore JN, Blackard WG. Increased transcapillary escape rate of albumin in nondiabetic men in response to hyperinsulinaemia. *Diabetes* 1990; **39**:1212–1217.

29. Smellie WSA, Warwick GL. Primary hyperlipidaemia is not associated with increased urinary albumin excretion. *Nephrol Dial Transplant* 1991; **6**:398–401.

30. Wiseman MJ, Hunt R, Goodwin A, Gross JL, Keen H, Viberti GC. Dietary composition and renal function in healthy subjects. *Nephron* 1987; **46**:37–42.

31. Shestakova MV, Mukhin NA, Dedov II, Titov VN, Warshavsky VA. Protein-loading test, urinary albumin excretion and renal morphology in diagnosis of subclinical diabetic nephropathy. *J Intern Med* 1992; **231**:213–217.

32. Hotz P, Pilliod J, Berode M, Rey F, Boillat M-A. Glycosaminoglycans, albuminuria and hydrocarbon exposure. *Nephron* 1991; **58**:184–191.

33. Boogard PJ, Caubo MEJ. Increased albumin excretion in industrial workers due to shift work rather than to prolonged exposure to low concentrations of chlorinated hydrocarbons. *Occ Envtl Med* 1994; **51**:638–641.

34. Kodama K, Tomioka M, Otani T, Shimizu S, Uchigata Y, Hirata Y. The range of albumin concentrations in the single-void first morning urine of 1090 healthy young children. *Diabetes Res Clin Pract* 1990; **9**:55–58.

4

Microalbuminuria in diabetes mellitus

Introduction

It has been recognised for many years that IDDM patients with persistent dip-stick positive proteinuria have a very much worse prognosis than patients who remain dip-stick negative. The relative mortality of proteinuric IDDM patients is 75–100 times that of the non-diabetic population, compared with 2–4 times for non-proteinuric patients[1]. Cardiovascular mortality is much more common in those patients with proteinuria than in those without[2], up to two thirds of proteinuric patients dying of cardiovascular disease and the remainder of renal complications. Conversely, few patients surviving for longer than 40 years with insulin-dependent diabetes have dip-stick positive proteinuria[3]. Thus, the sub-group of proteinuric IDDM patients have an exceptionally poor prognosis. Once proteinuria appears, the renal disease is irreversible, measures such as antihypertensive therapy and low protein diets reducing the rate of decline of the glomerular filtration rate rather than halting or reversing the process. There is thus a need to identify at a much earlier stage those patients who will later develop dip-stick positive proteinuria, in the hope that earlier intervention will completely halt or even reverse the renal and cardiovascular disease processes. The development of a specific and sensitive radioimmunoassay for urine albumin in 1963[4] opened up this prospect.

The Guy's group quickly followed this initial methodological paper with work showing that in some established IDDM patients without clinical proteinuria the albumin excretion rate was higher than in healthy non-diabetic individuals[5]. Other groups confirmed this work and, in addition, demonstrated that at diagnosis of IDDM the AER may be elevated but returns to normal as blood glucose is controlled[6]. In newly diagnosed NIDDM patients, albumin excretion rates measured during a 2 h, 50 g glucose toler-

53

ance test were noted to be higher than in non-diabetic individuals[7]. It was thus obvious that diabetic subjects without overt proteinuria could still exhibit increased albumin excretion above the normal range, and the term microalbuminuria was coined.

Significance of microalbuminuria in diabetes

Insulin-dependent diabetes

The significance of the above observations was not realised until 1982, when the first of several reports was published. In 1966–67, the Guy's group measured timed overnight albumin excretion rates in 87 IDDM patients without proteinuria. The patients were re-studied 14 years later, information on 63 of the original cohort being available[8]. Of the eight whose initial AER was ≥ 30 µg/min, seven had developed persistent proteinuria and three had died, whilst of the 55 with initial AER < 30 µg/min, five had died and only two developed proteinuria. Reassessment of the same cohort after a total of 23 years' follow-up[9] confirmed the higher risk of developing clinical proteinuria in the microalbuminuric patients and, in addition, demonstrated that they were also at increased risk of dying of a cardiovascular cause. The relative risk of clinical proteinuria was 9.3 and of cardiovascular death 2.9 compared with the normoalbuminuric patients. Recent papers from other groups have confirmed that microalbuminuric IDDM patients are at increased risk of large vessel disease, although this does not become clinically apparent until the patients have clinical proteinuria[10,11].

Several additional reports from different groups quickly confirmed these broad findings (Table 4.1). Although the types of urine collections, albumin assays, length of follow-up and predictive cut-off levels are different in each study, the overall conclusion is similar, namely that IDDM patients with microalbuminuria are at greatly increased risk of the later development of persistent proteinuria and of early death. Overall, approximately 80 % of patients with AER above the given cut-off develop persistent proteinuria, end-stage renal failure or die prematurely, whilst only 5 % of those below the cut-off do so.

Non-insulin-dependent diabetes

Microalbuminuria has a somewhat different significance in NIDDM patients. Jarrett and colleagues[17] studied 42 NIDDM patients, with urine negative to dip-stick, in 1966–67 and again in 1980. Of the 25 survivors,

Table 4.1 *Summary of the studies showing the predictive power of microalbuminuria in diabetes mellitus*

Reference	Type of urine sample	Length of follow-up (years)	Non-diabetic reference range	Discriminant value
Renal risk in IDDM				
Viberti[8]	Overnight	14	<12 µg/min	30 µg/min
Parving[12]	24 h	6	<40 mg/24 h	40 mg/24 h
Mogensen[13]	Short day-time	>7	<7.5 µg/min	15 µg/min
Mathiesen[14]	24 h	6	<20 µg/min	70 µg/min
MCS[15]	Overnight	4	<10 µg/min	10 µg/min
Mathiesen[16]	24 h	5	<15 mg/min	15 µg/min
Cardiovascular risk in NIDDM				
Mogensen[18]	EMU	9	<15 mg/l	15 mg/l
MacLeod[20]	Overnight	8	<10.6 µg/min	10.6 µg/min
Jarrett[17]	Overnight	14	<10 µg/min	10 µg/min
Neil[21]	Random	6.1	<15 mg/l	40 mg/l
Schmitz[19]	EMU	10	<15 mg/l	15 mg/l
Mattock[22]	Overnight	3.4	<20 µg/min	20 µg/min
Gall[23]	24 h	5	<30 mg/24 h	30 mg/24 h
Beatty[24]	Random	8	<35 mg/l	35 mg/l

EMU, early morning urine sample.

24 had initial AER ≤ 10 µg/min in an overnight collection, whilst of the 17 deceased, six had initial AER > 30 µg/min and ten > 10 µg/min. The mortality risk for subjects with AER > 30 and > 10 µg/min was 3.3 and 4.0 respectively. In a much larger study with a ten-year follow-up, increasing mortality was seen with rising albumin concentration in an early morning urine sample, mortality being increased 37 % above non-diabetic subjects in the diabetic subjects with albumin concentration < 15 mg/l, 76 % in those with albumin concentration 16-29 mg/l and 148 % in the group with albumin concentration 30–140 mg/l[18]. The predominant cause of death was cardiovascular disease in all groups. In addition, after nine years, those with initial albumin concentration 30–140 mg/l were more likely to have proteinuria (albumin concentration > 400 mg/l) than those with initially lower albumin concentrations, although only 17 out of 76 actually developed proteinuria. This gradient of increasing risk of early death with increased albumin concentration has been confirmed by other Danish workers (Fig. 4.1)[19]. Further work, summarised in Table 4.1 has confirmed that microalbuminuria is a risk marker for premature death in NIDDM, the relative risk being around two to three compared with normoalbuminuric NIDDM patients.

In all of the studies described above, the predominant cause of premature death was cardiovascular disease. One study compared 153 NIDDM patients with AER ≥10.5 µg/min in an overnight collection to 153 patients with AER < 10.5 µg/min, matched for age, gender and known duration of diabetes[20]. Ninety patients with elevated AER died during an 8 year follow-up, compared to 63 with normal albumin excretion. There was an excess of deaths due to large vessel disease (cardiovascular, peripheral vascular and cerebro-vascular disease combined) in those with elevated albumin excretion. The excess of vascular deaths was also seen in subgroups with AER 10.6–29.9 µg/min and > 29.9 µg/min. In this study and in most others, the increased risk associated with microalbuminuria has been shown to be independent of other established cardiovascular risk factors.

Thus, it would appear that in NIDDM, microalbuminuria identifies a subgroup with a particularly poor outlook, many dying prematurely, predominantly from large vessel disease. In addition, there does appear to be an increased risk of progression to clinical proteinuria, although for an individual patient, this risk is much smaller than in IDDM and is overshadowed by the cardiovascular risk.

Survival

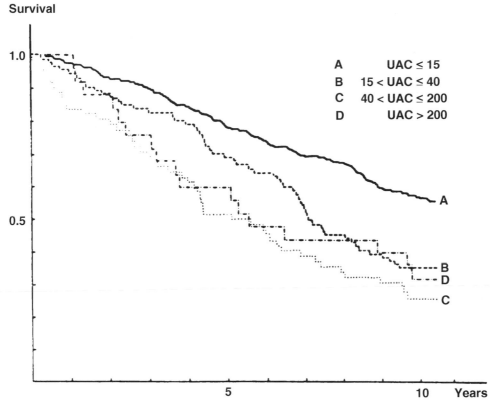

Fig. 4.1. Kaplan–Meier estimates of the survival curves for four levels of
   urinary albumin concentration (UAC, mg/l) measured in early
   morning urine samples obtained from 503 patients with non-
   insulin-dependent diabetes. Reproduced from reference 19 with
   permission (copyright John Wiley & Sons Limited).

Prevalence of microalbuminuria

The pathogenesis of microalbuminuria in diabetes appears more complex
than in the normoglycaemic population and will be discussed in detail later
in the chapter. It is clear, however, that the factors important in the pathophysiology of albuminuria in diabetes need to be taken account of in trying
to resolve the apparent inconsistencies when reviewing the literature on the
epidemiology of microalbuminuria. One of the key difficulties is that the vast
majority of surveys of the prevalence of microalbuminuria in diabetes is
hospital clinic based, where there is inevitable bias in patient selection. The
sample size in several studies, in particular of ethnic minorities, is often
woefully small. Those notable exceptions will be discussed in greater detail.
It is also necessary to consider the natural history of microalbuminuria in

Table 4.2 *Studies of the prevalence of microalbuminuria in NIDDM*

Study	Sample	Ethnic group	Number (M:F)	Age (years)	Duration of diabetes (years)	Sample	Prevalence (%)
Mogensen[25]	Clinic	Europid	601 (254:347)	60 (53–90)	5 (0–30[b])	EMU (× 2.9 samples)	> Pred 30 µg/ml: 13.7
Stiegler[26]	Population	Europid	290 (103:187)	64 (35–75)	8 (1–21)	EMU	> Ref 15 µg/ml: 39.6–49.5: > Pred 30 µg/ml: 20
Schmitz[19]	Clinic	Europid	503 (222:281)	66 (50–75)	7 (0–25)	EMU	> Ref 15 µg/ml: 30
Patrick[27]	Clinic	Europid	149 (87:62)	60 (36–86[a])	0	EMU	> Ref Alb:Cr > 2.5: 26
Gatling[28]	Population	Europid	329 (190:139)	? (5–98)	? (0–58)	Timed overnight	> Ref 7 µg/ml: 3: > Pred 30 µg/ml: 7.6
Marshall[29]	Clinic	Europid	524 (272:252)	65 (19–86)	8 (1–33)	Timed overnight	> Ref 10.5 µg/ml: 22.3: > Pred 30 µg/ml: 10
Mattock[30]	Clinic	Europid	141 (82:59)	56 (40–73[a])	5 (0–14[a])	Timed overnight	> Pred 30 µg/ml: 5
Damsgaard[31]	Population	Europid	211 (80:131)	68[+] (60–74)	7 (0–35)	Timed day time	> Ref 15 µg/ml: 55–68; > Pred 30 µg/ml: 30–45
Gall[32]	Clinic	Europidid	549 (296:253)	60 (35–76[a])	9 (0–20)	Timed 24 h	> Pred 21 µg/ml: 27
Collins[33]	Population	Polynesian	318 (142:176)	47 (20–65[b])	5 (0–21)	EMU	> Pred 30 µg/ml: 40
Erasmus[34]	Clinic	African (Ind)	113 (53:60)	51 (30–65)	5 (0–25)	Timed 24 h	> Pred 21 µg/min: 57
Tai[35]	Clinic	Chinese	63 (34:29)	55 (50–65[b])	10 (0–23)	Timed overnight	> Ref 8.6 µg/ml: 23.8
Cheung[36]	Clinic	Chinese	157 (45:112)	58 (21–88)	3 (1–21)	EMU	> Ref Alb:Cr > 2.5: 54.1
Haffner[37]	Clinic	Mex Amer	234 (105:129)	51 (25–64)	8 (7–10[a])	EMU	> Pred 30 µg/ml: 30.8
Allawi[38]	Clinic	Indian (Mig)	154 (93:61)	51 (28–65)	3 (0–22)	EMU	> Ref Alb:C > 2.0: 26.0
Gupta[39]	Clinic	Indian (Ind)	64 (34:30)	49 (26–60[a])	7 (0–18[a])	Timed day time	> Pred 20 µg/min: 26.6

Mex Amer: Mexican American, Ind: indigenous population, Mig: migrant population. Figures are mean or [b] median (range) or ([a] 95% confidence intervals of mean) concentrations or excretion rates. EMU: random untimed or early morning urine, Alb:Cr: albumin:creatinine ratio. > Ref: values outside non-diabetic reference range, > Pred: values outside cut-off predictive of complications.

diabetes (*vide infra*), in particular the influence of the duration of diabetes on the incidence of microalbuminuria.

Non-insulin-dependent diabetes

The prevalence of microalbuminuria in NIDDM in several studies is shown in Table 4.2. The essential difficulty in defining the precise duration of diabetes should be considered when assessing differences in the importance attributed to the impact of the duration of diabetes on microalbuminuria. Notwithstanding the additional problem of variable urine collection conditions, a broad consensus emerges with occasional exceptions. Microalbuminuria prevalence is expressed either as percentage prevalence outside a reference range, or as values greater than those predictive of morbidity and mortality end points. It is worth considering both. The majority of Europid population studies has been in older populations whose average age is 60–65 years, in contrast to those in other indigenous or migrant ethnic groups. The average proportion outside the reference range in Europids is around 25 %, with a wide scatter (20–68 %). When predictive cut-offs are used, the prevalence of excretion rates > 30 μg/min is around 10 % (range 8–45 %). The study of Damsgaard and Mogensen[31] focused on a slightly older cohort (average age 68 years) and confirmed that ageing is associated with a higher prevalence, outside the reference range in at least 55 %, and above the predictive cut-off in at least 30 % of cases. The vast majority of studies has confirmed a higher prevalence in men, although this difference seems less apparent in Chinese and African populations[34–36].

The only population-based studies of microalbuminuria prevalence in NIDDM are those of Gatling and coworkers[28], where detailed demographic data was not presented, or that of Stiegler and colleagues[26], where unfortunately a random non-timed single early morning urine specimen was used to assess urinary albumin concentration. Despite the fact that the study of Marshall and Alberti[29] focused on patients attending hospital clinics in Newcastle upon Tyne, it had the benefit of studying a large cohort of more than 500 subjects, and utilised apparently sterile timed overnight urine collections, thereby minimising variability and misclassification.

The data from Marshall and Alberti[29] are similar to that recorded by Gall and colleagues in Denmark[32], where a single timed 24 h collection was used, and microalbuminuria (excretion rates > 20 μg/min) was present in 27 % of cases, who were on average five years younger than the Newcastle cohort. The apparent higher prevalence of microalbuminuria in Denmark may not simply be the consequence of differing methods of sampling patients and

Table 4.3 *Studies of the prevalence of microalbuminuria in adult IDDM*

Study	Sample	Ethnic group	Number (M:F)	Age (years)	Duration of diabetes (years)	Sample	Prevalence (%)
Mogensen[25]	Clinic	Europid	481 (245:236)	30 (6–84[a])	8 (0–30[b])	EMU (2.9 samples)	> Pred 30 μg/ml: 9.4
Marshall[29]	Clinic	Europid	416 (215:201)	45 (14–87)	18 (1–55)	Timed overnight	> Ref 10.5 μg/mmin: 33.6: > Pred 30 μg/min: 7
Gatling[28]	Clinic	Europid	121 (70:51)	? (5–98)	? (0–58)	Timed overnight	> Ref 7.1 μg/min: 32; > Pred 30 μg/min: 5.0
McCance[42]	Clinic	Europid	210 (?)	25 (12–43)	10 (0–18)	Timed overnight	> Ref 20 μg/min: 8.1
Watts[43]	Clinic	Europid	172 (96:76)	30 (4–33[a])	16 (4–33[a])	Timed overnight	> Ref 15 μg/ml: 26.0
MCS[44]	Clinic	Europid	1888 (1059:829)	34 (16–60)	20 (1–39)	Timed overnight	> Pred 30 μg/min: 3.7
Berglund[45]	Clinic	Europid	102 (51:51)	36 (18–50)	22 (10–44)	Timed overnight	> Pred 20 μg/min: 16.0 (2 samples)
Parving[46]	Clinic	Europid	957 (514:443)	41 (18–71[a])	22 (5–48)	Timed 24 h	> Pred 21 μg/min: 22.0
Orchard[47]	Population	Europ/Af Amer	657 (332:325)	24 (8–48)	20 (5–30[b])	Timed 24 h	> Pred 20 μg/min: 21.0 (2 samples)
Descamps[48]	Clinic	Europid	413 (137:161)	39 ± 15	13±10	Timed 24 h	> Pred 20 μg/min: 21
Joner[49]	Population	Europid	351 (189:162)	20 (8–30)	11 (6–17)	Timed overnight	> Ref 15: 12.5 (> 3 samples)
Ramirez[50]	Clinic	?Europid	156 (77:79)	35 (17–25[a])	16 (5–25)	Timed overnight	> Pred 20 : 12.2
Kalk[51]	Clinic	Europid	127 (70:57)	20 (13–36[a])	20 (1–35[a])	Timed day time	> Ref 20 : 36.2
Haffner[37]	Clinic	Mex Amer	234 (105:129)	51 (25–64)	8 (7–10[a])	EMU	> Pred 30 : 30.8
Gupta[39]	Clinic	Ind Indian	38 (20:18)	22 (5–39[a])	6 (0–20)	Timed day time	> Ref 20 : 7.9

M:F (male:female), Mex Amer: Mexican American, Ind: indigenous, Af Amer: African American. Figures are mean or [b] median (range) or ([a] 95% confidence intervals of mean) concentrations or excretion rates. EMU: random untimed or early morning urine, Alb:Cr albumin: creatinine ratio. > Ref: values outside non-diabetic reference range, > Pred: values outside cut-off predictive of complications.

urine. Recent data on factors of potential importance for microalbuminuria such as the prevalence of hypertension, and the distribution of erythrocyte sodium lithium countertransport activity in both diabetic and control populations, raise the possibility of a genuine (genetic and/or environmental) difference between the epidemiology of microalbuminuria in England and Denmark.

In studies of non-white communities, between 25 and 75 % of urinary albumin values were outside reference ranges for African, Polynesian, Indian, Chinese and Mexican American NIDDM populations whose average age was 50–55 years, whilst the prevalence of values > 20 μg/min ranged from 26 % in Indians to 57 % in Nigerian Africans[33,34,37–41].

Insulin-dependent diabetes

The prevalence of microalbuminuria in adult IDDM is shown in Table 4.3. Whilst the criticism that a population-based approach is lacking could be made about all studies with the exception of Joner and colleagues[49] and Orchard and coworkers[47], it is still possible to distill a reasonable degree of consistency. The estimation of duration of diabetes in particular is more clearcut in IDDM compared with NIDDM, which may explain its importance as a determinant of microalbuminuria in most reports, the majority of which were in Europids. The most representative studies demonstrate that the prevalence of excretion rates outside the reference range is 20–30 % (cut offs respectively 10–15 μg/min on timed overnight collections), whilst 7–16 % had rates predictive of renal and vascular sequelae (reflecting overnight timed rates of 15–30 μg/min).

The ethnic aspect is less clear in IDDM. Orchard and colleagues[47] reported a higher prevalence of microalbuminuria in a group on average 20 years younger than those studied by Marshall and Alberti[29], but the likely inclusion of African Americans may in part explain the inconsistency. Another group to explicitly study non-white IDDM subjects recorded microalbuminuria in only 8 % of indigenous Indians, but the average duration of diabetes was only 6 years, and the sample size very small[39]. As suggested for NIDDM, the apparent higher prevalence of microalbuminuria in IDDM in Denmark (22 %), may reflect a true difference, as the patients had characteristics which suggested they were broadly representative of a population based sample[46]. The apparent consensus from the Microalbuminuria Collaborative Study Group of a 3.7 % prevalence (timed overnight excretion 30–250 μg/min) is an underestimate, since hypertensive subjects were excluded, and Norgaard and coworkers[52] have elegantly shown that increasing incidence of hypertension in IDDM is almost exclusively confined to those with microalbuminuria (Figure 4.2).

Studies of microalbuminuria in IDDM children to date have been carried out on predominantly (or exclusively) Europid clinic populations (Table 4.4)[53,58]. The largest study by Mortensen and colleagues[56] was performed in 22 paediatric clinics in 950 subjects, whose average duration of diabetes was only six years. The overall prevalence (on two to three timed overnight rates 20–150 µg/min) was 4.3 %, but was 13–14 % in adolescents, suggesting a joint impact of puberty and greater duration of diabetes as observed in

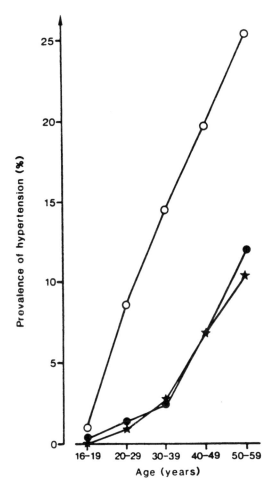

Fig. 4.2. Prevalence of hypertension in all insulin-dependent diabetic patients ($n = 1703$; o———o), in the Danish general population ($n = 10202$; ●———●) and in normoalbuminuric diabetic patients ($n = 1301$; *———*). Reproduced from reference 52 with permission (copyright Springer-Verlag).

Table 4.4 *Studies of the prevalence of microalbuminuria in children with IDDM*

Study	Sample	Ethnic group	Number (M:F)	Age (years)	Duration of diabetes (years)	Sample	Prevalence (%)
Mathiesen[53]	Clinic	Europid	97 (47:50)	15 (7–18)	10 (2–17)	Timed overnight	> Ref 14 µg/min: 20.0 (2 samples)
Ellis[54] Widstam-	Clinic						
Attorps[55]	Clinic	Europid	110 (69:41)	16[a] (5–98)	7 (2–19)	Timed day time	> Ref 20 µg/min: 15.0
Mortensen[56]	Clinic	Europid	950 (506:444)	13 (2–19)	6 (0–18)	Timed overnight	> Pred 20 µg/min: 4.3 (13–14 adolescents)
Davies[57]	Clinic	Europid	83 (43:40)	12 (1–18)	5 (0–14)	Timed overnight	> Ref 10 µg/ml: 15.7

M:F (male: female). Figures are mean or [a] median (range) concentrations or excretion rates. > Ref: values outside healthy reference range, > Pred: values outside cut-off predictive of complications.

other studies where the prevalence was greater. In children actual age thus appears a relatively more important correlate of microalbuminuria than in adults, and this is also the case for HbA_1 and body mass index. Blood pressure is usually related to microalbuminuria in children and, with metabolic control (females in particular), appears to exert a synergistic influence on the duration of diabetes, particularly in adolescents.

Determinants of microalbuminuria

Blood pressure

Blood pressure is one of the most important determinants of microalbuminuria and is discussed in detail later in this chapter and in Chapter 6.

Duration of diabetes

Several studies have suggested that microalbuminuria is rare in the first five years of IDDM[29,44]. However, in the large EURODIAB IDDM complications study[59], the overall prevalence of microalbuminuria was 20.7 %, and 19.3 % in those with duration of diabetes of one to five years. The prevalence of microalbuminuria and macroalbuminuria increased with increasing HbA_{1c}.

In NIDDM, there is general agreement that persistent microalbuminuria is present from diagnosis in a proportion, perhaps 10–20 %, of patients (*vide infra*).

Age

In children, there is a clear relationship of albumin excretion to age, which is compounded by the effects of puberty[53,57,58,60]. The relationship in adults is less readily apparent but still present.

Genetic factors

A full discussion of the genetic factors influencing the development of microalbuminuria and nephropathy is outwith the scope of this review. There is strong evidence for genetic susceptibility to nephropathy. In IDDM, sibling studies have suggested that siblings of probands with nephropathy are much more likely to develop nephropathy themselves than siblings of probands with normal albumin excretion[61,62]. The largest, and only prospective study has shown a difference of nearly 50 % in the risk to siblings, dependent on the probands' renal status, consistent with a major gene effect[63] (Fig. 4.3). In NIDDM, studies in Pima Indians also suggest a genetic component, with proteinuria being three times more likely in diabetic offspring whose parents both had proteinuria compared with offspring neither of whose parents had nephropathy[64].

A number of candidate genes have been studied, including elements of the renin–angiotensin system[65–67], ion countertransporters[68–74] and enzymes and proteins involved with basement membrane synthesis or structure[75–78]. As yet, no firm conclusions can be drawn. This area of research is developing rapidly and it is hoped that future studies will not be bedevilled by problems with small sample size and inappropriate subject selection.

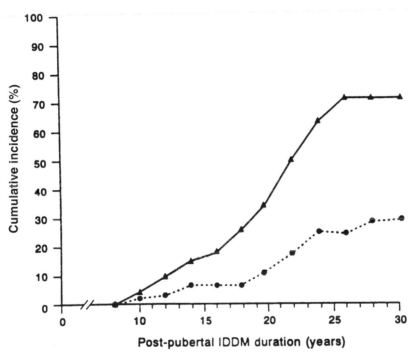

Fig. 4.3. Cumulative incidence of persistent proteinuria in IDDM siblings of
IDDM probands according to the proband's nephropathy status.
The higher curve is for siblings of probands with proteinuria (◄).
The lower curve is for siblings of probands with normoalbuminuria
or microalbuminuria (●). The difference in cumulative incidence
rate (risk difference) of nephropathy after 25 years of diabetes
post-puberty is 46.1 % (CI 20.2–72.0 %). Reproduced from reference 63 with permission (copyright Springer-Verlag).

Glycaemia

Ambient blood glucose levels are significantly higher in microalbuminuric than normoalbuminuric IDDM patients[79], although the relationship of current glycaemia does not necessarily relate to longer-term measures such as glycated haemoglobin, because acute hyperglycaemia may lead to acute increases in albumin excretion. However, in most cross-sectional studies of IDDM patients glycated haemoglobin values are also higher[14,49,56,79–82]. Several longitudinal, retrospective studies have also suggested that microalbuminuria develops in those patients with the poorest blood glucose control[83,84]. In a further retrospective large study in IDDM patients over six years, glycated haemoglobin values, both current and the mean of the previous six years, were higher in those with microalbuminuria defined as AER > 20 µg/min in a 24-h sample than in those with AER < 20 µg/min[42]. However, when those with microalbuminuria defined as AER > 20 µg/min in an overnight sample were studied, neither current nor previous glycated haemoglobin values were different in those with normoalbuminuria and microalbuminuria.

The contribution of glycaemia to microalbuminuria in NIDDM is less clear-cut, although associations have been reported which appear to be stronger in Europid than in other ethnic groups[85].

The role of blood glucose levels in the development and progression of microalbuminuria is discussed further later in this chapter.

Other microvascular complications

As in clinical proteinuria, the other microvascular complications are more common in microalbuminuric compared with normoalbuminuric diabetic patients. All retinopathy, including blindness and proliferative retinopathy[46] is more common[14,15,29,32,82,86]. Microalbuminuric patients are also more likely to have peripheral neuropathy[46,87] or foot ulceration[32]. Fernando and colleagues[88] found that in a mixed group of IDDM and NIDDM patients, vibration perception threshold and mean peak plantar foot pressure were elevated and peroneal motor conduction velocity reduced in patients with microalbuminuria compared with patients with normal albumin excretion.

IDDM patients with microalbuminuria have been shown to have enhanced contractility of hand veins to infusion of noradrenaline[89]. The vascular response to noradrenaline correlates with conduction velocity in the median and peroneal nerves, suggesting that damage to presynaptic inhibitory α_2-

adrenoreceptors is in part responsible[90]. The association of microalbuminuria to abnormalities of the endothelium is discussed in detail in Chapter 5.

In a cross-sectional study, detailed cardiovascular autonomic function tests were performed in ten IDDM patients with microalbuminuria (AER 30–200 µg/min) and in IDDM patients with normal albumin excretion, clinical proteinuria, renal insufficiency and end-stage renal disease matched for age, gender and duration of diabetes, and in non-diabetic control subjects[91]. Heart rate response to deep breathing and to standing, and Valsalva manoeuvre ratios were all significantly lower, and resting heart rates higher, in all the diabetic groups compared with the control subjects. However, only the Valsalva response ratio in the microalbuminuric group was significantly different to that in the normoalbuminuric diabetic group. Subjects with more advanced renal disease had progressively more marked abnormalities.

In a study looking from the converse aspect, Winocour and colleagues[92] found that IDDM patients with autonomic neuropathy had similar total 24-h and day-time albumin excretion rates, but their nocturnal excretion rates of albumin and sodium and urine volumes were significantly higher than in patients without autonomic changes. In a similar study, Spallone and colleagues[93] confirmed that the percentage day–night changes in systolic and diastolic blood pressure and AER were less in IDDM patients with autonomic neuropathy. In those with autonomic neuropathy, 2-h day, day and night AER all significantly correlated with day and night systolic BP. The authors suggested a causal relationship of autonomic neuropathy to nephropathy.

Macrovascular disease

As discussed above, microalbuminuria is a risk marker for cardiovascular disease in both IDDM and NIDDM. The presence of microalbuminuria also increases the likelihood of concurrent vascular disease, particularly in NIDDM. Coronary heart disease is more common in both Europid[30,32] and Asian microalbuminuric NIDDM populations[94], as is peripheral vascular disease[29].

The relationship of microalbuminuria to conventional cardiovascular risk factors, including dyslipidaemias, hypertension, obesity and smoking, is discussed in detail in Chapter 6.

Renal histological changes

Understandably, very few studies have examined the structural lesions associated with microalbuminuria in either insulin-dependent or non-insulin-dependent diabetes. Marked histological changes are seen in IDDM patients with and without clinical nephropathy, with arteriolohyalinosis, subcapsular fibrosis, glomerular mesangial expansion and capillary closure occurring in both groups[95]. However, the area of open capillaries appeared within normal limits in patients without nephropathy, but was markedly reduced in those with clinical evidence of renal impairment.

In a comparison of renal histological measures in IDDM patients with normal albumin excretion and blood pressure, microalbuminuria and normal blood pressure, and microalbuminuria and high blood pressure and/or decreased creatinine clearance, only those patients with microalbuminuria and high blood pressure and/or decreased creatinine clearance had consistently abnormal glomerular structure[96], with increased glomerular basement membrane thickness, fractional volume of mesangium and mesangial volume per glomerulus. However, in contrast another study has shown increased glomerular basement membrane thickness, fractional volume of mesangium, and matrix star volume in microalbuminuric compared with normoalbuminuric patients[97]. AER correlated positively with each of these three structural parameters and glomerular filtration rate and blood pressure were similar in the two groups.

In another small study of 15 IDDM patients, all with some degree of nephropathy, only four had AER < 300 µg/min[98]. However, significant correlations were found between an index of severity of clinical nephropathy (AER, GFR and blood pressure) and the severity of structural changes (basement membrane thickness, mesangial expansion and glomerular occlusion). The albumin excretion rate correlated with the percentage of the peripheral basement membrane carrying fluffy loose intrinsic fine structure. No relationship was found between histological parameters and blood pressure alone.

A small study of 17 adolescent IDDM patients with low levels of microalbuminuria (mean 32 µg/min) showed an increase in basement membrane thickness, mesangial volume fraction and matrix volume fraction compared with values measured in 11 healthy kidney donors[99]. Matrix star volume and thickness, interstitial volume fraction and mean capillary diameter were also increased. The increase in basement membrane thickness and matrix volume fraction per year of diabetes duration correlated with the mean HbA_{1c} over the year preceding biopsy.

One study has not found such consistent histological differences between groups of patients[100]. In microalbuminuric female IDDM patients with normal or reduced GFR, volume fraction of mesangium, index of arteriolar hyalinosis and percentage sclerosed glomeruli were increased compared with IDDM women with normal albumin excretion, as might have been expected from the above. However, similar morphometric changes were seen in women with low creatinine clearance rates and normal albumin excretion. The reasons for these observations are not clear, but it may be that estimation of glomerular filtration by endogenous creatinine clearance led to abnormally low results in this group of patients.

Thus in IDDM, the bulk of the evidence suggests that structural abnormalities are more marked in microalbuminuric patients (Fig. 4.4).

The situation is less clear-cut in NIDDM. Non-diabetic renal disease is said to be more common in proteinuric NIDDM than IDDM patients[101,102], although some authors have suggested that this apparent increase is due to bias in including patients with non-diabetic renal disease in the reported series[103]. One semi-quantitative study using light microscopy only demon-

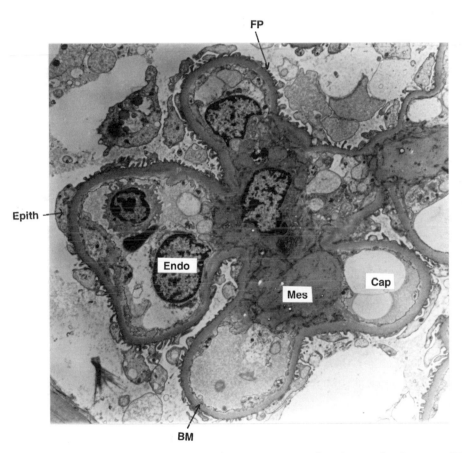

Fig. 4.4. Electron microscopic appearances of a glomerulus from an IDDM patient with microalbuminuria. Endo: Endothelium. Mes: Mesangium. Cap: Capillary. BM: Basement membrane. FP: Foot process. Epith: Epithelium.

strated that microalbuminuric NIDDM patients had greater glomerular volume, mesangial sclerosis and arteriolar hyalinosis compared with non-diabetic control subjects[104]. In a careful series of 34 apparently unselected microalbuminuric NIDDM patients of mean age 58 years, 10 were judged to have normal or near normal renal structure, 10 to have changes typical of diabetic nephropathy and 14 atypical changes[105]. Retinopathy was present in all patients with typical changes and in only 50–60 % of the others, whilst AER was similar in all three groups. Thus, NIDDM patients with micro-albuminuria may not demonstrate the classical features of diabetic nephro-pathy on histology. In these patients, it is perhaps conceivable that microalbuminuria is a reflection of renovascular disease.

Urinary excretion of other proteins

Glomerular proteinuria

The urinary excretion of other proteins is also abnormal in microalbumi-nuria. Cross-sectional studies have demonstrated an increased fractional excretion of IgG and albumin in microalbuminuric IDDM patients com-pared with normoalbuminuric controls[106], but with a decrease in the IgG:albumin clearance ratio when AER $>$ 30 µg/min. The clearance of albumin correlated with the clearance of IgG only in those patients with AER $<$ 60 µg/min, suggesting that increased intra-glomerular pressure is primarily responsible for low levels of microalbuminuria, but that higher levels are governed by a charge selectivity defect. Further cross-sectional work has extended and challenged these observations. Deckert and collea-gues[107] measured renal fractional clearances of albumin, total IgG, anionic IgG_4 and β_2-microglobulin in non-diabetic control subjects and IDDM patients with normal albumin excretion ($<$ 30 mg/24 h), early (30–100 mg/24 h) and late ($>$ 100 mg/24 h) microalbuminuria. In the normoalbuminuric patients, clearance of total IgG was high whilst clearance of anionic albumin and IgG_4 was similar to that in the non-diabetic population, suggesting an early increase in glomerular pore size or impairment of tubular reabsorption. In early microalbuminuria, fractional clearance of IgG was similar to nor-moalbuminuric patients, but clearance of albumin and IgG_4 was increased, supporting the concept of unchanged pore size but loss of anionic charge on the basement membrane. With more advanced albuminuria, fractional clear-ance of IgG increased to the same extent as clearance of albumin, suggesting that at this stage, an increase in pore size had occurred.

Further work from the Danish group[108] has shown that the IgG:IgG$_4$ selectivity ratio decreased in patients with low levels of microalbuminuria (30–100 mg/24 h) compared with normoalbuminuric IDDM patients, without differences in tubular function or renal haemodynamics (Figure 4.5). Size selectivity, as measured by clearance of neutral dextrans, was only altered in patients with clinical proteinuria and elevated serum creatinine (Figure 4.6).

Several groups have confirmed that the charge selectivity ratio (IgG/IgG$_4$) is decreased in patients with low levels of microalbuminuria[109,110] and one has demonstrated that following improvement in metabolic control, with a reduction in HbA$_{1c}$ of around 1.5 %, the selectivity index rose by around 50 %, without a change in albumin excretion rate.

Using the ratio of the clearance of pancreatic and the more anionic salivary amylase as an indicator of glomerular charge selectivity, Fox and colleagues[111] found similar ratios in non diabetic and normoalbuminuric diabetic subjects, but lower ratios in IDDM patients with micro- or macroalbuminuria. The molecular mass of amylase (56 kDa) is lower than albumin and IgG, and so its clearance may perhaps be less sensitive to size selectivity changes.

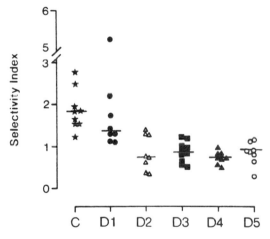

Fig. 4.5. Selectivity index (clearance of IgG/IgG4) in non-diabetic subjects (C), IDDM patients with normal albumin excretion (D1), IDDM patients with albumin excretion rate 30–100 mg/24 h (D2), IDDM patients with albumin excretion rate 101–300 mg/24 h (D3), IDDM patients with albumin excretion rate > 300 mg/24 h and serum creatinine < 110 μmol/l (D4) and IDDM patients with albumin excretion rate > 300 mg/24 h and serum creatinine ⩾ 110 μmol/l. Reproduced from reference 108 with permission (copyright Springer-Verlag).

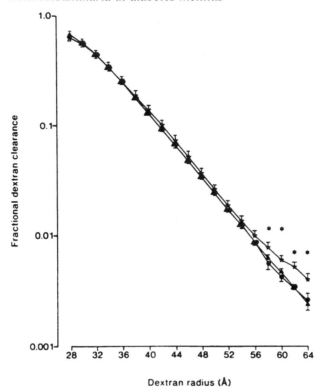

Fig. 4.6. Fractional clearance (mean ± SEM) of dextrans of different size (A) in insulin-dependent diabetic patients with normal urinary albumin excretion (< 30 mg/24 h; ●), patients with albumin excretion rate > 30 mg/24 h and GFR > 90 ml/min/1.73 m² (▲) and patients with albumin excretion rate > 30 mg/24 h and GFR < 90 ml/min/1.73 m² (♦). * $p < 0.05$. Reproduced from reference 108 with permission (copyright Springer-Verlag).

In a longitudinal study over approximately eight years of IDDM patients with normoalbuminuria, intermittent microalbuminuria or persistent micro-albuminuria, albumin clearance correlated closely with transferrin, IgG and total protein clearance in the whole group[112]. In most subjects with inter-mittent microalbuminuria or who progressed from normoalbuminuria to persistent microalbuminuria, increases in albumin excretion were associated with increases in transferrin and IgG clearance, supporting the concept that the 'microproteinuria' is of glomerular origin, arising because of increased intra-glomerular pressure. Further analysis, however, suggested a triphasic development of proteinuria. In the first phase of normoalbuminuria or early microalbuminuria, proteinuria is non-selective with IgG clearance equal to or greater than transferrin or albumin clearance. As microalbuminuria develops, there is a progressive increase in selectivity, reflecting the preferential excretion of albumin and transferrin compared with IgG. In clinical proteinuria, there is a return to non-selective proteinuria[113].

All of this work suggests that initially in diabetes there is an unselective loss of protein in the urine, consequent to increased intra-glomerular pressure. As microalbuminuria develops, the loss becomes progressively more selective, with preferential excretion of transferrin and albumin compared with IgG. As has been documented previously, as albuminuria advances further to the macroproteinuric stage, selectivity is lost and the IgG:albumin clearance ratio rises[114]. Selectivity at the stage of microalbuminuria is thought to relate to loss of glomerular basement membrane charge, in particular with loss of anionic heparan sulphate proteoglycan from the basement membrane[115]. In later stages, the glomerular pore size increases, as demonstrated by increased clearance of all sizes of neutral dextrans[114], so that charge selectivity becomes less important and IgG can again escape. One study has shown a loss of erythrocyte anionic charge (sialic acid and acidic glycosaminoglycan content) which correlates with increasing albuminuria in the normo- and micro-albuminuric range[116], suggesting that loss of charge is widespread, although another found no difference in non-diabetic and in IDDM subjects with normal albumin excretion, micro- and macroalbuminuria[117].

Tubular proteinuria

Abnormalities in tubular proteinuria may be present in diabetes regardless of the albumin excretion rate. A cross-sectional study in IDDM patients has shown a correlation between urinary excretion rates of albumin and transferrin, and albumin and N-acetyl-β-D-glucosaminidase excretion[118]. All patients with elevated albumin excretion had increased transferrin excretion but, in addition, 78 % of those with normal albumin excretion had increased transferrin excretion. The authors suggested that elevated transferrin excretion may be a marker for renal dysfunction, but this is likely to be tubular rather than glomerular dysfunction, perhaps reversible with improved glycaemic control and not necessarily indicative of subsequent decline in glomerular function. In children with and without diabetes, urinary excretion of transferrin correlates with indices of proximal tubular function (α-1-microglobulin and N-acetyl-β-D- glucosaminidase excretion) and with urinary glucose and albumin excretion[119]. Urinary transferrin excretion was significantly higher in the diabetic children whereas albumin excretion was not statistically different.

A longitudinal study over eight months confirmed the relationship of changes in microalbuminuria to changes in total protein excretion, and also demonstrated by SDS-PAGE electrophoresis that microalbuminuria is accompanied by persistent excretion of a variety of low molecular weight proteins, thought to be of tubular origin[120]. Cross-sectional studies have also suggested that proteinuria of glomerular and tubular origin may co-exist at the stage of microalbuminuria. Significant increases in excretion of retinol binding protein have been observed in both normo-[121–123] and micro-albuminuric IDDM patients[122,123]. The excretion of both retinol binding protein and albumin correlates with systolic and diastolic blood pressure[124] and is influenced by glycaemic control. Excretion of retinol binding protein increased by ten-fold during a hyperinsulinaemic, euglycaemic insulin clamp in normoalbuminuric IDDM patients[121], suggesting that acute changes in glycaemia may lead to acute changes in tubular function. Longer-term changes in blood (and urinary) glucose levels may lead to reductions in excretion of retinol binding protein and other tubular proteins[125].

A longer-term study has followed changes in urinary excretion of N-acetyl-ß-D-glucosaminidase (NAG) and albumin excretion in 36 IDDM patients over five years[126]. Urinary albumin and creatinine concentrations were measured in a first morning urine sample, and the fractional albumin excretion rate calculated as the ratio between the albumin clearance and the creatinine clearance multiplied by 10^{-3}. Initial albumin concentration was 14 ± 1 mg/l rising to 127 ± 53 mg/l after five years, the urinary excretion of NAG remaining constant (0.58 ± 0.07 vs 0.62 ± 0.08 U/mmol creatinine). The urinary excretion of NAG was similar at baseline and after five years in the nine patients who developed nephropathy and in those who did not. Thus, urinary excretion of NAG does not appear to predict the later development of diabetic nephropathy.

Plasma activity of NAG appears to be related to glycaemic control[127]. In 28 newly presenting NIDDM patients, plasma NAG activity was elevated at presentation and fell over the following three months as glycaemic control was improved by dietary measures. The change in NAG activity correlated with changes in fasting plasma glucose and glycated haemoglobin. Interestingly, plasma levels of NAG were also elevated in eight poorly controlled IDDM patients, but after four days' normoglycaemia induced by insulin infusion, NAG activity did not fall significantly.

Development and progression of microalbuminuria

Insulin-dependent diabetes

Albumin excretion is elevated at diagnosis of diabetes, in both insulin-dependent[6,128] and non-insulin dependent patients[27,129–132]. The changes in albumin excretion are generally small, day-time AER falling from around 18 µg/ min at diagnosis of IDDM to around 5 µg/min after insulin treatment[6]. However, on occasions, much larger changes may be observed. In the vast majority of IDDM patients, our current knowledge suggests that with good metabolic control, AER returns to within the normal range: in the only study so far published, three to six months after diagnosis of IDDM, when glycaemic control was stable, only 4 out of 52 patients had a 24-h albumin excretion rate in the range 30–300 mg/24 h[133]. One of these had exceedingly poor glycaemic control at the time of the urine collection, one had sustained a myocardial infarction seven years before the onset of diabetes, and the remaining two were adolescent boys where the day-time but not the night-time AER was elevated, suggesting that orthostatic proteinuria accounted for their apparent microalbuminuria.

After these changes around diagnosis and stabilisation, albumin excretion remains normal in the majority of patients for many years, although it may rise transiently because of acute deterioration in glucose control or as a response to exercise (Fig. 4.7). Parving and coworkers[128] studied 10 IDDM patients of short duration (less than four years) before and after insulin

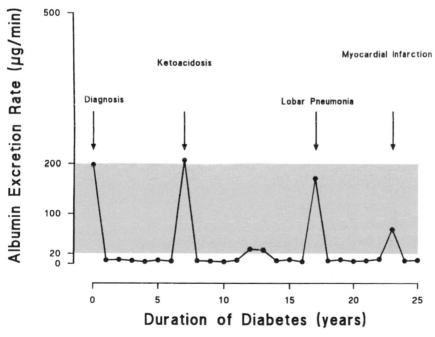

Fig. 4.7. Fluctuations in albumin excretion rate in IDDM patients who do not develop clinical proteinuria. Reproduced from reference 161 with permission (copyright John Wiley & Sons Limited).

withdrawal. Insulin withdrawal was accompanied by a 125 % increase in albumin excretion, to a mean of 16.0 mg/24 h. This short-term fluctuation in AER with blood glucose control suggests a functional rather than structural cause for the albuminuria.

Several studies failed to find microalbuminuria in IDDM patients in stable blood glucose control for up to five years from diagnosis[29,44], although more recent reports from much larger populations suggest that microalbuminuria may occur in around 20 % of patients with diabetes of one to five years' duration[59]. The reasons for this difference may simply reflect the difference in numbers studied, or may represent better glycaemic control in the initial, smaller studies. It remains to be established from long-term prospective studies whether those patients with persistent microalbuminuria soon after diagnosis are those who will eventually progress to proteinuria and end-stage disease or whether the microalbuminuria will regress with improved glycaemic control.

At some point within the first ten years of IDDM, AER will begin to rise in those patients destined eventually to develop nephropathy (Fig. 4.8). Progression from normal albumin excretion to microalbuminuria has not

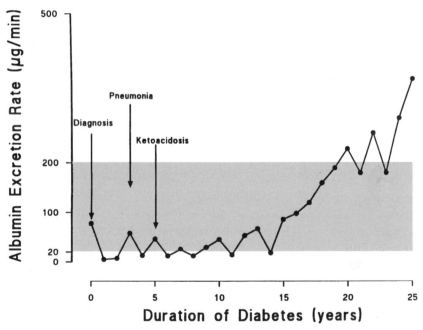

Fig. 4.8. The development of microalbuminuria and proteinuria in an IDDM patient. Reproduced from reference 161 with permission (copyright John Wiley & Sons Limited).

been well characterised but in one detailed study of IDDM patients with initial overnight AER less than 30 µg/min[134] the cumulative incidence of persistent microalbuminuria (AER > 30 µg/min) was 11 % in seven years, equivalent to 1.6 % per annum. This compares closely with the results of a Danish cohort of 205 IDDM patients followed for five years[16] and to the incidence of 16 % in nine years in the intensively treated group of the Diabetes Control and Complications Trial[135] although, in the DCCT, patients with intermittent microalbuminuria are included in this incidence.

In a detailed prospective five year study of 62 young people (initial age 5.8–20.9 years) followed from diagnosis, 21 % had microalbuminuria (24 h AER > 20 µg/min) after five years, with similar incidence in boys and girls[136]. None had hypertension (as defined by age-specific limits) and in the whole microalbuminuric group, five-year mean glycated haemoglobin was similar to that in the normoalbuminuric patients. However, glycated haemoglobin was significantly higher in the girls with microalbuminuria compared to the normoalbuminuric females.

Several studies suggest that those patients with AER in the 'borderline area' between the upper limit of the non-diabetic reference range (approximately 10 µg/min in an overnight sample) and the lower limit of AER which by consensus defines microalbuminuria (20 µg/min) progress through the borderline range to true microalbuminuria in a few years[16,134,137]. As there have been no longitudinal studies from diagnosis, it is not clear whether these patients have elevated albumin excretion from diagnosis, which does not fall to normal with good glycaemic control, or whether the excretion is initially normal and then becomes abnormal. This is an important point, as it may mean that individuals who will subsequently develop nephropathy could be identified soon after the diagnosis of diabetes. As discussed above, the only study addressing this point would suggest that albumin excretion is normal in almost all patients initially[133]. There also appears to be a state of 'intermittent microalbuminuria', where AER may fluctuate between the normal and abnormal ranges for some time, before microalbuminuria becomes persistent. Poor glycaemic control, systemic blood pressure and the initial albumin excretion rate all appear to influence the progression from normal albumin excretion to microalbuminuria[134].

Progression of microalbuminuria to proteinuria again is not well studied, most reports being of albumin excretion at two time points rather than serial measurements. The initial prospective studies suggest that approximately 80 % of IDDM patients with microalbuminuria will progress to persistent proteinuria, end-stage renal disease or death in 8–14 years. Studies of individuals are not well documented. In an eight month study, in 12 IDDM patients with initial AER $>$ 50 mg/24 h, AER increased from a mean of around 160 to 220 mg/24 h, whilst in those with initial AER $<$ 50 mg/24 h, AER did not change during follow-up[120]. This rate of increase is somewhat faster than reported by others. Christensen and Mogensen[138] reported a mean increase in AER in ten microalbuminuric (AER $>$15 µg/min in a short-term collection) male patients of 19 % per annum. However, the rate of change varied greatly from person to person, the range being −7.3 to +58.5 %.

More recent studies have suggested that the numbers progressing from microalbuminuria to proteinuria and the rate of progression are lower than these initial studies suggested. The Steno group followed 118 microalbuminuric IDDM patients, matched for gender, age and duration of diabetes to normoalbuminuric patients, for five years[139]. Initial classification was done on the basis of only one 24 h urine collection. Those with microalbuminuria were more likely to progress to clinical proteinuria, but only 20 % of the microalbuminuric patients progressed, compared to 2 % of the normoalbuminuric group. After five years, 33 % of the microalbuminuric group had normoalbuminuria, 48 % were microalbuminuric and 19 % had developed proteinuria. In the normoalbuminuric group, 8 % had developed microalbuminuria, 2 % clinical proteinuria and 90 % remained normoalbuminuric. Of the 79 patients with persistent microalbuminuria, only 46 % had an annual increase in their 24-h urine albumin excretion rate of $>$ 5 %. These so-called progressors had higher mean HbA_{1c} and mean blood pressure over the five years, and more developed proliferative retinopathy. Smoking was more prevalent in those with persistent microalbuminuria.

In keeping with the above study, in the conventionally treated groups of both the DCCT[135] and the UK Microalbuminuria studies[140], approximately one third of initially microalbuminuric patients reverted to persistent normoalbuminuria, half remained microalbuminuric and one sixth developed proteinuria. Microalbuminuric IDDM patients with duration of diabetes $>$15 years also appear to be at lower risk of progression to proteinuria[141]. In all of these more recent studies, general improvements in diabetes care, particularly in glycaemic and blood pressure control, may have led to this apparent decline in the rate of progression of microalbuminuria.

Non-insulin-dependent diabetes

As in IDDM, albumin excretion is elevated at presentation of NIDDM[27,129–132,142–146]. In most patients, the increase is minimal and albumin excretion remains within the non-diabetic reference range[27,130,142]. However, approximately 20–30 % of patients have albumin excretion rates outwith the normal range[27,129,132]. At diagnosis of NIDDM, albumin excretion correlates with age, smoking, systolic blood pressure, HbA_{1c}, serum triglyceride levels and the presence of peripheral vascular disease[132,142,145].

With control of glycaemia by diet or diet and oral hypoglycaemic agents, albumin excretion falls in the majority of patients, whether initially 'normoalbuminuric', microalbuminuric or proteinuric[27,130,131,142–144,146]. However, in a proportion of patients with microalbuminuria at presentation, albumin excretion remains abnormal. Patrick and colleagues[27] followed for one year from diagnosis 39 NIDDM patients who had an initial albumin:creatinine ratio >2.5 mg/mmol. In ten patients, the albumin:creatinine ratio fell to < 2.5 mg/mmol as blood glucose control improved: these patients had significantly higher glycated haemoglobin values at presentation than the 21 with persistent microalbuminuria. Martin and colleagues[131] followed 20 newly diagnosed NIDDM patients for two years. At diagnosis, eight patients had AER in timed overnight collection >15 µg/min, with six of these >30 µg/min. By two months, only three patients had AER > 30 µg/min, with one additional patient > 15 µg/min. At two years, one microalbuminuric patient had died from cerebrovascular disease and only two patients remained microalbuminuric. No patient who had AER < 15 µg/min at diagnosis developed microalbuminuria in the two-year follow-up. Several other small studies have confirmed persistence of microalbuminuria from diagnosis in NIDDM[129,143]. In one study, male patients with AER >35 mg/24 h at diagnosis had significantly lower creatinine clearance than patients with AER < 35 mg/24 h[129].

All of this work suggests that, at presentation of NIDDM, microalbuminuria may reflect functional abnormalities related to hyperglycaemia and be reversible in the majority of patients. However, in others, microalbuminuria may represent established, irreversible structural renal changes and thus may persist even after good glycaemic control is achieved.

The rate of progression from normal albumin excretion to microalbuminuria and from microalbuminuria to proteinuria in NIDDM appears to be at least as fast as in IDDM. In a three-year follow-up study of NIDDM patients, 16 % with initial urinary albumin concentration <15 mg/l developed micro- or macroalbuminuria (albumin concentration >30 mg/l)[26], whilst in 55 % of those with initial albumin concentration 15–30 mg/l, the albumin concentration rose > 30 mg/l, despite the fact that blood glucose and lipid control improved over the follow-up period. In those who progressed, final but not initial systolic blood pressure, serum triglycerides and C-peptide were higher than in those patients in whom the albumin concentration remained < 15 mg/l. Microalbuminuric patients also had higher prevalence of peripheral vascular disease and carotid artery stenosis.

In a five-year follow-up study from diagnosis, less than half of those patients with microalbuminuria at diagnosis still had microalbuminuria after five years[147]. Approximately one third of patients progressed from normal to abnormal albumin excretion. The follow-up HbA_1 level was higher in those who had progressed to microalbuminuria than in those with persistent normoalbuminuria, and both baseline and five-year fasting serum insulin levels were closely related to the follow-up AER. In a small study over 3.4 years, 24 normoalbuminuric and 13 microalbuminuric patients, with similar baseline characteristics apart from the AER, were studied[148]. There was a small but significant increase in AER, from a geometric mean of 6.8 to 11.4 μg/min in the normoalbuminuric group, with 9 patients developing microalbuminuria. The only parameter found to be related to changes in AER was systolic blood pressure, the mean of the baseline and follow-up AER correlating to the mean systolic blood pressure. The mean rate of fall of GFR was around 1.4 ml/min/1.73 m^2, although there was wide inter-individual variation. The rate of decline observed in this study does not seem to be much different from that reported in non-diabetic individuals of similar age[149]. The fall rate in GFR also correlated to initial and mean systolic blood pressure.

In a large study of Indian patients with NIDDM, albumin excretion was measured yearly, and expressed as the mean of two 24-h collections[150]. After five years, 241 of the initial 349 patients with normal albumin excretion were available for follow-up; 169 were still normoalbuminuric, whilst 62 had developed microalbuminuria and 10 macroproteinuria. The baseline AER was significantly higher in those who progressed (8.5 ± 6 versus 5.3 ± 4 μg/min), and more had hypertension at baseline. A significant increase in systolic blood pressure was seen in those who progressed from normo- to micro-albuminuria. Of the 62 patients with baseline microalbuminuria, 23 developed macroproteinuria, 29 remained microalbuminuric and 9 became normoalbuminuric.

In the Pima Indians, a group of 456 normoalbuminuric (albumin:creatinine ratio < 30 mg/g; < 2.73 mg/mmol) NIDDM subjects have been followed for a maximum of 11.6 (median 4.7) years[151]; 192 developed elevated albumin excretion, with 172 of these being microalbuminuric (albumin:creatinine ratio 30–299 mg/g; 2.73–272 mg/mmol). The cumulative incidence of abnormal albumin excretion was 17 % after five years. The appearance of high albumin excretion was associated with the development of retinopathy, type of diabetes treatment, longer duration of diabetes, lower body mass index and higher values of mean arterial pressure, HbA_1, and fasting and 2-h plasma glucose concentration at baseline.

Factors related to the development and progression of microalbuminuria

The demonstration above that even at the very early stages of microalbuminuria there are small but distinct differences particularly in glycaemic control, blood pressure and blood lipid levels compared with normoalbuminuric subjects, has suggested that these abnormalities may not be secondary to advanced renal disease as had previously been thought, but may be highly important in the initiation and progression of early diabetic kidney disease. Obviously, once the process has begun, a self-fuelling circle is created with, for example, rising blood pressure accelerating the progression of renal disease which leads to further elevation of the blood pressure.

Glycaemic control

The evidence that hyperglycaemia is important in progression from normoalbuminuria to microalbuminuria has come mainly from the cross-sectional and retrospective studies described above. One prospective, longitudinal study followed IDDM patients who had an initial overnight AER < 30 µg/min for seven years[134]. Glycated haemoglobin levels were higher at baseline and throughout the study in those in whom the AER rose. In a further prospective study over a mean of 2.1 years, a significant relationship was demonstrated between change in AER at low levels of albumin excretion and glycated haemoglobin levels[137]. In those patients with AER initially in the 'borderline' area 7.6 30.0 µg/min, the mean glycated haemoglobin value in the year preceding the final AER measurement was lowest in those who regressed from borderline to normoalbuminuria, intermediate in those who remained in the borderline area and highest in those who progressed from borderline to frank microalbuminuria. A third, large study of 209 initially normoalbuminuric IDDM patients found that initial AER and glycated haemoglobin levels were independently related to the final AER measured about 5 years later[16].

In one careful, longitudinal study, 156 children with IDDM were followed up from diagnosis for up to 15 years[152]. Albumin excretion and glycated haemoglobin were measured three monthly from diagnosis and arterial blood pressure three monthly after five years of diabetes. Persistent microalbuminuria developed in 17 children, giving a cumulative incidence of 24.2 %

at 15 years. Eleven patients developed microalbuminuria after five years' duration and in these patients the five year mean glycated haemoglobin was the only factor which independently predicted the development of microalbuminuria. In those children who developed microalbuminuria within five years of onset of diabetes, glycated haemoglobin did not influence the transition.

All of these studies suggest that at levels of albumin excretion which are below the consensus definition of 20 µg/min, glycaemic control is important in determining which patients develop frank microalbuminuria.

Once microalbuminuria is present, one study has demonstrated that the rate of change of AER correlates with HbA_{1c}, the AER in patients with HbA_{1c} < 7.0 % being likely to stabilise rather than increase[153]. However, in other studies[140], the importance of glycaemic control in the progression of microalbuminuria appears less strong and is outweighed by the effects of blood pressure.

Blood pressure

There has been much debate as to whether blood pressure is elevated before the development of microalbuminuria. As discussed above, most studies have shown that microalbuminuric patients have systolic and diastolic blood pressure levels higher than their normoalbuminuric peers, although the numeric differences are small. Few prospective, longitudinal studies have been sufficiently detailed to dissect out the relative time course of the development of microalbuminuria and raised blood pressure. In a careful study of 209 initially normoalbuminuric (24-h AER < 30 µg/min) IDDM patients over five years, Mathiesen and coworkers[16] demonstrated that a significant rise in blood pressure occurred in the third year after the AER had risen into the microalbuminuric range. However, this study may be criticised on the grounds that blood pressure was only measured once per year in the outpatient clinic by several observers, whilst AER was quantified three times a year. Thus subtle changes in blood pressure, such as may have been observed by 24-h monitoring, may have been missed. A similar study has shown that IDDM patients with AER 10–30 µg/min will progress in seven years to true microalbuminuria (AER > 30 µg/min), and that their systolic blood pressure is higher at baseline than in those with initial AER < 10 µg/min[134], suggesting that blood pressure may rise before the development of microalbuminuria. In a third, less rigorous, study over a mean of 6.6 years, the relationship of 'high normal' blood pressure (> 90th centile for age) to the development of microalbuminuria was assessed[154]. Of 60 patients who developed microalbuminuria (overnight AER > 30 µg/min) during the study, the blood pressure rose before microalbuminuria developed in 26, microalbuminuria appeared before borderline hypertension in 27 and in 7 microalbuminuria and borderline hypertension appeared together or the data was insufficient to interpret. Overall, it would appear that increases in systemic blood pressure are very closely linked to rises in albumin excretion and may precede a rise in AER.

The role of blood pressure in the progression of microalbuminuria to proteinuria has also been studied. In a small study of 10 microalbuminuric (AER > 15 µg/min in a short-term collection) IDDM men followed for a mean of 4.9 years, systolic and diastolic blood pressures were both elevated at baseline compared to matched normoalbuminuric patients[138]. However, a further significant increase in diastolic blood pressure was only seen in those microalbuminuric patients followed for more than four years. In the UK Microalbuminuria Collaborative Study[140], a mean arterial blood pressure above the group mean (93.6 mmHg) predicted progression to clinical proteinuria (relative risk 4.2, 95% CI 1.3–13.0; Fig. 4.9). In NIDDM, the rate of change of AER is related to systolic blood pressure[148].

Lipids

Numerous cross-sectional studies described above have demonstrated an excess of dyslipidaemias in microalbuminuric diabetic patients, as discussed

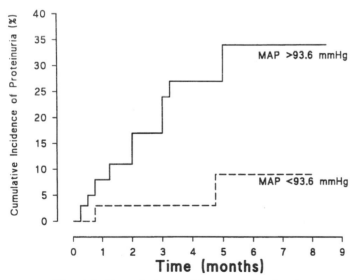

Fig. 4.9. Cumulative incidence of the development of proteinuria in IDDM patients with mean arterial pressure < 93.6 mmHg (– –) and > 93.6 mmHg (—). Data derived from reference 140.

fully in Chapter 6. It has been suggested that dyslipidaemias may be important in the initiation and progression of renal disease rather than a consequence of kidney damage. However, there is little direct evidence to support
this hypothesis in diabetic nephropathy. In a five year follow-up of 113
NIDDM patients, serum lipid profiles were similar at baseline in normoalbuminuric and microalbuminuric subjects[155]. However, after five years, significant increases in VLDL-cholesterol and VLDL- and LDL-triglyceride
levels, and a decrease in HDL-cholesterol, were seen in the microalbuminuric
subjects, suggesting that microalbuminuria predates and predicts the development of dyslipidaemia.

Initial AER

Several large, longitudinal studies have demonstrated that in the progression
of normoalbuminuria to microalbuminuria, the initial AER is an important
independent determinant of the final AER[16,134]. The level of albumin excretion also appears to be an important determinant in progression of microalbuminuria to clinical proteinuria, the risk of progression being greatest if
AER > 70 µg/min[14].

Smoking

Smoking does seem to accelerate the rate of progression of microalbuminuria
and proteinuria[156,157]. In a rather complex study of hypertensive IDDM
patients with microalbuminuria or proteinuria, Sawicki and colleagues[156]
found that progression was less common in non-smokers than in smokers
or ex-smokers. Cigarette pack years was an independent risk factor for progression, along with 24-h sodium excretion and glycated haemoglobin.

Albumin excretion and pregnancy in diabetes

The physiological changes in albumin excretion in normal pregnancy are
discussed in Chapters 1 and 7. Few studies have examined the effect of
pregnancy on albumin excretion in diabetic women. In one study of 30
IDDM women with initially normal AER, albumin excretion rose non-significantly in the first and second trimesters, but increased 3.8 fold to a mean
of 43.7 µg/min in the third trimester[158]. However, by 12 weeks after delivery,
AER had returned to pre-pregnancy levels. McCance and colleagues[159] also
reported an increase in albumin excretion in normoalbuminuric IDDM and
non-diabetic women during the third trimester, the excretion rates in the

diabetic women being higher than in the non-diabetic control subjects from 36 weeks onwards. In both groups, the peak AER occurred one week post-partum, but by 12 weeks excretion rates in both groups had returned to pre-pregnancy values. In 12 women with pre-existing microalbuminuria, the pattern of increase in AER appears to be an exaggeration of the increase in non-diabetic and normoalbuminuric IDDM women[158] (Fig. 4.10): the peak rise in excretion rate is seen in the third trimester, AER increasing from a mean of 63.2 µg/min before conception to 482 µg/min in the third trimester. Again, values return to pre-pregnancy levels within 12 weeks post-partum.

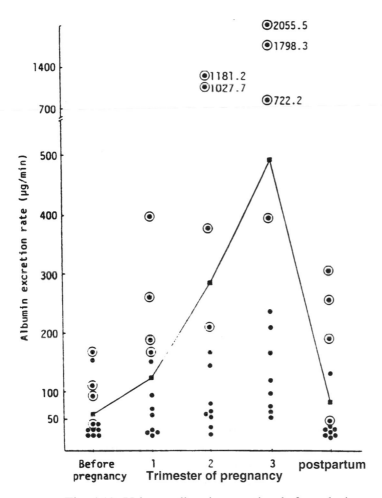

Fig. 4.10. Urinary albumin excretion before, during and after pregnancy in diabetic women with pre-existing microalbuminuria: — mean. Four women with transient nephrotic syndrome ⊙ showed the highest albumin excretion rates during pregnancy. Reproduced from reference 158 with permission (copyright Springer-Verlag).

The physiological increase in creatinine clearance was observed in the micro-albuminuric women. In this small series, 4 of 12 women with pre-existing microalbuminuria developed transient nephrotic syndrome (protein excretion > 3 g/24 h), although nephrotic syndrome has also been reported in IDDM women with initially normal AER[160]. Thus pregnancy does not appear to cause a permanent increase in urinary albumin excretion. Although the reported series have been small, there is also no suggestion that the outcome for the fetus of a mother with microalbuminuria but preserved glomerular filtration is any different to that of a fetus of a normoalbuminuric mother.

References

1. Borch-Johnsen K, Andersen PK, Deckert T. The effect of proteinuria on relative mortality in Type 1 (insulin-dependent) diabetes mellitus. *Diabetologia* 1985; **28**:590–596.
2. Borch-Johnsen K, Kreiner S. Proteinuria: value as predictor of cardio-vascular mortality in insulin-dependent diabetes mellitus. *Br Med J* 1987; **294**:1651–1654.
3. Oakley WG, Pyke DA, Tattersall RB, Watkins PJ. Long-term diabetes. A clinical study of 92 patients after 40 years. *Q J Med* 1974; **169**:145–156.
4. Keen H, Chlouverakis C. An immunoassay method for urinary albumin at low concentrations. *Lancet* 1963; **2**:913–914.
5. Viberti GC, Jarrett RJ, McCartney M, Keen H. Increased glomerular permeability to albumin induced by exercise in diabetic subjects. *Diabetologia* 1978; **14**:293–300.
6. Mogensen CE. Urinary albumin excretion in early and long-term juvenile diabetes. *Scand J Clin Lab Invest* 1971; **28**:183–193.
7. Keen H, Chlouverakis C, Fuller J, Jarrett RJ. The concomitants of raised blood sugar: studies in newly-detected hyperglycaemics. *Guy's Hosp Rep* 1969; **118**:247–254.
8. Viberti GC, Hill RD, Jarrett RJ, Argyropoulos A, Mahmud U, Keen H. Microalbuminuria as a predictor of clinical nephropathy in insulin-dependent diabetes mellitus. *Lancet*, 1982; **2**:1430–1432.
9. Messent J, Elliott TG, Hill RG, Jarrett RJ, Keen H, Viberti GC. Prognostic significance of microalbuminuria in insulin-dependent diabetes mellitus: a twenty-three year follow-up study. *Kidney Int* 1992; **41**:836–839.
10. Deckert T, Yokoyama H, Mathiesen E, Ronn B, Jensen T, Feldt-Rasmussen B, *et al*. Cohort study of predictive value of urinary albumin excretion for atherosclerotic vascular disease in patients with insulin dependent diabetes. *Br Med J* 1996; **312**:871–874.
11. Rossing P, Hougaard P, Borch-Johnsen K, Parving HH. Predictors of mortality in insulin dependent diabetes: 10 year observational follow up study. *Br Med J* 1996; **313**:779–784.
12. Parving HH, Oxenboll B, Svendsen PAa, Sandahl Christiansen J, Andersen AR. Early detection of patients at risk of developing diabetic nephropathy. A longitudinal study of urinary albumin excretion. *Acta Endocrinol* 1982; **100**:550–555.
13. Mogensen CE, Christensen CK. Predicting diabetic nephropathy in insulin-dependent patients. *N Engl J Med* 1984; **311**:89–93.

14. Mathiesen ER, Oxenboll B, Johansen K, Svendsen PAa, Deckert T. Incipient nephropathy in Type 1 (insulin-dependent) diabetes. *Diabetologia* 1984; **26**:406–410.
15. Microalbuminuria Collaborative Study Group, United Kingdom. Risk factors for development of microalbuminuria in insulin dependent diabetic patients: a cohort study. *Br Med J* 1993; **306**:1235–1239.
16. Mathiesen ER, Ronn B, Jensen T, Storm B, Deckert T. Relationship between blood pressure and urinary albumin excretion in development of microalbuminuria. *Diabetes* 1990; **39**:245–249.
17. Jarrett RJ, Viberti GC, Argyropoulos A, Hill RD, Mahmud U, Murrells TJ. Microalbuminuria predicts mortality in non-insulin dependent diabetes. *Diabet Med* 1984; **1**:17–19.
18. Mogensen CE. Microalbuminuria predicts clinical proteinuria and early mortality in maturity-onset diabetes. *N Engl J Med* 1984; **310**:356–360.
19. Schmitz A, Vaeth M. Microalbuminuria: a major risk factor in non-insulin-dependent diabetes. A 10-year follow-up study of 503 patients. *Diabet Med* 1988; **5**:126–134.
20. MacLeod JM, Lutale J, Marshall SM. Albumin excretion and vascular deaths in NIDDM. *Diabetologia* 1995; **38**:610–616.
21. Neil HAW, Thorogood M, Hawkins M, Cohen D, Potok M, Mann J. A prospective population-based study of microalbuminuria as a predictor of mortality in NIDDM. *Diabetes Care* 1993; **16**:996–1003.
22. Mattock MB, Morrish NJ, Viberti GC, Keen H, Fitzgerald AP, Jackson G. Prospective study of microalbuminuria as predictor of mortality in NIDDM. *Diabetes* 1992; **41**:736–741.
23. Gall M-A, Borch-Johnsen K, Hougaard P, Nielsen FS, Parving H-H. Albuminuria and poor glycaemic control predict mortality in NIDDM. *Diabetes* 1995; **44**:1303–1309.
24. Beatty OL, Ritchie CM, Bell PM, Hadden DR, Kennedy L, Atkinson B. Microalbuminuria as identified by a spot morning urine specimen in non-insulin-treated diabetes: an eight year follow-up study. *Diabet Med 1995;* **12**:261–266.
25. Mogensen CE. A complete screening of urinary albumin concentration in an unselected diabetic out-patient clinic population. *Diabet Nephropath* 1983; **2**:11–18.
26. Stiegler H, Standl E, Schulz K, Roth R, Lehmacher W. Morbidity, mortality and albuminuria in Type 2 diabetic patients: a three-year prospective study of a random cohort in general practice. *Diabet Med* 1992; **9**:646–653.
27. Patrick AW, Leslie PJ, Clarke BF, Frier BM. The natural history and associations of microalbuminuria in Type 2 diabetes during the first year after diagnosis. *Diabet Med* 1990; **7**:902–908.
28. Gatling W, Knight C, Mullee MA, Hill RD. Microalbuminuria in diabetes: a population study of the prevalence and an assessment of three screening tests. *Diabet Med* 1987; **5**:343–347.
29. Marshall SM, Alberti KGMM. Comparison of the prevalence and associated features of abnormal albumin excretion in insulin-dependent and non-insulin-dependent diabetes. *Q J Med* 1989; **261**:61–71.
30. Mattock MB, Keen H, Viberti GC, El-Gohari MR, Murrells TJ, Scott GS *et al*. Coronary heart disease and urinary albumin excretion rate in Type 2 (non-insulin-dependent) diabetic patients. *Diabetologia* 1988; **31**:82–87.
31. Damsgaard EM, Mogensen CE. Microalbuminuria in elderly hyperglycaemic patients and controls. *Diabet Med* 1986; **3**:430–435.

32. Gall MA, Rossing P, Skott P, Damsbo P, Vaag A, Bech K *et al*. Prevalence of micro- and macroalbuminuria, arterial hypertension, retinopathy and large vessel disease in European Type 2 (non-insulin-dependent) diabetic patients. *Diabetologia* 1991; **34**:655–661.

33. Collins VR, Dowse GK, Finch CF, Zimmet PZ, Linnane AW. Prevalence and risk factors for micro- and macroalbuminuria in diabetic subjects and entire population of Nauru. *Diabetes* 1989; **38**:1602–1610.

34. Erasmus RT, Oyeyinka G, Arije A. Microalbuminuria in non-insulin-dependent (type 2) Nigerian diabetics: relation to glycaemic control, blood pressure and retinopathy. *Postgrad Med J* 1992; **68**:638–642.

35. Tai T-Y, Chuang L-M, Tseng T-H, Wu H-P, Chen M-S, Lin BJ. Microalbuminuria and diabetic complications in Chinese non-insulin-dependent diabetic patients: a prospective study. *Diabetes Res Clin Pract* 1990; **9**:59–63.

36. Cheung CK, Yeung YTF, Cockram CS, Swaminathan R. Urinary excretion of albumin and enzymes in non-insulin-dependent Chinese diabetics. *Clin Nephrol* 1990; **34**:125–130.

37. Haffner SM, Morales PA, Gruber MK, Hazuda HP, Stern MP. Cardiovascular risk factors in non-insulin-dependent diabetic subjects with microalbuminuria. *Arteriosclerosis Thrombosis* 1993; **13**:205–210.

38. Allawi J, Rao PV, Gilbert R, Scott G, Jarrett RJ, Keen H. Microalbuminuria in non-insulin dependent diabetes: its prevalence in Indian compared with Europid patients. *Br Med J* 1988; **296**:462–464.

39. Gupta DK, Verma LK, Khosla PK, Dash SC. The prevalence of microalbuminuria in diabetes: a study from North India. *Diabetes Res Clin Pract* 1991; **12**:125–128.

40. Lunt H, Lim CW, Crooke MJ, Smith RBW. Comparison of urinary albumin excretion between Maoris, Pacific Island Polynesians and Europeans with non-insulin-dependent diabetes. *Diabetes Res Clin Pract* 1990; **8**:45–50.

41. Dasmahapatra A, Bale A, Raghuwanshi MP, Reddi A, Byrne W, Suarez S., *et al*. Incipient and overt diabetic nephropathy in African Americans with NIDDM. *Diabetes Care* 1994; **17; 297–304.**

42. McCance DR, Hadden DR, Atkinson AB, Johnston H, Kennedy L. The relationship between long-term glycaemic control and diabetic nephropathy. *Q J Med* 1992; **82**:53–61.

43. Watts GF, Harris R, Shaw KM. The determinants of early nephropathy in insulin-dependent diabetes mellitus: a prospective study based on the urinary excretion of albumin. *Q J Med* 1991; **79**:365–378.

44. Microalbuminuria Collaborative Study Group. Microalbuminuria in Type 1 diabetic patients. *Diabetes Care* 1992; **15**:495–501.

45. Berglund J, Lins P-E, Adamson U, Lins L-E. Microalbuminuria in long-term insulin-dependent diabetes mellitus. *Acta Med Scand* 1987; **222**:333–338.

46. Parving HH, Hommel E, Mathiesen ER, Skott P, Edsberg B, Bahnsen M *et al*. Prevalence of microalbuminuria, arterial hypertension, retinopathy and neuropathy in patients with insulin dependent diabetes. *Br Med J* 1988; **296**:156–160.

47. Orchard TJ, Dorman JS, Maser RE, Becker DJ, Drash AL, Ellis D *et al*. Prevalence of complications in IDDM by sex and duration. Pittsburgh Epidemiology of Diabetes Complications Study II. *Diabetes* 1990; **39**: 1116–1124.

48. Descamps O, Buysschaert M, Ketelslegers JM, Hermasn M, Lambert AE. Etude de la microalbuminurie dans une population de 653 patients diabetique de Type 1 et 2. *Diabete Metab* 1991; **17**:469–475.

49. Joner G, Brinchmann-Hansen O, Torres CG, Hanssen KF. A nationwide cross-sectional study of retinopathy and microalbuminuria in young Norwegian Type 1 (insulin-dependent) diabetic patients. *Diabetologia* 1993; **35**:1049–1055.

50. Ramirez L, Rosenstock J, Arauz C, Hellenbrand D, Raskin P. Low prevalence of microalbuminuria in normotensive patients with insulin-dependent diabetes mellitus. *Diabetes Res Clin Pract* 1991; **12**:85–90.

51. Kalk WJ, Osler C, Taylor D, Panz VR, Esse JD, Reinach SG. The prevalence of microalbuminuria and glomerular hyperfiltration in young patients with IDDM. *Diabetes Res Clin Pract* 1990; **8**:145–153.

52. Norgaard K, Feldt-Rasmussen B, Borch-Johnsen K, Saelen H, Deckert T. Prevalence of hypertension in Type 1 (insulin-dependent) diabetes mellitus. *Diabetologia* 1990; **33**:407–410.

53. Mathiesen ER, Saurbrey N, Hommel E, Parving HH. Prevalence of microalbuminuria in children with Type 1 (insulin-dependent) diabetes mellitus. *Diabetologia* 1986; **29**:640–643

54. Ellis D, Becker DJ, Daneman D, Lobes L, Drash AL. Proteinuria in children with insulin-dependent diabetes: relationship to duration of disease, metabolic control and retinal changes. *J Pediat* 1983; **102**:673–680.

55. Widstam-Attorps U, Berg U. Urinary protein excretion and renal function in young people with diabetes mellitus. *Nephrol Dial Transplant* 1992; **7**:487–492.

56. Mortensen HB, Martinelli K, Norgaard K, Main K, Kastrup KW, Ibsen KK, *et al.* A nation-wide cross-sectional study of urinary albumin excretion rate, arterial blood pressure and blood glucose control in Danish children with Type 1 diabetes mellitus. *Diabet Med* 1990; **7**:887–897.

57. Davies AG, Price DA, Postlethwaite RJ, Addison GM, Burn JL, Fielding BA. Renal function in diabetes mellitus. *Arch Dis Child 1985;* **60**:299–304.

58. Marshall SM, Hackett A, Court S, Parkin M, Alberti KGMM. Albumin excretion in children and adolescents with insulin-dependent diabetes. *Diabetes Res* 1986; **3**:345–348.

59. EURODIAB IDDM Complications Study Group. Microvascular and acute complications in IDDM patients: the EURODIAB IDDM Complications Study. *Diabetologia* 1994; **37**:278–285.

60. Rowe DJF, Hayward M, Bagga H, Betts P. Effect of glycaemic control and duration of disease on overnight albumin excretion in diabetic children. *Br Med J* 1984; **289**:957–959.

61. Seaquist ER, Goetz FC, Rich S, Barbosa J. Familial clustering of diabetic kidney disease. *N Engl J Med* 1989; **320**:1161–1165.

62. Borch-Johnsen K, Norgaard K, Hommel E, Mathiesen ER, Jensen JS, Deckert T, Parving H-H. Is diabetic nephropathy an inherited complication? *Kidney Int.* 1992; **41**:719–722.

63. Quinn M, Angelico MC, Warram JH, Krolewski AS. Familial factors determine the development of diabetic nephropathy in patients with IDDM. *Diabetologia* 1996; **39**:940–945.

64. Pettitt DJ, Saad MF, Bennett PH, Nelson RG, Knowler WC. Familial predisposition to renal disease in 2 generations of Pima Indians with type 2 (non-insulin dependent) diabetes mellitus. *Diabetologia* 1990; **33**:438–443.

65. Marre M, Bernadette P, Gallois Y, Savagner F, Guyene T, Hallab M, *et al.* Relationships between angiotensin 1 converting enzyme gene polymorphism, plasma levels and diabetic retinal and renal complications. *Diabetes* 1994; **43**:384-388.

66. Tarnow L, Cambien F, Rossing P, Nielsen FS, Hansen BV, Lecerf L, *et al.* Lack of relationship between an insertion/deletion polymorphism in the angiotensin 1 converting enzyme gene and diabetic nephropathy and proliferative retinopathy in IDDM patients. *Diabetes* 1995; **44**:489–494.

67. Chowdhury TA, Dronsfield MJ, Kumar S, Gough SLC, Gibson SP, Khatoon A, *et al.* Examination of two genetic polymorphisms within the renin–angiotensin system: no evidence for an association with nephropathy in IDDM. *Diabetologia* 1996; **39**:1108–1114.

68. Mangili R, Bending JJ, Scott G, Li LK, Gupta A, Viberti GC. Increased sodium–lithium countertransport activity in red cells of patients with insulin-dependent diabetes in nephropathy. *N Engl J Med* 1988; **318**:146–150.

69. Krolewski AS, Canessa M, Warram JH, Laffel LMB, Christlieb AR, Knowler WC, Rand LI. Predisposition to hypertension and susceptibility to renal disease in insulin-dependent diabetes mellitus. *N Engl J Med* 1988; **318**:140–145.

70. Jensen JS, Mathiesen ER, Norgaard K, Hommel E, Borch-Johnsen K, Funder J *et al.* Increased blood pressure and erythrocyte sodium–lithium countertransport activity are not inherited in diabetic nephropathy. *Diabetologia* 1990; **33**:619–624.

71. Elving LD, Wetzels JFM, de Nobel E, Berden JHM. Erythrocyte sodium–lithium countertransport is not different in type I (insulin dependent) diabetic patients with and without diabetic nephropathy. *Diabetologia* 1991; **34**:126–128.

72. Gall M-A, Rossing P, Jensen JS, Funder J, Parving H-H. Red cell Na^+ Li^+ countertransport in non-insulin-dependent diabetics with diabetic nephropathy. *Kidney Int* 1991; **39**:135–40.

73. Ng LL, Simmons D, Frighi V, Garrido MC, Bomford J, Hockaday TDR. Leucocyte Na^+/H^+ antiport activity in type I (insulin dependent) diabetic patients with nephropathy. *Diabetologia* 1990; **33**:371–377.

74. Trevisan R, Li LK, Messent J, Tariq T, Earle K, Walker JD, Viberti GC. Na/H antiport activity in cell growth in cultured skin fibroblasts of IDDM patients with nephropathy. *Diabetes* 1992; **41**:1239–1246.

75. Kofoed-Enevoldsen A. Inhibition of glomerular glucosaminyl N/deacetylase in diabetic rats. *Kidney Int* 1992; **41**:763–767.

76. Deckert T, Horowitz I, Kofoed-Enevoldsen A, Kjellen L, Deckert M, Lykkelund L *et al.* Possible genetic defects in the regulation of glycosaminoglycans in patients with diabetic nephropathy. *Diabetes* 1991; **40**:764–770.

77. Kallunki P, Eddy R, Byers M, Kestila M, Shows T, Tryggvason K. Cloning of the human heparan sulphate proteoglycan core protein, assignment of the gene (HSPG 2) to 1p 36.1/p35 and identification of a BAMH1 restriction fragment length polymorphism. *Genomics* 1991; **11**:389–396.

78. Krolewski A, Tryggvason K, Stanton V, Houseman D. Diabetic nephropathy (DN) and polymorphism in cDNA of the alpha-1 chaintype IV collagen. *J Am Soc Nephrol* 1990; **1**:634 (abstract).

79. Wiseman M, Viberti G, Mackintosh D, Jarrett RJ, Keen H. Glycaemia, arterial hypertension and microalbuminuria in Type 1 (insulin-dependent) diabetes mellitus. *Diabetologia* 1984; **26**:401–405.

80. Bangstad HJ, Hanssen KF, Kierulf P, Parsen S, Dahl-Jorgensen K, Joe GB, Aegenaes O. Elevated albumin excretion rate is common among poorly controlled adolescent insulin-dependent diabetics. *Diabetes Res* 1987; **6**:43–46.

81. Jay RH, Jones SL, Hill CE, Richmond W, Viberti GC, Rampling MW. Blood rheology and cardiovascular risk factors in Type 1 diabetes: relationships with microalbuminuria. *Diabet Med* 1991; **8**:662–667.

82. Molitch ME, Steffes MW, Cleary PA, Nathan DM. Baseline analysis of renal function in the Diabetes Control and Complications Trial. *Kidney Int* 1993; **43**:668–674.

83. Norgaard K, Storm B, Graae M, Feldt-Rasmussen B. Elevated albumin excretion and retinal changes in children with Type 1 diabetes are related to long-term poor blood glucose control. *Diabet Med* 1988; **6**:325–328.

84. Bangstad HJ, Hanssen KF, Dahl-Jorgensen K, Aagenaes O. Microalbuminuria is associated with long term poor glycaemic control in adolescent insulin dependent diabetics. *Diabetes Res* 1989; **12**:71–74.

85. Metcalf PA, Baker JR, Scragg RKR, Dryson E, Scott AJ, Wild CJ. Microalbuminuria in a middle-aged workforce: effect of hyperglycaemia and ethnicity. *Diabetes Care* 1993; **16**:1485–1493.

86. Vigstrup J, Mogensen CE. Proliferative diabetic retinopathy: at risk patients identified by early detection of microalbuminuria. *Acta Ophthalmol* 1985; **63**:530–543.

87. Bell DSH, Ketchum CH, Robinson CA, Wagenknecht LE, Williams BT. Microalbuminuria associated with diabetic neuropathy. *Diabetes Care* 1992; **15**:528–531.

88. Fernando DJS, Hutchison A, Veves A, Gokal R, Boulton AJM. Risk factors for non-ischaemic foot ulceration in diabetic nephropathy. *Diabet Med* 1991; **8**:223–225.

89. Bodmer CW, Patrick AW, How TV, Williams G. Exaggerated sensitivity to NE-induced vasoconstriction in IDDM patients with microalbuminuria. *Diabetes* 1992; **41**:209–214.

90. Bodmer CW, Masson EA, Savage MW, Benbow S, Patrick AW, Williams G. Asymptomatic peripheral nerve dysfunction and vascular reactivity in IDDM patients with and without microalbuminuria. *Diabetologia* 1994; **37**:1056–1061.

91. Zander E, Schulz B, Heinke P, Grimmberger E, Zander G, Gottschling HD. Importance of cardiovascular autonomic dysfunction in IDDM subjects with diabetic nephropathy. *Diabetes Care* 1989; **12**:259–264.

92. Winocour PH, Dhar H, Anderson DC. The relationship between autonomic neuropathy and urinary sodium and albumin excretion in insulin-treated diabetics. *Diabet Med* 1986; **3**:436–440.

93. Spallone V, Gambardella S, Maiello MR, Barini A, Frontoni S, Menzinger G. Relationship between autonomic neuropathy, 24-h blood pressure profile and nephropathy in normotensive IDDM patients. *Diabetes Care* 1994; **17**:578–584.

94. Tindall H, Martin P, Nagi D, Pinnock S, Stickland M, Davies JA. Higher levels of microproteinuria in Asian compared with European patients with

diabetes mellitus and their relationship to dietary protein intake and diabetic complications. *Diabet Med* 1994; **11**:37–41.

95. Frokjaer Thomson O, Andersen AR, Sandahl Christiansen J, Deckert T. Renal changes in long-term Type 1 (insulin-dependent) diabetic patients with and without clinical nephropathy: a light microscopic, morphometric study of autopsy material. *Diabetologia* 1994; **26**:361–365.
96. Chavers BM, Bilous RW, Ellis EN, Steffes MW, Mauer SM. Urinary albumin excretion as a predictor of renal structure in type 1 diabetic patients without overt proteinuria. *N Engl J Med* 1989; **320**:966–970.
97. Walker JD, Close CF, Jones SL. Glomerular structure in type 1 (insulin dependent) diabetic patients with normo- and microalbuminuria. *Kidney Int* 1992; **41**:741–748.
98. Osterby R. Glomerular structural changes in type 1 (insulin dependent) diabetes. Consequences, causes and prevention. *Diabetologia* 1992; **35**: 803–812.
99. Bangstad H-J, Osterby R, Dahl-Jorgensen K, Berg KJ, Hartmann A, Nyberg G, *et al*. Early glomerulopathy is present in young, Type 1 (insulin dependent) diabetic patients with microalbuminuria. *Diabetologia* 1993; **36**:523–529.
100. Lane PH, Steffes MW, Mauer SM. Glomerular structure in IDDM women with low glomerular filtration rate and normal urinary albumin excretion. *Diabetes* 1992; **41**:581–586.
101. Parving HH, Gall MA, Skott P, Jorgensen HE, Lokkegaard H, Jorgensen F *et al*. Prevalence and causes of albuminuria in non-insulin dependent diabetes. *Kidney Int* 1992; **41**:758–762.
102. Gambara V, Mecca G, Remuzzi G, Bertani T. Heterogeneous nature of renal lesions in type II diabetes. *J Am Soc Nephrol* 1993; **3**:1458–1466.
103. Olsen S, Mogensen CE. How often is NIDDM complicated with non-diabetic renal disease? An analysis of renal biopsies and the literature. *Diabetologia* 1996; **39**:1638–1645.
104. Bertani T, Gambara V, Remuzzi G. Structural basis of diabetic nephropathy in microalbuminuric NIDDM patients: a light microscopy study. *Diabetologia* 1996; **39**:1625–1628.
105. Fioretto P, Mauer M, Brocco E, Velussi M, Frigato F, Muollo B *et al*. Patterns of renal injury in NIDDM patients with microalbuminuria. *Diabetologia* 1996; **39**:1569–1576.
106. Viberti GC, MacKintosh D, Keen H. Determinants of the penetration of proteins through the glomerular barrier in insulin-dependent diabetes mellitus. *Diabetes* 1983; **32: suppl 2**:92–95.
107. Deckert T, Feldt-Rasmussen B, Djurup R, Deckert M. Glomerular size and charge selectivity in insulin-dependent diabetes mellitus. *Diabetologia* 1988; **33**:100–106.
108. Deckert T, Kofoed-Enevoldsen A, Vidal P, Norgaard K, Andreasen HB, Feldt-Rasmussen B. Size- and charge-selectivity of glomerular filtration in Type 1 (insulin-dependent) diabetic patients with and without albuminuria. *Diabetologia* 1993; **36**:244–251.
109. Bangstad H-J, Kofoed-Enevoldsen A, Dahl-Jorgensen K, Hanssen KF. Glomerular charge selectivity and the influence of improved glucose control in Type 1 (insulin-dependent) diabetic patients with microalbuminuria. *Diabetologia* 1992; **35**:1165–1169.

110. Pietravalle P, Morano S, Cristina G, de Rossi MG, Mariani G, Cotroneo P *et al*. Charge selectivity of proteinuria in Type 1 diabetes explored by Ig subclass clearance. *Diabetes* 1991; **40**:1685–1690.

111. Fox JG, Quin JD, Paterson KR, O'Reilly D StJ, Smith MP, Boulton-Jones JM. Glomerular charge selectivity in Type 1 (insulin-dependent) diabetes mellitus. *Diabet Med* 1995; **12**:387–391.

112. Jerums G, Cooper ME, Seeman E, Murray RML, McNeil JJ. Spectrum of proteinuria in Type 1 and Type 2 diabetes. *Diabetes Care* 1987; **10**:419–427.

113. Jerums G, Allen TJ, Cooper ME. Triphasic changes in selectivity with increasing proteinuria in Type 1 and Type 2 diabetes. *Diabet Med* 1989; **6**: 772–779.

114. Meyers BD, Winetz JA, Chul F, Michaels AS. Mechanisms of proteinuria in diabetic nephropathy: a study of glomerular barrier function. *Kidney Int* 1982; **21**:633–641.

115. Viberti GC, Keen H. The patterns of proteinuria in diabetes mellitus. Relevance to pathogenesis and prevention of diabetic nephropathy. *Diabetes* 1984; **33**:686–692.

116. Gambaro G, Baggio B, Cicerello E, Mastrosimone S, Marzaro G, Borsatti A, Grepaldi G. Abnormal erythrocyte charge in diabetes mellitus: link with microalbuminuria. *Diabetes* 1988; **37**:745–748.

117. Mathiesen ER, Smith C, Lauritzen M, Hommel E, Levin M, Parving H-H. Surface charge of red blood cells in insulin-dependent diabetic patients with incipient and overt nephropathy. *Diabet Med* 1987; **4**:431–433.

118. O'Donnell MJ, Martin P, Florkowski CM, Toop MJ, Chapman C, Holder R. Urinary transferrin excretion in Type 1 (insulin-dependent) diabetes mellitus. *Diabet Med* 1991; **8**:657–661.

119. Martin P, Walton C, Chapman C, Bodansky HJ, Stickland MH. Increased urinary excretion of transferrin in children with Type 1 diabetes mellitus. *Diabet Med* 1990; **7**:35–40.

120. Pun KK, Ho P, Lau P, Wong FH. Eight-month longitudinal study of urinary excretion of albumin and tubular proteins in diabetic subjects. *Am J Nephrol* 1990; **10**:475–481.

121. Catalano C, Winocour PH, Gillespie S, Gibb I, Alberti KGMM. Effect of posture and acute glycaemic control on the excretion of retinol binding protein in normoalbuminuric insulin-dependent diabetic patients. *Clin Sci* 1993; **84**:461 467.

122. Rowe DJF, Anthony F, Polak A, Shaw K, Ward CD, Watts GF. Retinol binding protein as a small molecular weight marker of renal tubular function in diabetes mellitus. *Ann Clin Chem* 1987; **24**:477–482.

123. Holm J, Hemmingsen L, Nielsen NV. Relationship between the urinary excretion of albumin and retinol binding protein in insulin-dependent diabetics. *Clin Chim Acta* 1988; **177**:101–106.

124. Holm J, Hemmingsen L, Nielsen NV. Arterial blood pressure related to degree of albuminuria and low-molecular weight proteinuria in IDDM. *Diabetes Care* 1990; **13**:443–446.

125. Catalano C, Winocour PH, Parlongo S, Gibb I, Gillespie S, Alberti KGMM. Measures of tubular function in normoalbuminuric insulin-dependent diabetic patients and their relationship with sodium lithium countertransport activity. *Nephron* 1996; **73**:613–618.

126. Agardh CD, Tallroth G, Hultberg B. Urinary N-acetyl-β-D-glucosaminidase activity does not predict development of diabetic nephropathy. *Diabetes Care* 1987; **10**:604–606.
127. Poon PYW, Davies TME, Dornan TL, Turner RC. Plasma N-acetyl-β-D-glucosaminidase activities and glycaemia in diabetes mellitus. *Diabetologia* 1983; **24**:433–436.
128. Parving HH, Noer I, Deckert T, Evrin PE, Nielsen SL, Lyngsoe J, *et al.* The effect of metabolic regulation on microvascular permeability to small and large molecules in short-term juvenile diabetics. *Diabetologia* 1976; **12**: 161–166.
129. Uusitupa M, Siitonen O, Penttila I, Aro A, Pyorala K. Proteinuria in newly diagnosed Type 2 diabetic patients. *Diabetes Care* 1987; **10**:191–194.
130. Mohamed A, Wilkin T, Leatherdale BA, Rowe D. Response of urinary albumin to submaximal exercise in newly diagnosed non-insulin dependent diabetes. *Br Med J* 1984; **288**:1342–1343.
131. Martin P, Hampton KK, Walton C, Tindall H, Davies JA. Microproteinuria in Type 2 diabetes mellitus from diagnosis. *Diabet Med* 1990; **7**:315–318.
132. Olivarius NdeF, Andreasen AH, Keiding N, Mogensen CE. Epidemiology of renal involvement in newly-diagnosed middle-aged and elderly diabetic patients. Cross-sectional data from the population-based study 'Diabetes Care in General Practice'. *Diabetologia* 1993; **36**:1007–1016.
133. Lind B, Jensen T, Feldt-Rasmussen B, Deckert T. Normal urinary albumin excretion in recently diagnosed Type 1 diabetic patients. *Diabet Med* 1989; **6**:682–684.
134. Marshall SM on behalf of the Microalbuminuria Collaborative Study Group, UK. Factors involved in the transition from normoalbuminuria to microalbuminuria in IDDM. *Diabet Med* 1996; **13: suppl 3**:S14.
135. The Diabetes Control and Complications Trial Research Group. The effect of intensive treatment of diabetes on the development and progression of long term complications of insulin dependent diabetes mellitus. *N Engl J Med* 1993; **329**:977–986.
136. d'Antonio JA, Ellis D, Doft BH, Becker DJ, Drash AL, Kuller LH, Orchard T. Diabetes complications and glycaemic control. The Pittsburgh prospective insulin-dependent diabetes cohort study status report after 5 years of IDDM. *Diabetes Care* 1989; **12**:694–700.
137. Chase HP, Marshall G, Garg SK, Harris S, Osberg I. Borderline increases in albumin excretion rate and the relation to glycaemic control in subjects with Type 1 diabetes. *Clin Chem* 1991; **37**:2048–2052.
138. Christensen CK, Mogensen CE. The course of incipient diabetic nephropathy: studies of albumin excretion and blood pressure. *Diabet Med* 1985; **2**:97–102.
139. Almdal T, Norgaard K, Feldt-Rasmussen B, Deckert T. The predictive value of microalbuminuria in IDDM. *Diabetes Care* 1994; **17**:120–125.
140. Microalbuminuria Study Group, UK. Intensive therapy and progression to clinical albuminuria in patients with insulin dependent diabetes and microalbuminuria. *Br Med J* 1995; **311**:973–977.
141. Forsblom CM, Groop P-H, Ekstrand A, Groop LC. Predictive value of microalbuminuria in patients with insulin dependent diabetes of long duration. *Br Med J* 1992; **305**:1051–1053.
142. UK Prospective Diabetes Study (UKPDS). X. Urinary albumin excretion over 3 years in diet-treated Type 2 (non-insulin-dependent) diabetic patients

and association with hypertension, hyperglycaemia and hypertryglyceridaemia. *Diabetologia* 1993; **36**:1021–1029.

143. Vasquez B, Flock EV, Savage PJ, Nagulesparan M, Bennion LJ, Baird HR, Bennett PH. Sustained reduction of proteinuria in Type 2 (non-insulin-dependent) diabetes following diet-induced reduction of hyperglycaemia. *Diabetologia* 1984; **26**:127–133.

144. Schmitz A, Hvid Hansen H, Christensen T. Kidney function in newly diagnosed Type 2 (non-insulin-dependent) diabetic patients before and during treatment. *Diabetologia* 1989; **32**:434–439.

145. Standl E, Stiegler H. Microalbuminuria in a random cohort of recently diagnosed Type 2 (non-insulin-dependent) diabetic patients living in the Greater Munich Area. *Diabetologia* 1993; **36**:1017–1020.

146. Vora JP, Dolben J, Williams JD, Peters JR, Owens DR. Impact of initial treatment on renal function in newly-diagnosed Type 2 (non-insulin-dependent) diabetes mellitus. *Diabetologia* 1993; **36**:734–740.

147. Niskanen L, Voutilainen R, Terasvirta M, Lehtinen J, Teppo AM, Groop L, Uusitupa M. A prospective study of clinical and metabolic associates of proteinuria in patients with Type 2 diabetes mellitus. *Diabet Med* 1993; **10**:543–549.

148. Nielsen S, Schmitz A, Rehling M, Mogensen CE. Systolic blood pressure relates to the rate of decline of glomerular filtration rate in Type 2 diabetes. *Diabetes Care* 1993; **16**:1427–1432.

149. Rowe JW, Andres R, Tobin JD, Norris AH, Shock NW. The effect of age on creatinine clearance in men: a cross-sectional and longitudinal study. *J Gerontol* 1976; **31**:155–163.

150. John L, Sunder Rao PSS, Kanagasabapathy AS. Rate of progression of albuminuria in Type 2 diabetes. Five year prospective study from South India. *Diabetes Care* 1994; **17**:888–890.

151. Nelson RG, Knowler WC, Pettitt DJ, Hanson RL, Bennett PH. Incidence and determinants of elevated urinary albumin excretion in Pima Indians with NIDDM. *Diabetes Care* 1995; **18**:182–187.

152. Rudberg S, Ullman F, Dahlquist G. Relationship between early metabolic control and the development of microalbuminuria – a longitudinal study in children with Type 1 (insulin-dependent) diabetes mellitus. *Diabetologia* 1993; **36**:1309–1314.

153. Feldt-Rasmussen B, Mathiesen ER, Deckert T. Effect of two years of strict metabolic control on progression of incipient nephropathy in insulin-dependent diabetes. *Lancet* 1986; **2**:1300–1304.

154. Chase HP, Garg SK, Harris S, Hoops SL, Marshall G. High-normal blood pressure and early diabetic nephropathy. *Arch Intern Med* 1990; **150**:639–641.

155. Niskanen L, Uusitupa M, Sarland H, Siitonen O, Voutilainen E, Penttila I, Pyorala K. Microalbuminuria predicts the development of serum lipoprotein abnormalities favouring atherogenesis in newly diagnosed Type 2 (non-insulin-dependent) diabetic patients. *Diabetologia* 1990; **33**:237–243.

156. Sawicki P, Didjurgeit U, Mulhauser I, Bender R, Heinemann L, Berger M. Smoking is associated with progression of diabetic nephropathy. *Diabetes Care* 1994; **17**:126–131.

157. Chase PH, Garg SK, Marshall G, Berg C, Harris S, Jackson WE, Hamman RE. Cigarette smoking increases the risk of albuminuria among subjects with Type 1 diabetes. *J Am Med Ass* 1991; **265**:614–617.

158. Biesenbach G, Zazgornik J, Stoger H, Graflinger P, Hubmann R, Kaiser W *et al.* Abnormal increases in urinary albumin excretion during pregnancy in IDDM women with pre-existing microalbuminuria. *Diabetologia* 1994; **37**:905–910.
159. McCance DR, Traub AI, Harley JMG, Hadden DR, Kennedy L. Urinary albumin excretion in diabetic pregnancy. *Diabetologia* 1989; **32**:236–239.
160. Biesenback G, Zazgornik J. Incidence of transient nephrotic syndrome during pregnancy in diabetic women with and without pre-existing microalbuminuria. *Br Med J* 1989; **299**:366–367.
161. Bilous R, Marshall SM. Diabetic Nephropathy: Clinical Aspects. In *International Textbook of Diabetes Mellitus*, 2nd edn, ed KGMM Alberti, P Zimmet, R deFronzo, H Keen, pp. 1363–1412. John Wiley, Chichester, UK. 1997.

Notes added in proof

Genetic factors

An important prospective study of 159 normoalbuminuric IDDM subjects with over five years' follow-up found that the 79 with consistently higher levels of erythrocyte sodium–lithium counter-transport activity (SLC) had a much greater incidence ($p < 0.01$) of microalbuminuria (22.3%), in comparison with those with lower SLC (5.2%).

Monciotti CG, Semplicini A, Morocutti A, Maioli M, Cipollina MR, Barzon I, *et al.* Elevated sodium–lithium countertransport activity in erythrocytes is predictive of the development of microalbuminuria in IDDM. *Diabetologia* 1997; **40**: 654–661.

A recent meta-analysis of 4773 diabetic subjects from 18 studies shows that insertion–deletion polymorphism of the gene for angiotensin I-converting enzyme significantly increases the risk of nephropathy (but not retinopathy) in both NIDDM and IDDM.

Fujisawa T, Ikegami H, Kawaguchi Y, Hamada Y, Ueda H, Shintani M, *et al.* Meta-analysis of association of insertion/deletion polymorphism of angiotensin I-converting enzyme with diabetic nephropathy and retinopathy. *Diabetologia* 1998; **41**: 47–53.

A nested case-control study suggests that polymorphism of the angiotensin II type 1 receptor gene can interact with an index of severe hyperglycaemia over the first decade of IDDM to increase the relative risk of nephropathy twelve-fold.

Doria A, Onuma T, Warram JH, Krolewski AS. Synergistic effect of angiotensin II type 1 receptor genotype and poor glycaemic control on risk of nephropathy in IDDM. *Diabetologia*, 1997; **40**: 1293–1299.

5

Microalbuminuria as a marker of endothelial dysfunction

The relationship between microalbuminuria and cardiovascular disease will be dealt with at length in Chapter 6, but one compelling view is that glomerular dysfunction leading to microalbuminuria may reflect a more widespread dysfunction of all vascular endothelium. Before discussing the evidence for, and the difficulties with this hypothesis, it is important to consider the intricate nature of normal vascular endothelial cell function.

The vascular endothelium may be regarded as a complex regulatory 'organ system' with endocrine, paracrine and autocrine function. It is closely integrated with underlying structures, which themselves may vary in their composition and function in different organ systems, for example between the retina and the glomerulus. This concept of local variation in function is further demonstrated by experimental evidence of endothelial function operating within a 'microenvironment', by which focal regulatory function in response to a given stimulus takes place within a limited area of the vascular bed. This immediately highlights the difficulty of extrapolating information on endothelial function from, for example, the systemic to the coronary, or from the venous to the arterial circulation, or from large arteries to arterioles.

Furthermore endothelial function differs between the venous and arterial components of the circulation, and drawing parallels between *in vitro* and *in vivo* findings may be quite inappropriate. Many *in vivo* studies to date have been cross-sectional in nature, and thus have been limited in their ability to define pathophysiology. There are other imponderables such as gender variation in endothelial function, and awareness that basal endothelial tone may not reflect local responsiveness to various stimuli. Of additional importance is the impact of the many abnormalities in the circulating constituents (discussed in Chapter 6). Drugs such as oral contraceptives seem to reprogramme the level at which procoagulatory and fibrinolytic balance is set[1]. Current

Table 5.1. *Endothelial cell constituents and functions*

Vasomotor tone
Nitric oxide (endothelium-derived relaxing factor)
Endothelin-1
Angiotensin-converting enzyme

Coagulation and fibrinolysis
Prostacyclin (PGI$_2$)
Thromboxanes
von Willebrand factor
Thrombomodulin
Tissues plasminogen activator (tPA)
Plasminogen activator inhibitor (PAI-1)
Fibronectin

Growth and repair of endothelium and underlying tissues
Platelet-derived growth factor (PDGF)
Fibroblast growth factor (FGF)
Transforming growth factor-β (TGF-β)
Insulin-like growth factor 1 (IGF-1)

Permeability
Transcapillary escape of albumin and fibrinogen
?Microalbuminuria

knowledge of normal endothelial function in the intact human is therefore incomplete.

Accepting these limitations, the vascular endothelium serves four major regulatory functions (Table 5.1), which are best reviewed with reference to the relationship to surrounding structures and circulating components (Fig. 5.1).

Vasomotor tone

The main area of interest is the impact of endothelial function in arteries and precapillary resistance vessels as, here, altered function has most relevance to the putative link between glomerular and atherosclerotic disease. In the resting state it is thought that normal basal tone is predominantly vasodilatory. The key substance implicated in larger vessel function is endothelial derived relaxing factor (EDRF), which is now known to be nitric oxide. This is produced by endothelial cells following stimulation of muscarinic receptors, although the receptors are also responsive to other substances such as histamine, thrombin and platelet derived growth factor[2]. Non-muscarinic triggers are important as acetylcholine does not circulate *in vivo*. In view of the very short half life of EDRF (6 seconds), it essentially has a paracrine function.

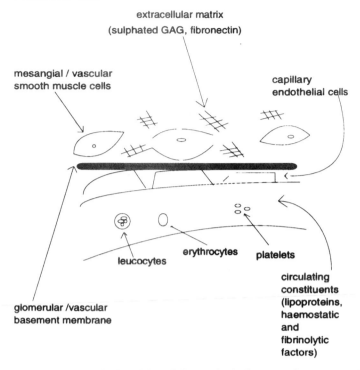

Fig. 5.1. The relationship of the endothelium to the surrounding structures.

EDRF is formed from L-arginine (Fig. 5.2) and acts on underlying smooth muscle by elevating cyclic GMP (Fig. 5.3). In addition to this action, EDRF also has antiproliferative effects (e.g. on mesangial cells), and inhibits platelet adhesion and aggregation, acting in synergy with prostacyclin (*vide infra*). Haemoglobin and free radicals such as superoxide can inactivate EDRF, but this may be partially offset by the action of superoxide dismutase.

More recently, an endothelial derived hyperpolarising factor (EDHF) has been reported. This is distinct from EDRF in that it relaxes smooth muscles by opening potassium channels, without activation of cGMP. In contrast to EDRF, EDHF may exert more influence on arterioles[3].

The endothelins are a group of substances with vasoconstrictor activity. They are a good example of a family of vasoactive substances which are produced not only by endothelial cells, but by other cell types, for example mesangial cells in the kidney. The predominant molecule is ET-1, which is proteolytically activated in the endothelium from 'big Endothelin', and has potent paracrine effects (Fig. 5.3). Whether or not circulating ET-1 has any endocrine role is not yet clear, but *in vitro* it is the most potent pressor agent yet described, some ten times as powerful as angiotensin II. In addition to

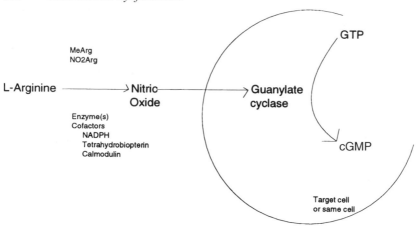

Fig. 5.2. The formation of nitric oxide (endothelium-derived relaxing factor) from L-arginine. A terminal guanidino nitrogen of L-arginine is transformed into nitric oxide by an oxidation pathway requiring the co-factors NADPH, tetrahydrobiopterin and calmodulin. Nitric oxide stimulates guanylate cyclase in the same cell or in a target cell, which converts guanosine triphosphate (GTP) into cyclic guanosine monophosphate (cGMP), thus causing the concentration of cGMP to rise. The conversion of L-arginine to nitric oxide is inhibited by the arginine antagonists N^{G}-monomethyl-L-arginine (MeArg) or N^{W}- nitro-L-arginine (NO$_2$Arg).

its effect on local vascular tone, ET-1 may regulate intra-renal blood flow, mesangial and other cell growth, and stimulate mRNA involved in expression of collagen and laminin (*vide infra*). As a potent hypertensive agent, it normally remains in balance with EDRF, which limits its activity. ET-1 acts through activation of phospholipase C, with the subsequent release of diacylglycerol and inositol trisphosphate, and activation of protein kinase C[4]. Expression of ET-1 is regulated at the level of gene transcription, and induced by stimuli such as thrombin, aldosterone, catecholamines, interleukin-1, angiotensin II, transforming growth factor ß (TGFß) and vasopressin.

The vasoconstrictor angiotensin II is activated within endothelial cells by the action of angiotensin converting enzyme (ACE). The activity of the enzyme varies in different endothelial beds, being particularly high in the glomerulus, and is further subject to genetic variation.

Coagulation and fibrinolytic factors

The endothelium is crucially implicated in the fine balance of intra-vascular coagulation and fibrinolysis, through the production of many substances

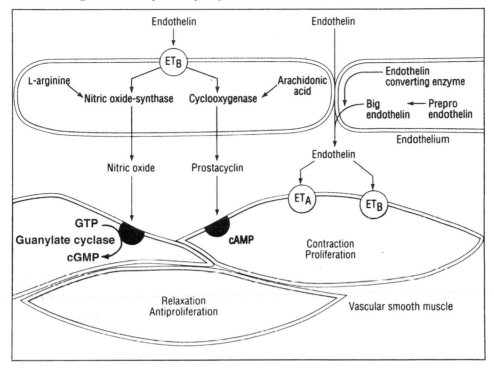

Fig. 5.3. Endothelium dilating and contracting factors. Nitric oxide (NO) is a short-acting gas produced by endothelial nitric oxide synthase from endogenous arginine. It diffuses into the underlying vascular smooth muscle cells where it stimulates guanylate cyclase to produce cyclic GMP. Endothelin is a long-acting and powerful vaso-constrictor which acts on a cell surface receptor causing increased calcium release within the muscle cell. Reproduced from reference 44 with permission.

which respond within the localised microenvironment to allow repair and turnover of the endothelium. This enables the 'response to injury' (haemo-dynamic or toxic) to be measured and localised, and, when uncontrolled, is hypothesised to be the initiating factor in atherosclerosis.

Many of the substances secreted by the endothelium have complex roles, being involved not only in haemostatic balance, but also in vascular tone and growth.

Prostacyclin (PGI_2) is an eicosanoid, the principal product of cyclo-oxyge-nase action on arachidonic acid, and a powerful vasodilator through ablum-inal smooth muscle relaxation. Its biosynthetic pathway and balance with thromboxane is shown in Fig. 5.4. PGI_2 also inhibits platelet aggregation, reduces platelet derived growth factor (PDGF) production from both plate-

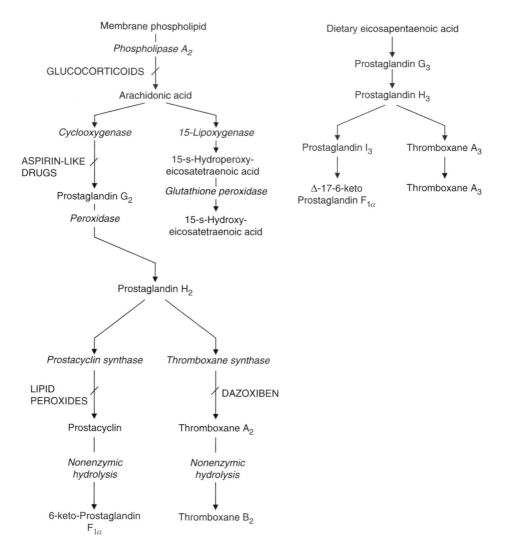

Fig. 5.4. The metabolism of arachidonic acid and eicosapentaenoic acid in
endothelial cells. Prostacyclin and thromboxane A_2 are formed
from arachidonic acid, with the endoperoxides and prostaglandins
G_2 and H_2 as intermediates. They are unstable and break down into
the stable and less active 6-keto-prostaglandin F_1 and thromboxane
B_2. Glucocorticoids, by inhibiting phospholipase A_2, and aspirin-
like drugs, by inhibiting cyclooxygenase, reduce the synthesis of
prostacyclin and thromboxane A_2. High concentrations of lipid
peroxides inhibit prostacyclin synthase, whereas the thromboxane-
synthesis inhibitor dazoxiben prevents thromboxane formation and
shunts endoperoxidases, thus increasing prostacyclin production.
15-Lipoxygenase metabolises arachidonic acid to 15-s-hydroperoxy-
eicosatetraenoic acid and then to 15-s-hydroxy-eicosatetraenoic
acid. Eicospentaenoic acid is transformed by cyclooxygenase into
prostaglandin metabolites with three double bonds.

lets and endothelial cells and blocks glycoprotein receptors for fibrinogen and von Willebrand factor. It exerts mainly paracrine effects by inhibiting vascular growth and smooth muscle cholesterol ester metabolism. It is generated by a host of substances such as kinins, thrombin, serotonin, IL-1 and PDGF itself. PGI_2 has a sophisticated inter-relationship with the many endothelial factors, operating with checks and counter-balances in order to maintain homeostasis and prevent thrombosis or haemorrhage. In contrast to PGI_2, thromboxane B_2 induces local platelet aggregation and vasoconstriction.

Thrombomodulin is a specific endothelial cell surface receptor which modulates the coagulation cascade. It acts as a co-factor in the thrombin-catalysed activation of protein C (Fig. 5.5). Activated protein C is a natural anticoagulant which inhibits coagulation factors V, VIII and platelet aggregation, and enhances fibrinolysis. Whilst it can be detected in plasma, the physiological and possible pathological significance of circulating thrombomodulin is not presently known.

Von Willebrand factor is a glycoprotein derived from the endothelium which is part of the factor VIII complex, and which may serve a procoagulatory function. It may also stimulate platelet adhesion to exposed subendothelium[5]. In contrast to many of the other endothelial products, raised

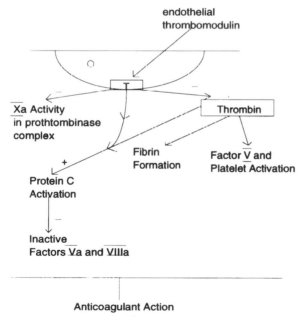

Fig. 5.5. Endothelial thrombomodulin and the coagulation and anticoagulation pathways. + : stimulation; – : inhibition.

circulating vWF levels may indicate generalised endothelial dysfunction, and itself promote haemostasis.

Both tissue plasminogen activator (tPA) and plasminogen activator inhibitor (PAI-1) are endothelial derived components of the fibrinolytic process. tPA is a serine protease whose concentration is the rate limiting step in fibrinolysis (Fig. 5.6). It is resistant to denaturation and involved in PAI-1 production when bound to specific cell receptors, but when free in the circulation is inactivated by PAI-1; thus it more clearly operates as a paracrine substance. tPA gene expression is inhibited by fibroblast growth factor (FGF), histamine and transforming growth factor β (TGFß). PAI-1 is produced by liver and endothelium, and stored in the α-granules of platelets. Increased circulating concentrations may reflect endothelial damage, and inhibit fibrinolysis.

Fibronectin is an endothelial α_2-glycoprotein which *in vitro* and *in vivo* has a role in reducing erythrocyte deformability, and in enhancing erythrocyte and platelet adhesion to subendothelial collagen.

Growth factors

The vascular endothelium secretes a variety of growth factors although their nomenclature makes it clear that they do not originate solely from endothelial cells. These include platelet derived growth factor, fibroblast growth factor, insulin-like growth factor 1 (IGF1) and transforming growth factor β. Whilst they exert a paracrine effect on cell growth and repair, in turn controlled by the aforementioned endothelial products, they also affect underlying cell and supporting connective tissue structures.

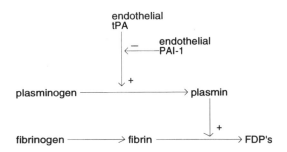

Fig. 5.6. The fibrinolytic cascade. tPA: tissue plasminogen activator; PAI-1: plasminogen activator inhibitor 1; FDP's: fibrin degradation products. +: stimulation; −: inhibition

Endothelial permeability

Glomerular endothelium permeability was discussed in detail in Chapter 1. The basis of the connection between renal dysfunction (suggested by micro-albuminuria) and widespread vasculopathy is that a similar permeability to macromolecules may take place in other vascular systems. Support for this comes mainly from *in vivo* animal experimentation, but isotopic methods in humans have suggested that in addition to retinal vascular permeability (exemplified by exudative diabetic retinopathy), transcapillary escape of albumin and fibrinogen takes place in healthy individuals.

Structure and function of the sub-endothelial structures

Permeability reflects not just endothelial function, but also that of the under-lying basement membrane, a structure containing both collagenous and non-collagenous glycoprotein components such as laminin P1. Structural changes in these molecules account for the basement membrane thickening character-istic of diabetic microangiopathy, and increased circulating concentrations of these as well as endothelial derived substances may reflect extensive damage to the endothelium–basement membrane complex.

Beyond the basement membrane, the extra-cellular matrix and mesenchy-mal derived cells (mesangium and vascular smooth muscle) are in intimate contact. One of the major components of the extracellular matrix are the proteoglycans, macromolecules with glycosaminoglycan (GAG) side-chains, which serve several functions. GAGs are also present on the basement mem-brane and include heparan sulphate (HS) and chondroitin sulphate, which by anionic charge maintain structural integrity and control basement membrane and endothelial permeability. In addition they exert anti-proliferative, anti-thombogenic and anti-lipaemic effects.

Sulphation of GAGs is a key factor in conferring activity, and this is controlled by the enzyme N-deacetylase. Animal models have suggested that genetic polymorphism in this enzyme may alter HS content and conse-quently affect the efficient control of trans-vascular molecular passage[6]. Enzyme activity may also be vulnerable to other influences such as hypergly-caemia. In addition, glycated collagen turnover may be reduced and binding of HS-PG to glycated collagen hindered[7].

The cells of mesenchymal origin have contractile properties which deter-mine vascular reactivity, and which are mediated by both α_1 and α_2 adrener-gic receptors. These may interact with other vasoactive factors such as EDRF, and the relative influence of the two receptors may vary between different vascular beds. Evidence has recently suggested that α_2-adrenorecep-tors may play a significant role in intraglomerular vasoconstriction[8].

Endothelial dysfunction and microalbuminuria in disease

Before summarising the evidence that markers of endothelial function may be linked to microalbuminuria and altered in certain conditions, the role of the endothelium in atherosclerosis will be discussed. The 'response to injury' hypothesis is supported by a wealth of *in vitro* and *in vivo* evidence, which in essence suggests that non-specific endothelial damage leads to denudation, exposure of underlying structures, and medial damage and dissection. The many endothelial substances previously alluded to may then trigger athero-sclerosis, through smooth muscle proliferation, fibroblast transformation to foam cells, and a prothrombotic state. Certain factors may increase the vulnerability of the underlying structures to transform and proliferate (vide infra). Alternatively, endothelial defence mechanisms such as EDRF and PGI_2 may stabilise the lesions and allow re-endothelialisation to take place.

It appears that the degree of endothelial damage depends on the intensity and duration of the injury. In later discussion of the impact of hypertension, hyperglycaemia, smoking and hyperlipidaemia on endothelial function, there may be the potential for either stabilisation or even reversal of those pro-cesses which have led from endothelial dysfunction to established atheroma.

Within the endothelium, several regulatory proteins are encoded for by genes with a single signalling pathway. Endothelial synthesis of adhesion molecules such as intercellular adhesion molecule-1 (ICAM-1) and vascular cell adhesion molecule-1 (VCAM-1), and vasoactive factors such as PAI-1, may be upregulated in response to various leucocyte-derived stimuli, such as superoxide and other free radicals, tumour necrosis factor-1 (TNF-1) and interleukin-1 (IL-1). Effectively the phenotype of the endothelium can then change from a basal state of vasodilation, anti-thrombosis, anti-proliferation and impermeability, to one of vasoconstriction, inflammation, coagulation, proliferation and permeability. The response to injury hypothesis suggests that endothelial leakage of albumin through glomerular endothelial cells into the urinary space is paralleled by increased permeability of athero-thrombo-tic substances and leucocytes through larger vascular beds. Leucocytes inter-act with endothelial receptors known as selectins and adhesion molecules such as ICAM, and are then implicated in atherosclerosis. There is support-ing evidence from animal models demonstrating that coronary permeability is increased by the paracrine effects of ET-1, and antagonised by PGE_1.

It will be evident from the initial discussion that the impact of dysfunction of the endothelium and the subendothelial structures in human disease can only be hinted at indirectly, usually by surrogate measures in cross-sectional studies.

Blunted peripheral vasodilation in response to acetylcholine has been demonstrated in essential hypertension, hypercholesterolaemia, smokers and in homocysteinuria. In advanced atherosclerosis, paradoxical vasospasm to such stimuli has been observed[3].

In essential hypertension various markers have been examined in order to further investigate these phenomena. Abnormal EDRF induced relaxation has been reported[9]. Perhaps not unexpectedly, only a minority of studies have documented increased serum ET-1 concentrations, and the pathological relevance is unclear in that most ET-1 is released locally and abluminally, and as yet there is no standardised assay. Most experimental studies would suggest that any alteration of ET-1 is the consequence rather than the cause of essential hypertension, since the abnormalities described appear reversible in *in vitro* experimentation but not *in vivo*. There are no longitudinal studies of EDRF or ET-1 and their relation to albuminuria in essential hypertension[10].

Raised serum concentrations of other endothelial components such as ACE and vWF have also been reported in essential hypertension. Concentrations of vWF correlated with microalbuminuria and blood pressure, but not with left ventricular mass or forearm vascular resistance[11]; the significance is therefore uncertain, particularly as in another study vWF and fibrinogen concentrations were increased in microalbuminuric hypertensive subjects, but only increased body mass index was related to microalbuminuria in multivariate analyses[12]. There was no increase in PAI-1 or the thrombin–antithrombin complex, and obesity appeared to be the common link between microalbuminuria and endothelial-derived haemostatic factors. As yet there have been no direct comparisons of vWF and acetyl choline-induced vasodilation in essential hypertensive subjects with and without microalbuminuria.

As diabetes mellitus is associated with hypertension and dyslipidaemia, often alongside smoking and hyperglycaemia, this combination of factors might be most likely to result in objective evidence of endothelial and vascular dysfunction. This should be most apparent amongst microalbuminuric diabetic subjects, if, as hypothesised, excessive glomerular albumin loss is a reflection of a widespread loss of vascular integrity, since these vascular risk factors often co-aggregate in these patients (vide infra)[13,14].

Synthesis of EDRF is inhibited by N-monomethyl-L-arginine (NMMA), and the acute forearm vasoconstrictor response to NMMA infusion has been evaluated as an indirect estimate of generalised EDRF synthesis and function. Under euglycaemic conditions in IDDM, basal and nitroprusside-induced and carbachol-induced vasodilatory responses were similar in control and diabetic subjects with and without microalbuminuria, but NMMA did not reduce the vasodilator response in microalbuminuric subjects[15]. As nitroprusside breaks down spontaneously to EDRF, the conclusion of this rather complex series of studies was that microalbuminuric IDDM subjects have reduced EDRF (nitric oxide) synthesis.

The impact of chronic hyperglycaemia on EDRF has been suggested by elegant *in vitro* studies where advanced glycation products accumulated on basement membrane collagen, then inactivated EDRF, and enhanced aortic smooth muscle and renal mesangial cell proliferation[16]. Serum concentrations of the basement membrane component laminin P1 are not increased in microalbuminuric diabetic subjects, whereas they are increased in diabetes complicated by macroalbuminuria or renal failure[17].

Altered EDRF activity may in turn influence catecholamine-induced vascular reactivity in the dorsal hand veins of microalbuminuric IDDM patients. A series of experiments by Bodmer and colleagues established that vascular reactivity to noradrenaline and clonidine was exaggerated in microalbuminuric IDDM patients, but that the response to phenylephrine was comparable amongst patients with and without microalbuminuria. This was associated with asymptomatic peripheral nerve dysfunction, but not with central cardiovascular autonomic dysfunction[18,19]. It was suggested that peripheral autonomic dysfunction of pre-synaptic inhibitory α_2-adrenoreceptors could account for this, since noradrenaline acts on both pre- (vasodilator) and post-synaptic (vasoconstrictor) α_2-adrenoreceptors, as well as post-synaptic (vasoconstrictor) α_1-adrenoreceptors, whereas phenylephrine specifically stimulates post-synaptic α_1-vasoconstrictor receptors, and clonidine is a selective α_2-vasoconstrictor agonist[8].

Smoking appears to attenuate the enhanced vasoconstrictor responses just described, perhaps by inducing catecholamine surges and receptor down-regulation[20].

As mentioned earlier, ET-1 is a potent vasoconstrictor, but it is not clear whether it exerts more than local paracrine effects. Serum and urine concentrations have been examined in several cross-sectional studies in diabetic subjects with conflicting results, partly through differing methodology for ET-1 measurement. Certain assays will cross-react with other endothelins, particularly the larger inactive precursor. Thus, higher concentrations have been observed in comparison to normoglycaemic controls in some[21] but not all studies[22]. Although it might be conceivable that metabolic control and blood pressure could affect ET-1 levels, several studies have found no association[21-24]. A similar lack of consensus is apparent in diabetic patients with complications. Raised ET-1 levels have been recorded in advanced atherosclerosis in normoglycaemic subjects[25], but not in relation to more modest degrees of angiopathy in diabetes[21,22]. The relationship between microalbuminuria and ET-1 is also unclear, with a modest association in one small study in IDDM[23], no relationship in others in NIDDM[21,22], but the suggestion that both serum and urine ET-1 concentrations are elevated in macroalbuminuric subjects. The overriding impression is that abnormal ET-1 is a late marker of major vascular or renal damage, and is unlikely to play an important aetiological role in hypertension, nephropathy or atherosclerosis.

Adhesion molecules such as ICAM and VCAM may be increased in diabetes, but as with ET-1 appear unrelated to possible influencing factors such as hyperglycaemia and microalbuminuria[26]. The co-factor thrombomodulin appears to have a local anticoagulant function. A sole report[27] of progressively increasing thrombomodulin concentrations in NIDDM between normo-, micro- and macroalbuminuric subjects, suggests it to be a rather insensitive marker of established small vessel disease, whose secretion may be partly compensatory. Alternatively delayed renal clearance of thrombomodulin could have accounted for the findings.

Although increased circulating levels of vasoactive substances implies endothelial disease, and the molecules themselves may further this process, documented increased transcapillary escape of macromolecules more clearly demonstrates endothelial dysfunction, and supports the notion that microalbuminuria is but one manifestation of this process.

Increased transcapillary escape (TER) of both albumin and fibrinogen has been documented in microalbuminuric IDDM patients, NIDDM subjects and also in elderly non-diabetic smokers[28-31]. The methodology involved radio-isotopic labelling and reinfusion of labelled molecules, and may be relatively insensitive[32]. The impact of hypertension, hyperglycaemia and ageing on increased TER is disputed: thus in one study whilst TER was greater in microalbuminuric IDDM subjects regardless of hypertension, it was apparently no different in healthy controls and normoalbuminuric normoglycaemic subjects with moderate essential hypertension[33]. Another report[34] suggested that severe essential hypertension (diastolic blood pressure > 120 mmHg) did lead to an increased TER of albumin. Non-enzymatic glycation of albumin seems to have a minimal impact *in vivo* on TER, if anything reducing it[35,36]. The interpretation of these data is that as with so many of the other markers, alterations of TER seem to parallel rather than determine the development of microalbuminuria.

Urinary excretion of chondroitin sulphate (CS) and GAGs has been evaluated in diabetic patients, with the objective of suggesting a role *in vivo* for the sub-endothelial extra-cellular matrix in nephropathy and atherosclerosis[37]. Significant univariate correlations were recorded between excretion of CS and GAGs and both total and LDL cholesterol, particularly in microalbuminuric and hypercholesterolaemic subjects. There was no correlation between microalbuminuria and CS or GAGs in this report. Therefore, a reasonable conclusion from this cross-sectional data would be that altered excretion of these molecules appears a late secondary phenomenon of renal and vascular disease processes, rather than an early feature of an inherent abnormality in those predisposed to microalbuminuria.

The most consistent and well documented abnormality of endothelial function associated with microalbuminuria is raised circulating concentrations of von Willebrand factor. This was first reported by Jensen[31] in 1989 in microalbuminuric IDDM patients, and has subsequently been confirmed in microalbuminuric NIDDM and essential hypertensive subjects[11,38,39]. However, the most important reports are longitudinal studies which have evaluated the impact of basal vWF on subsequent nephropathy and cardiovascular disease, taking account of other integral factors such as albuminuria and lipoproteins.

The studies which have evaluated vWF have relied on immunological assays which detect vWF antigen, and express vWF as a percentage of values in 'normal pooled plasma' (usual reference range 50–150 %). This will not necessarily reflect true functional activity, and there are precedents of immunologically active, but biologically inactive, molecules whose importance may be overstated. It is not clear at present whether vWF concentrations give a reliable quantitative as opposed to qualitative measure of endothelial damage, or whether concentrations reflect the degree (i.e. marked triple vessel coronary artery disease) or the extent (e.g. widespread mild atherosclerosis) of atherosclerotic disease. vWF also has a significant diurnal variation of at least 10 %, and is susceptible to elevations through the use of a tourniquet during venepuncture. Finally, the several reports have used RIA, ELISA or immunoelectrophoretic methods. Thus, without standardisation it is difficult to make comparisons between studies.

Notwithstanding these considerations, vWF has clearly been correlated with blood pressure, blood glucose and albuminuria in diabetic subjects. In the most important study to date, the relationship between microalbuminuria and vWF was put into perspective. Stehouwer and colleagues[40] studied 94 subjects with NIDDM, of whom 66 had normoalbuminuria and 28 microalbuminuria at entry to the study. The average duration of follow up was 36–

41 months, during which time albumin excretion became abnormal in 33 (50 %) of those who originally were normoalbuminuric. In those who remained normoalbuminuric, vWF remained stable, but it rose amongst those who became microalbuminuric (where activity almost doubled), and also amongst those who initially were microalbuminuric. Most importantly, an increased risk of fatal and non-fatal cardiovascular events was only seen amongst microalbuminuric subjects where vWF activity initially was greater than 133 %. The relative risk of new cardiovascular events was highest (relative risk 5.7) when there was a past history of cardiovascular disease. The cardiovascular risk from microalbuminuria was further independently modified by low HDL cholesterol (< 1.1 mmol/l).

Thus, the presence of several markers together greatly magnified the risk of coronary heart disease. There are several important caveats in interpretation of the data. An earlier study demonstrated similar vWF concentrations in microalbuminuric and macroalbuminuric subjects[5], and the incidence of coronary heart disease is much greater amongst macroalbuminuric subjects, so in this sense the raised vWF only acts as a qualitative categorical risk marker. Changing activity of the order of 50–100 % was observed in persistently normoalbuminuric subjects in the longitudinal study, and the significance of this is uncertain in isolation. In addition other markers of endothelial/ haemostatic dysfunction, such as factor VIII antigen, did not appear to parallel vWF in the longitudinal study which predicted macroproteinuric diabetic nephropathy[40].

It would appear that the role of vWF (and HDL) is to magnify and better categorise the risk attributable to microalbuminuria. This is clearly vital if reproduced in other studies as it may enable proper early targeting for intervention with ACE inhibitors, aspirin and lipid-lowering therapy.

Aspects of treatment of microalbuminuria will be covered in detail in Chapter 8, but with regard to microalbuminuria as a marker of widespread endothelial dysfunction it is understood that standard antihypertensive therapy and specific ACE inhibitor therapy will influence this as well as vascular resistance. Other strategies have been examined more recently, including subcutaneous unfractionated and low molecular heparin therapy twice daily in microalbuminuric IDDM patients. After three months, albuminuria fell in comparison to those given placebo saline injections[41]. Increased synthesis and sulphation of heparan sulphate proteoglycan, lipolytic and antithrombotic action may all be implicated, and further research in this area is clearly necessary.

Other experimental strategies have suggested that albuminuria may be reduced by infused sulodexide (a synthetic glycosaminoglycan)[42] or by the somatostatin analogue octreotide, which also may reduce markers of endothelial dysfunction such as vWF[43]. Twenty first century strategies such as genetic modification of endothelial proteins with recombinant viral DNA may also be feasible at an early stage of subclinical disease.

Despite the many difficulties involved in '*in vivo*' evaluation of the interaction between microalbuminuria and endothelial dysfunction in the intact human, a longitudinal interventional study of microalbuminuric diabetic and essential hypertensive subjects with and without raised vWF levels, should be feasible. Prior to that, many other questions need to be addressed. These include whether or not the measurement of other endothelial markers alongside vWF (e.g. PAI-1 and ACE) confers any extra risk (additive or synergistic) or no extra risk, and whether the several markers exert an 'all-or-none', or graded influence on vascular risk.

Longer-term data on reproducibility of endothelial markers is important, particularly in determining whether 'acute phase' transient responses may have longer-term pathogenetic implications.

References

1. Petersen KR, Skouby SO, Sidelmann J, Jespersen J. Assessment of endothelial function during oral contraception in women with insulin-dependent diabetes mellitus. *Metabolism* 1994; **43**:1379–1383.
2. Meidell RS. Southwestern Internal Medicine Conference: endothelial dysfunction and vascular disease. *Am J Med Sci* 1994; **307**:378–389.
3. Vanhoutte PM, Scott-Burden T. The endothelium in health and disease. *Texas Heart Inst J* 1994; **21**:62–67.
4. Vane JR, Anggard EE, Botting RM. Regulatory functions of the vascular endothelium. *N Engl J Med* 1990; **323**:27–36.
5. Stehouwer CDA, Stroes ESG, Hackeng HL, Mulder PGH, Den Ottolander GJH. Von Willebrand factor and development of diabetic nephropathy in IDDM. *Diabetes* 1991; **40**:971–976.
6. Deckert T, Horowitz IM, Kofoed-Enevoldsen A, Kjellen L, Deckert M, Lykkelund C, Burcharth F. Possible genetic defects in regulation of glycosaminoglycans in patients with diabetic nephropathy. *Diabetes* 1991; **40**:764–770.
7. Van Den Born J, van Kraats AA, Bakker MAH, Assmann KJM, van den Heuvel LPWJ, Veerkamp JH, Berden JHM. Selective proteinuria in diabetic nephropathy in the rat is associated with a relative decrease in glomerular basement membrane heparan sulphate. *Diabetologia* 1995; **38**:161–172.
8. Bodmer CW, Schaper NC, Janssen M, De Leeuw PW, Williams G. Selective enhancement of α_2-adrenoreceptor-mediated vasoconstriction in insulin-dependent diabetic patients with microalbuminuria. *Clin Sci* 1995; **88**:421–426.
9. Panza JA, Quyyumi AA, Brush JE, Epstein SE. Abnormal endothelium-dependent vascular relaxation in patients with essential hypertension. *N Engl J Med* 1990; **323**:22–27.

10. Luscher TF. The endothelium in hypertension: bystander, target or mediator? *J Hypertension* 1994; **12** suppl 10: S105–S116.
11. Pedrinelli R, Giampietro O, Carmassi F, Melillo E, Dell'Ormo G, Catapano G *et al.* Microalbuminuria and endothelial dysfunction in essential hypertension. *Lancet* 1994; **344**:14–18.
12. Agewall S, Fagerberg B, Attvall S, Ljungman S, Ursanavicius V, Tengbon L, Wikstrand J. Microalbuminuria, insulin sensitivity and haemostatic factors in non-diabetic treated hypertensive men. *J Int Med* 1995; **237**:195–203.
13. Deckert T, Kofoed-Enevoldsen A, Norgaard K, Borch-Johnsen K, Feldt-Rasmussen B, Jensen T. Microalbuminuria. Implications for micro- and macrovascular disease. *Diabetes Care* 1992; **15**:1181–1191.
14. Deckert T, Feldt-Rasmussen B, Borch-Johnsen K, Jensen T, Kofoed-Enevoldsen A. Albuminuria reflects widespread vascular damage. The Steno hypothesis. *Diabetologia* 1989; **32**: 219–226.
15. Elliot TG, Cockroft JR, Groop P-H, Viberti GC, Ritter JM. Inhibition of nitric oxide synthesis in forearm vasculature of insulin-dependent diabetic patients: blunted vasoconstriction in patients with microalbuminuria. *Clin Sci* 1993; **85**:687–693.
16. Hogan M, Cerami A, Bucala R. Advanced glycosylation endproducts block the antiproliferative effect of nitric oxide. Role in the vascular and renal complications of diabetes mellitus. *J Clin Invest* 1992; **90**:1110–1115.
17. Pietschmann P, Schernthaner G, Schnack CH, Gaube S. Serum concentrations of laminin P1 in diabetics with advanced nephropathy. *J Clin Path* 1988; **41**:929–932.
18. Bodmer CW, Patrick AW, How TV, Williams G. Exaggerated sensitivity to NE-induced vasoconstricion in IDDM patients with microalbuminuria: possible etiology and diagnostic implications. *Diabetes* 1992; **41**:209–214.
19. Bodmer CW, Masson EA, Savage MW, Benbow S, Patrick AW, Williams G. Asymptomatic peripheral nerve dysfunction and vascular reactivity in IDDM patients with and without microalbuminuria. *Diabetologia* 1994; **37**:1056–1061.
20. Bodmer CW, Valentine DT, Masson EA, Savage MW, Lake D, Williams G. Smoking attenuates the vasoconstrictor response to noradrenaline in Type 1 diabetic patients and normal subjects: possible relevance to diabetic nephropathy. *Eur J Clin Invest* 1994; **24**:331–336.
21. Takahashi K, Ghatei MA, Lam HC, O'Halloran DJ, Bloom SR. Elevated plasma endothelin in patients with diabetes mellitus. *Diabetologia* 1990; **33**:306–310.
22. Bertello P, Veglio F, Pinna G, Gurioli L, Molino P, Alban S, Chiandussi L. Plasma endothelin in NIDDM patients with and without complications. *Diabetes Care* 1994; **17**:574–577.
23. Collier A, Leach JP, McLellan A, Jardine A, Morton JJ, Small M. Plasma endothelin like immunoreactivity levels in IDDM patients with microalbuminuria. *Diabetes Care* 1992; **15**:1038–1040.
24. Lee Y-J, Shin S-J, Tsai J-H. Increased urinary endothelin-1-like immunoreactivity excretion in NIDDM patients with albuminuria. *Diabetes Care* 1994; **17**:263–266.
25. Lerman A, Edwards BS, Hallett JW, Heublein DM, Sandberg SM, Burnett JC. Circulating and tissue endothelin immunoreactivity in advanced atherosclerosis. *N Engl J Med* 1991; **325**:997–1001.

26. Steiner M, Reinhardt KM, Krammer B, Ernst B, Blann AD. Increased levels of soluble adhesion molecules in type 2 (non-insulin dependent) diabetes mellitus are independent of glycaemic control. *Thromb Haemostasis* 1994; **72**:979–984.

27. Iwashima Y, Sato T, Watanabe K, Ooshima E, Hiraishi S, Ishii H, *et al.* Elevation of plasma thrombomodulin level in diabetic patients with early diabetic nephropathy. *Diabetes* 1990; **39**:983–988.

28. Feldt-Rasmussen B, Jensen T. Microalbuminuria. Implications for micro- and macrovascular disease. *Diabetes Care* 1992; **15**:1181–1191.

29. O'Hare JA, Ferriss JB, Twomey B, O'Sullivan DJ. Poor metabolic control, hypertension, and microangiopathy independently increase the transcapillary escape rate of albumin in diabetes. *Diabetologia* 1983; **25**:260–263.

30. Jensen EW, Espersen K, Knudsen JH, Nielsen SL. Increased transcapillary escape rate of albumin in elderly subjects due to long-term smoking habits. *Clin Physiol* 1995; **15**:159–167.

31. Jensen T. Increased plasma concentration of von Willebrand factor in insulin dependent diabetics with incipient nephropathy. *Br Med J* 1989; **298**:27–28.

32. Valensi P, Attali JR, Behar A, Sebaoun J. Isotopic test of capillary permeability to albumin in diabetic patients : effects of hypertension, microangiopathy, and duration of diabetes. *Metabolism* 1987; **36**:834–839.

33. Norgaard K, Jensen T, Feldt-Rasmussen B. Transcapillary escape rate of albumin in hypertensive patients with type 1 (insulin-dependent) diabetes mellitus. *Diabetologia* 1993; **36**:57–61.

34. Parving HH, Gyntelberg F. Transcapillary escape rate of albumin and plasma volume in essential hypertension. *Circ Res* 1973; **32**:643–651.

35. Bent-Hanson L, Deckert T. Metabolism of albumin and fibrinogen in type 1 (insulin-dependent) diabetes mellitus. *Diabetes Res* 1988; **7**:159–164.

36. Bent-Hansen L, Feldt-Rasmussen B, Kverneland A, Deckert T. Transcapillary escape rate and relative metabolic clearance of glycated and non-glycated albumin in Type 1 (insulin-dependent) diabetes mellitus. *Diabetologia* 1987; **30**:2–4.

37. Colette C, Etienne P, Percheron C. Glycosaminoglycan excretion in diabetes mellitus: relation with atherosclerosis and glomerulosclerosis. *Diabet Nutr Metab* 1994; **7**:295–301.

38. Neri S, Bruno CM, Raciti C, D'Angelo G, D'Amico R, Cristaldi R. Alteration of oxide reductive and haemostatic factors in type 2 diabetics. *J Intern Med* 1994; **236**:495–500.

39. Stehouwer CDA, Nauta JJP, Zeldenrust GC, Hackeng WHL, Donker AJM, Den Ottolander GJH. Urinary albumin excretion, cardiovascular disease and endothelial dysfunction in non-insulin-dependent diabetes mellitus. *Lancet* 1992; **340**:319–323.

40. Stehouwer CDA, Fischer HRA, van Kuijk AWR, Polak BCP, Donker AJM. Endothelial dysfunction precedes development of microalbuminuria in IDDM. *Diabetes* 1995; **44**:561–564.

41. Myrup B, Hansen PM, Jensen T, Kofoed-Enevoldsen A, Feldt-Rasmussen B, Gram J, *et al.* Effect of low-dose heparin on urinary albumin excretion in insulin-dependent diabetes mellitus. *Lancet* 1995; **345**:421–422.

42. Solini A, Carraro A, Barzon I, Crepaldi G. Therapy with glycosaminoglycans lowers albumin excretion rate in non-insulin dependent diabetic patients with macroalbuminuria. *Diabet Nutr Metab* 1994; **7**:304–307.

43. Dullaart RPF, Meijer S, Marbach P, Sluiter WJ. Effect of a somatostatin analogue, octreotide, on renal haemodynamics and albuminuria in acromegalic patients. *Eur J Clin Invest* 1992; **22**:494–502.
44. Brown MJ. Hypertension. *Br Med J* 1997; **314**:1258–1261.

6

Microalbuminuria, cardiovascular risk factors and cardiovascular disease

The relationship between microalbuminuria and cardiovascular disease (CVD) was first noted in NIDDM, but has since been documented in IDDM and non-diabetic populations. The exact nature of the association is not fully resolved, but at least three major factors are of importance.

(1) The observation that microalbuminuria is often manifest in subjects who also have other features which, in their own right, put them at risk of atherosclerotic vascular disease.

(2) The attractive hypothesis that microalbuminuria reflects generalised loss of endothelial integrity, affecting not only glomerular capillaries, but also arterial and arteriolar intimal function, thereby promoting transvascular escape of atherogenic molecules.

(3) The suggestion that in many cases, microalbuminuria is simply the consequence of established cardiovascular disease.

These three concepts are by no means mutually exclusive, and together may well explain why the development of microalbuminuria carries such a poor long-term prognosis. The hypothesis that microalbuminuria is a marker of generalised endothelial dysfunction has already been discussed in Chapter 5.

The present chapter will focus on the interaction between microalbuminuria, cardiovascular risk factors, and atherosclerotic and non-atherosclerotic cardiovascular disease. These will be discussed in diabetic and non-diabetic subjects. One important practical point is that microalbuminuria and several other vascular risk factors often cluster within individuals, more particularly amongst those with diabetes mellitus. This pattern magnifies considerably the likelihood of cardiovascular morbidity and mortality, even though the absolute levels of the various factors are often only modestly disturbed.

In this situation microalbuminuria appears to exert a synergistic effect. The additional impact of diabetes is to double the attributable risk of other cardiovascular risk factors, by accelerating the course of early atherosclerosis, as opposed to directly initiating it. This is likely to be the consequence of the key metabolic disturbances of diabetes – hyperglycaemia, insulin insensitivity, non-enzymatic protein glycation, and development of advanced glycation end products – which may modify intravascular lipoprotein metabolism, haemostasis, renal function, arterial structure and tone, cellular transport mechanisms, and free radical activity.

Microalbuminuria and hypertension

Microalbuminuria was first documented in essential hypertension in 1974[1], but its clinical importance in this setting is still not established at present. It is by no means ubiquitous in essential hypertension, but there are very few population-based studies of the prevalence of microalbuminuria in essential hypertension, or vice versa. Estimates of urinary albumin concentration > 20 mg/l in 7.8 % in our own community based study of 100 Europids with previously diagnosed hypertension[2] compare reasonably well with the 5 % > 10.6 mg/l recorded in the 223 hypertensive subjects of mixed ethnic background in New Zealand[3].

Agewall and colleagues[4] suggested that microalbuminuria (overnight excretion > 10 µg/min) was present in 25 % of treated hypertensive subjects whose average age was 66 years. In this report microalbuminuria was associated more frequently with evidence of cardiovascular damage. Mild-to-moderate hypertension has been associated with microalbuminuria in 40 % of 123 cases[5], but selection bias may have a role in explaining this higher than expected prevalence.

Difficulties in definitions of both microalbuminuria and hypertension limit further clarification of the nature of the relationship between the variables. The definition of blood pressure according to WHO criteria is systolic > 160 mmHg and/or diastolic blood pressure > 95 mmHg and/or ongoing antihypertensive treatment. This limited categorisation is based on previous epidemiological studies which have demonstrated attributable cardiovascular risk and a response to treatment at or beyond these levels of blood pressure. They take no account of the normal age and gender differences in blood pressure distribution. Thus, blood pressures $> 140/90$ mmHg in younger adults may be well outside the 90th centile population distribution, and should also be considered to be abnormal, although this would not be recognised by current WHO criteria. This is important with regard to the relationship with microalbuminuria in the light of the suggestion that the relationship between blood pressure and albuminuria is not linear, and is only apparent at diastolic pressures ≥79 mmHg, with pressure-dependent albuminuria a feature at values > 140/90 mmHg[6].

The early report by Parving and coworkers[1] demonstrated that microalbuminuria was only a feature of moderate (mean 182/112 mmHg) as opposed to mild (mean 143/89 mmHg) hypertension. A more recent study has supported this concept, with the observation that white coat hypertension is associated with microalbuminuria less often than established hypertension[7]. The relative importance of systolic as opposed to diastolic pressure on albuminuria has been examined. Diastolic pressure has been found to be more important in some reports[3], whilst equivalent importance was suggested in others[2,8]. It has been suggested that day-time ambulatory diastolic pressure correlates more closely with microalbuminuria than casual diastolic readings in mild essential hypertension (> 140/90 and < 160/95 mmHg)[9]. These factors have a bearing on the likely natural history of microalbuminuria in essential hypertension (*vide infra*).

Ethnic origin also appears to influence the impact of hypertension on albumin excretion. In contrast to suggestions that microalbuminuria was seen in less than 10 % of Europids with essential hypertension, urine albumin concentrations > 30 mg/l were found in 20.6 % of normoglycaemic Polynesian inhabitants of the Pacific island of Nauru whose blood pressure was > 140/90 but < 160/95 mmHg, and in 44 % of those with hypertension according to WHO criteria[10]. A paper from New York[11] actually suggested that hypertensive Europids were five times more likely to have microalbuminuria than hypertensive Hispanics, but the sample size was small (60 subjects), and the findings were contrary to the knowledge that hypertensive renal disease is more common amongst such non-White communities. In non-diabetic Chinese subjects, multivariate analyses suggested that systolic blood pressure in men and diastolic blood pressure in women, are independent contributors to increasing albumin:creatinine ratios, and exclusion of mildly hypertensive subjects (> 140/90 mmHg) abolished any such relationship[12].

On balance therefore, after taking account of published information in non-White diabetic subjects, it appears that the impact of hypertension on albuminuria is greater in non-Europids, particularly in association with obesity and more recent acculturation to a Western lifestyle. Obesity may also infuence microalbuminuria independent of hypertension[13], but whether this is solely due to insulin resistance (*vide infra*) is presently unknown.

These differences lead on to a discussion of the pathogenesis of albuminuria in hypertension, and the perennial argument as to whether genetic or environmental factors assume greater importance. Proponents of the genetic theory have suggested that a family history of hypertension and coronary heart disease is more likely amongst those with essential hypertension complicated by microalbuminuria. Furthermore, albumin excretion rates > 20 μg/min have been recorded in 57 % of non-obese hypertensive individuals with raised *in vitro* activity of erythrocyte sodium lithium countertransport (SLC) activity, a putative genetic marker for essential hypertension, in contrast to 18 % with normal SLC and equivalent levels of blood pressure[14]. Those with elevated SLC also had a host of additional cardiorenal and metabolic abnormalities, including increases in glomerular filtration rates, kidney volume, left ventricular mass, total exchangeable sodium, serum triglyccrides, and reductions in HDL cholesterol and renal lithium clearance (a marker of tubular dysfunction). The difficulty in deciding whether or not these associations are causal is in part that seen with any cross-sectional study in small numbers, namely a chance observation in a group with more complications of hypertension. Just as important is the increasing recognition that SLC activity is susceptible to many biological factors such as circulating levels of lipids and insulin, and that information on the kinetics of ion transport could be more informative[15,16]. An early suggestion that 65 % of SLC activity is genetically determined[17], may therefore be misleading. Microalbuminuria does appear to be related to body mass index, waist:hip ratio, and serum insulin in treated hypertension, all factors reflecting insulin insensitivity[4], but another report suggested that microalbuminuria was not related to hyperinsulinaemia in non-diabetic atherosclerotic subjects, of whom 60 % were hypertensive[18]. A recent report has demonstrated a more than two-fold increase in albumin excretion rates amongst salt-sensitive hypertensive patients. Albuminuria was correlated with the estimated increased intraglomerular pressure amongst salt-sensitive patients[19]. Of course, the uncertainty still remains as to whether the prime mover in these processes are predominantly genetically or environmentally mediated.

Further support for a genetic basis to account for microalbuminuria in only a proportion of subjects with essential hypertension was suggested by the finding of microalbuminuria in seven out of ten normotensive subjects with a history of hypertension in a first degree relative, in contrast to none with no family history[20]. This preliminary observation requires confirmation before too much credibility is assigned to this hypothesis. The observation that microalbuminuria precedes hypertension has been discussed earlier in the context of diabetes (see Chapter 4), but it seems an unlikely scenario in essential hypertension. The suggestion that microalbuminuria is pressure dependent beyond a threshold blood pressure is a reasonably consistent finding, and in keeping with the concept that the primary mechanism is predominantly haemodynamic, the consequence of raised intraglomerular pressure.

Altered glomerular pore permselectivity may also play a role, based on the observation by Cottone and Cerasola[21], that nocturnal fractional clearance of albumin was increased in microalbuminuric hypertensive subjects, despite no appreciable difference in overnight glomerular filtration in comparison to normoalbuminuric hypertensive patients. Unfortunately this study only evaluated renal filtration by estimation of creatinine clearance, and an apparently non-significant mean difference of 11 mmHg in diastolic pressure was noted between the two groups. Parving and colleagues[1] found no alteration of β_2-microglobulin excretion in essential hypertension, and suggested that tubular dysfunction did not therefore appear to be implicated in the albuminuria of essential hypertension. A later study recorded increased ß$_2$-microglobulin excretion in both benign and accelerated hypertension[22]. Since that time, however, the role of this protein as a marker of tubular dysfunction has been somewhat discredited, but increased excretion of the smaller molecular weight retinol binding protein has been noted in essential hypertension in conjunction with microalbuminuria[23]. The possibility thus remains that tubular disease and dysfunction could also contribute to albuminuria in essential hypertension.

The rapid reduction in albuminuria with blood pressure lowering (*vide infra*) suggests that there is a large functional component to the relationship, at least early in the course of hypertension, prior to establishment of hypertensive nephrosclerosis.

Hypertension is not a mandatory prerequisite for the development of microalbuminuria. Several studies[2,24,25] demonstrated that diagnosed and treated hypertension was a finding in only 25–37 % of individuals with microalbuminuria. Hypertension does however seem to operate as a contributory factor which interacts with genetic and environmental components.

Exposure to hydrocarbons in organic solvents is one possible example of an environmental cause of albuminuria. Hotz and colleagues[26] found that mildly hypertensive (> 140/90 mmHg) floor layers and printers exposed to water-based glues and toluene had increased fractional albumin clearance, in comparison to mildly hypertensive roadmen whose exposure to hydrocarbons was slight. Hypertension may therefore promote albuminuria in subjects with glomerular membrane damage from hydrocarbons, a fact supported by the group's earlier observation of erythrocyturia in these same workers. By contrast, Yaqoob and colleagues[27] have recently demonstrated that urinary protein and enzyme markers of tubular dysfunction were increased with chronic hydrocarbon exposure, but there was no associated increase in urinary albumin excretion. No comment was made, however, about the possibility of any interaction with coincidental hypertension.

Most recently, Pedrinelli and coworkers[28] suggested that microalbuminuria in essential hypertension was independently associated with increased concentrations of von Willebrand antigen, a marker of endothelial dysfunction, as well as increased plasma fibrinogen and smoking.

Microalbuminuria and hypertension in IDDM

Despite extensive work in this area, at present there is no clear consensus as to the extent or the nature of the relationship between albuminuria and blood pressure in IDDM. This is partly because of different definitions of microalbuminuria (cut-off points varying between 10 and 70 µg/min have been found to predict subsequent renal and cardiovascular disease), and the failure to consider hypertension in relative terms which take account of age-related norms. Other factors such as glycaemia, glycation and hyperinsulinaemia are intrinsic to IDDM, and themselves may affect albuminuria. The pathogenesis of hypertension in IDDM may itself have a bearing on the relationship with albuminuria, but at present controversy surrounds the suggestion that a genetic predisposition to hypertension and altered cellular ion transport is implicated in hypertension and diabetic nephropathy. There is no doubt, however, regarding the intimate relationship between hypertension and albuminuria in IDDM.

The reported prevalence of hypertension in microalbuminuric IDDM patients has possibly been underestimated at 30 %, since WHO criteria were used for the diagnosis of hypertension (systolic > 160 mmHg and/or diastolic > 95 mmHg and/or current antihypertensive therapy) and albumin excretion rates > 21 µg/min were diagnostic of microalbuminuria in this study[29]. It is clear that the prevalence of hypertension in microalbuminuria changes with increasing duration of diabetes (from 11 % after 5–9 years, to 53 % after 30–34 years)[29]. These data, however, are from a tertiary referral centre with a major interest in early diabetic renal disease, so the representativeness of the population is not certain. The prevalence of hypertension by whatever diagnostic criteria increases with the degree of microalbuminuria, and is increased two-fold when the excretion rates are 70–200 µg/min, as opposed to 20–69 µg/min.

The prevalence of microalbuminuria amongst hypertensive IDDM patients is not stated explicitly, but is likely to be of the order of at least 80 %, bearing in mind the observation by Norgaard and colleagues[29] that the prevalence of hypertension amongst normoalbuminuric IDDM patients aged 40–50 years is of the order of 12 %, analogous to an age-matched non-diabetic population, in contrast to 30 % amongst microalbuminuric IDDM subjects of similar age. The prevalence of microalbuminuria (> 20 μg/min in timed overnight collections) amongst normotensive (< 140/90 mmHg) IDDM patients has been estimated at 12–16 %[30-32]. Marshall and Alberti[32] demonstrated that univariate and multivariate relationships with albuminuria are evident when systolic blood pressure exceeds 140 mmHg.

The broad consensus from earlier cross-sectional studies in IDDM suggested that day-time resting diastolic pressure, as opposed to systolic blood pressure, was the clearer discriminator of microalbuminuric from normoalbuminuric subjects. This appeared most notably in studies where the greater proportion of subjects were less than 40 years of age. Part of the explanation for the observation is simply mathematical, in that absolute differences in blood pressure would have greater significance for diastolic blood pressure, because of less spread of values. This is supported by scrutiny of the age- and gender-based centile charts (Fig. 6.1)[33] where, in contrast to systolic blood pressure, the 90th centile line for diastolic blood pressure is quite flat at ages < 40 years. In pathophysiological terms the greater importance of diastolic pressure would suggest that intrinsic renal vascular tone may be more important than the systemic effect of left ventricular outflow in determining glomerular protein loss. Gender differences in 'normal' patterns of blood pressure also need consideration. Under the age of 45 years, the 90th centile of diastolic pressure for women is 4–5 mmHg less than in men. This could suggest that if early increases in blood pressure above reference ranges are associated with microalbuminuria, for any given modest increase of blood pressure in IDDM, women may be more susceptible to albuminuria than men.

One additional point in assessing the impact of early rises in blood pressure is to look at ethnic variations in age- and gender-based normative ranges. Below the age of 35 years, there appears to be no difference between Europid and African Americans, in either men or women. Thereafter, a significant difference emerges, with 7–12 mmHg higher 90th centile cut-offs in Black compared with White men, and 6–22 mmHg higher 90th centile cut-offs in Black compared with White women[34]. The implications of this are either that a higher threshold for attributable risk could operate in Blacks (and possibly other ethnic groups), in comparison with Europids, or alternatively that the

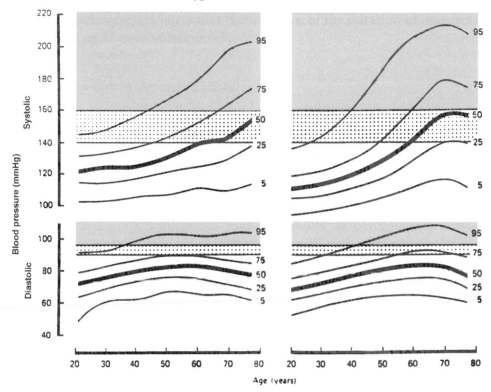

Fig. 6.1. Age and gender centile charts for systolic (upper panels) and diastolic (lower panels) blood pressure in men (left) and women (right). Borderline hypertension by WHO criteria is depicted by large dotted area and definite hypertension by small dotted area. Data derived from reference 34 and reproduced from reference 33 with permission (copyright John Wiley & Sons Limited).

approach of using centile cut-offs to define normality may require downward revision in these populations, in recognition of the fact that they are more susceptible to both hypertension and its sequelae. Although the impact of ethnic variation on glomerular protein loss to a given systemic blood pressure in IDDM is not totally clear, it is known that the incidence of end stage diabetic renal disease is greater amongst African Americans than Europids[35]. The approach of lowering the centile for abnormality in non-Europids, to equate to the absolute value of the 90th centile for diastolic blood pressure in Europids, may therefore prove to be appropriate.

An area of active debate is whether increases in blood pressure precede microalbuminuria or vice versa. This has focused on the possibility that early diabetic nephropathy evolves in those with a genetic predisposition to essential hypertension, characterised by increased erthyrocyte SLC activity, and accelerated by the impact of hyperglycaemia, smoking, and possibly glomer-ular hyperfiltration[36]. Under these circumstances early changes in blood pressure and mild sustained intraglomerular hypertension would be the driving force behind the microalbuminuria. Protagonists of this hypothesis have documented that the 8–15 % incidence of microalbuminuria (> 20 or > 30 µg/min in overnight timed collections) over four years in IDDM patients with mean age 33 years is preceded by a relative increase in resting day-time systolic and diastolic blood pressure (138/82 versus 124/73 mmHg)[37]. The suggestion that raised SLC activity was a genetic marker for familial essential hypertension and subsequent renal dysfunction[38-42] has not, however, been supported by several projects which have taken care to avoid the study of patients with confounding variables such as dyslipidaemia and persistent albuminuria[43-45]. We have documented that raised SLC activity is not associated with altered tubular reabsorptive activity or total exchangeable sodium in IDDM uncomplicated by overt nephropathy[46].

The contrary view of the relationship between blood pressure and the evolution of albuminuria has been expounded by Mathiesen and collea-gues[47,48]. During a prospective follow-up study of > 5 years' duration, the 15 of 205 subjects with initial and follow up albumin excretion rates respec-tively < 21 and > 21 µg/min, had comparable rested seated blood pressure at baseline, in comparison to the majority of 190 whose albumin excretion rate remained < 21 µg/min (122/80 versus 126/79 mmHg, respectively). At follow-up, both systolic and diastolic blood pressure were greater amongst those who developed microalbuminuria. It was concluded that established early nephropathy initiated hypertension.

The dilemma may be resolved in part by acknowledging that overnight albumin excretion rates > 15 µg/min are also in fact elevated; thus, there would be some with early nephropathy in the original cohort, and in the bulk whose AER remained < 21 µg/min. A more attractive and likely expla-nation rests with information from 24-h ambulatory monitoring, which effec-tively demonstrates that resting day-time blood pressure does not always reflect overnight blood pressure control. This is particularly pertinent in microalbuminuric IDDM patients, since even in the absence of relative or absolute hypertension as defined by WHO, the normal attenuation of blood pressure whilst supine at night is not seen[49,50] (Fig. 6.2). Furthermore this is associated with increased resting nocturnal heart rates[49], in keeping with the suggestion that autonomic dysfunction may be implicated in the phenom-enon[51-53]. One of us has suggested a complementary finding in an earlier report, namely that nocturnal increases in albumin excretion rates were more apparent amongst those with early diabetic autonomic dysfunction[54].

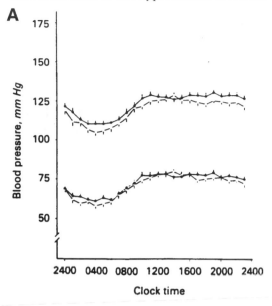

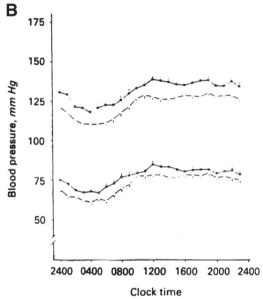

Fig. 6.2. A 24-h profile of mean systolic and diastolic blood pressure for: (A) normoalbuminuric IDDM patients (solid circles) and non-diabetic control subjects (open circles); (B) microalbuminuric IDDM patients (solid circles) and non-diabetic control subjects (open circles). Reproduced from reference 55 with permission.

Some reports have documented altered nocturnal blood pressure patterns which are reflected in random blood pressure measures in microalbuminuria[50], whereas the majority did not discern the altered pattern by reference to day-time measures[49,55,56]. The phenomenon does appear to be age related, in that the physiological nocturnal blood pressure fall is preserved in children < 14 years old with IDDM, and only nocturnal systolic pressure is elevated in microalbuminuric IDDM adolescents aged 15–20 years, whereas both nocturnal systolic and diastolic blood pressure are elevated in microalbuminuric IDDM subjects aged 21–37 years[56]. The interesting and reasonably consistent difference between day-time and nocturnal BP associations with microalbuminuria is that both nocturnal systolic and diastolic blood pressure are increased in, and correlate closely with, the degree of albuminuria. The observation that nocturnal blood pressure is increased in 50 % of cases with normal day-time blood pressure and albumin excretion rates < 15 µg/min lends support to the suggestion that blood pressure is literally the driving force behind early microalbuminuria[50]. Nocturnal increases in blood pressure were not related to day-time glomerular filtration rates in this study. However altered nocturnal control of autonomic tone, blood pressure and renal blood flow could be determining intraglomerular hypertension, thereby leading to increased microalbuminuria.

The marked day-time variability in albuminuria and blood pressure[57] suggests that future prospective studies of the pathogenesis of microalbuminuria and hypertension in IDDM should focus on the supine nocturnal control of systemic and renal haemodynamics.

The potential impact of insulin insensitivity (*vide infra*) on the relationship between microalbuminuria and hypertension requires consideration, in the light of its recent documentation in a cross-sectional study of microalbuminuric IDDM patients[58]. Whether this is an epiphenomenon or the prime factor in the development of hypertension, nephropathy, an atherogenic lipoprotein profile, and later cardiovascular disease, can only be answered by longitudinal studies.

Microalbuminuria and hypertension in NIDDM

In contrast to IDDM, the relationship between blood pressure and albuminuria in NIDDM is less direct. The reasons for this are varied. Hypertension and NIDDM may share a common aetiological factor, explaining why hypertension is a feature in at least 50 % of patients with NIDDM, and why over 40 % of obese treated hypertensive non-diabetic women develop NIDDM over the ensuing 12 years[59]. However the frequent difficulty in timing the exact onset of NIDDM means that information on the early natural history of albuminuria and its relation to hypertension in NIDDM is imprecise. Various other factors implicated in albuminuria may be more apparent in NIDDM than IDDM – namely established cardiovascular disease and co-existent non-diabetic renal disease.

Thus hypertension (WHO criteria) may still be a feature in 48 % of normoalbuminuric Europid NIDDM patients, and in 68 % with microalbuminuria (24-h excretion rates 21–208 µg/min)[60]. The corollary is that microalbuminuria (overnight > 10 µg/min) was present in less than 70 % of Europids with NIDDM with systolic blood pressure $\geq$220 mmHg[32].

There is possibly a further interaction with gender, in that microalbuminuria (overnight > 20 µg/min) accompanies hypertension less frequently in women than in men, such that the prevalence of hypertension (WHO criteria) amongst microalbuminuric men with NIDDM appears to be twice that of women[61,62].

Patrick and colleagues[63] have shown that microalbuminuria (early morning albumin:creatinine ratio > 2.5 mg/mmol) is present at diagnosis of NIDDM in up to 24 % of patients with treated hypertension, with the prevalence unchanged one year after diagnosis, raising the question as to the nature of the relationship between blood pressure and albuminuria. This substantiated the earliest observation of microalbuminuria in newly diagnosed NIDDM associated with hypertension[64]. There are at least three longitudinal studies (in non-Europids) which demonstrate that early relative hypertension precedes microalbuminuria in NIDDM by a period of three to five years[65–67], and increases in blood pressure accompanied the development of microalbuminuria over a three-year period in a study of Europids with NIDDM[68].

The relative importance of systolic and diastolic blood pressure in microalbuminuric NIDDM patients contrasts with the situation in IDDM. The majority of studies supporting a role for hypertension in microalbuminuric NIDDM patients has demonstrated that the association is strongest for systolic blood pressure[32,60,63,68–70]. This may be partly because of the greater incidence of isolated systolic hypertension due to arteriosclerosis in NIDDM.

There are reports, however, which have found either diastolic blood pressure to be more important[71], or have not found any difference in hypertension prevalence between NIDDM patients with or without microalbuminuria[63,72,73]. Likewise, 24-h albumin excretion rates were no different in at least one study in NIDDM comparing those with and without hypertension[74]. This emphasises the multifaceted pathogenesis of microalbuminuria, particularly in NIDDM. There is clear evidence, however, that the relationship between blood pressure and albuminuria is graded and is particularly evident at higher levels of blood pressure and clinical proteinuria[61,62,70].

As in IDDM, ambulatory blood pressure monitoring has been employed to evaluate the relationship with albuminuria, and 24 hour mean systolic pressures correlated best with albuminuria[72]. There is also evidence of reversed circadian rhythmn, that is attenuation of the normal nocturnal reduction in mean blood pressure, in ostensibly normotensive NIDDM subjects which was closely correlated with albuminuria[75].

The relationship between evolving hypertension and albuminuria might suggest that at least a component of the association could be predetermined, as has been suggested in essential hypertension and in IDDM. Raised SLC activity has been noted in cross-sectional studies in proteinuric NIDDM patients[76], and a similar phenomenon has been noted in a small study of microalbuminuric NIDDM patients. Insulin resistance is another associated feature of NIDDM which may be confined to those with both microalbuminuria and hypertension, and which itself may have played a part in the development of these complications[77,78]. However, the criticism of similar findings in IDDM could also be proposed in NIDDM, namely the presence of co-existent confounding variables such as dyslipidaemia, which could affect SLC and insulin sensitivity. In addition, there is uncertainty whether abnormal SLC activity predates the evolution of hypertension and albuminuria, although one report demonstrated that they may be preceded by insulin resistance[78]. In this study normoalbuminuric normotensive NIDDM subjects with impaired insulin-induced glucose uptake by extrahepatic tissue more frequently developed both microalbuminuria and hypertension during a six-year follow-up, in comparison with those with normal insulin sensitivity.

Many studies have been carried out in non-Europid ethnic groups, which demonstrate broadly similar associations to all those just described. There is the possibility, however, that hypertension may exert a greater influence on the presence and evolution of microalbuminuria in certain ethnic groups. In the Japanese, pre-existing hypertension was reported in 72.7 % of those who developed microalbuminuria (> 15 μg/min over 24 h) over the ensuing five years, in comparison with 17.4 % with persistent normoalbuminuria. More specific was the observation that the annual incidence of microalbuminuria was three times that previously reported in Europids[65].

Hypertensive British Asian Indians with NIDDM also appear more prone to microalbuminuria than their Europid counterparts. Allawi and colleagues[79] showed that the prevalence of microalbuminuria (early morning albumin:creatinine ratio > 2 mg/mmol) was more than doubled in those with hypertension (44 %), in comparison with those without (16%). Furthermore the comparable prevalence was also double that of hypertensive Europids (22 %). An increased incidence of hypertension amongst non-diabetic Asian Indians and the Japanese is well recognised, which could have a bearing on the disparity. Alternatively, the impact of hypertension on intraglomerular haemodynamics and glomerular permeability may differ.

Pre-existing hypertension (WHO criteria) has also been associated with a higher prevalence of microalbuminuria (overnight > 8.6 µg/min) in Chinese NIDDM subjects, in comparison with those without hypertension (40.0 % compared with 22.6 %, respectively)[67]. Progression from normo- to micro-albuminuria was also evident amongst those with hypertension[67]. Cheung and coworkers[80] recorded no difference in hypertension amongst Hong Kong Chinese with or without microalbuminuria (untimed random albu-min:creatinine ratio > 2.5 mg/mmol), although differences were evident amongst those with clinical nephropathy (albumin:creatinine ratio > 26.8 mg/mmol).

The hypothesis of an ethnic predisposition to albuminuria in hypertensive NIDDM patients might also appear to be contradicted by Lunt and colleagues[81], who observed that the correlation between hypertension and increased urinary albumin excretion was in fact stronger in Europids than Polynesians. Scrutiny of the data reveals that patient selection could explain the discrepancy, since more than 50 % of the Europids were hypertensive, in contrast to less than 30 % of the Polynesians. However if Polynesians actually have a higher prevalence of microalbuminuria but less hypertension than Europids, as may be inferred from other reports[10], then the observation by Lunt and coworkers[81] would be sound and would suggest that blood pressure is less important than other factors in determining microalbuminuria in Pacific Islanders.

Nigerian Africans with NIDDM are another population with a high prevalence of microalbuminuria bearing little relationship to hypertension[82], and Mexican Americans with microalbuminuria (> 30 mg/l) have on average higher systolic and diastolic blood pressures than normoalbuminuric subjects, although again surprisingly no greater prevalence of hypertension[25].

The inconsistencies reflect partly the evidently different classifications of microalbuminuria, as well as true phenomenology, and the possibility that non-diabetic renal disease such as pyelonephritis, glomerulonephritis, or renovascular hypertension, could play a more important role than diabetes in hypertension and albuminuria in non-Europids. More longitudinal studies with definitive information on renal structure and function could help resolve these issues.

Microalbuminuria, hyperlipidaemia and dyslipoproteinaemia

The concept that microalbuminuria could be associated with alterations in lipoprotein metabolism derives from observations of hyperlipidaemia in the nephrotic syndrome and chronic renal failure[83–85], and increasing knowledge that the kidney itself plays an important role in lipoprotein handling. The impact of minor disturbances of renal function is likely to be much more subtle, but it is also necessary to consider other factors in the context of microalbuminuria, which could modify lipoproteins. The association between albuminuria and dyslipidaemia could be the result of a common unrelated factor, for example endothelial lipolytic function, or the consequence of the effects of concomitant antihypertensive therapy on lipid metabolism. The alternative sequence of events – dyslipidaemia as a mediator of microalbuminuria – does not appear to be a likely scenario[86].

At present there are remarkably few reports of lipoproteins in microalbuminuric non-diabetic subjects, but the alterations appear to be less evident than those reported in diabetes. In discussion of the impact of microalbuminuria on lipoprotein metabolism, one has to consider the population base, in recognition of the underlying variable patterns of lipid distribution in the healthy population, and the underlying prevalence of other factors of pathophysiological significance, such as obesity and hypertension.

Our own study[87] predominantly concentrated on Europids, where the prevalence of hypercholesterolaemia (fasting > 6.5 mmol/l) was 32 %. This is broadly comparable to other population-based studies in the United Kingdom. Of the other factors likely to have made an impact on the association with microalbuminuria, 10 % were obese (body mass index > 30 kg/m^2) but the prevalence of hypertension (according to WHO criteria) was only 10.3 %. In this group, microalbuminuria (> 20 mg/l and albumin:creatinine ratio > 3.5 mg/mmol) was associated with significant increases and reductions respectively in the low density lipoprotein (LDL) cholesterol:apoB and the high density lipoprotein (HDL) cholesterol:apoA1 ratios, and a marginal reduction in HDL cholesterol. A further univariate correlation was observed between albumin:creatinine ratios and both total and LDL cholesterol. Specific isolation and full characterization of lipoprotein composition was not carried out in this study, so that the suggestion of altered lipoprotein composition can only be inferred from cholesterol:protein ratios. However similarities can be noted with other studies.

The much larger study of Metcalf and colleagues[3,88] also focused on a mainly Europid (10 % Polynesian and Asian) population with a low prevalence of hypertension (4 %), but a higher prevalence of obesity (20 %). The prevalence of hypercholesterolaemia was not stated and those whose fasting serum triglycerides were > 2.5 mmol/l were excluded. Both urinary albumin concentration and albumin:creatinine ratio were correlated directly to serum cholesterol and triglycerides and inversely to HDL cholesterol. Multivariate analysis determined that the association with triglycerides was stronger although it was inferred that combined hyperlipidaemia (albeit mild) was an accompaniment of microalbuminuria. The association with HDL cholesterol in part reflected the close correlation between HDL and triglycerides, and importantly was lost after correction for body mass index. Nosadini and coworkers[14] provide support for the suggestion that dyslipoproteinaemia accompanies albuminuria in hypertension by the observation of reduced HDL in essential hypertension complicated by microalbuminuria, with increased serum triglycerides confined to those with increased erythrocyte SLC activity.

Studies in Nauruans and Mexican Americans have also demonstrated mean differences of 0.2–0.3 mmol/l in fasting triglycerides between those with and without microalbuminuria, with less significant differences in HDL cholesterol. Between 50 and 60 % of these populations had obesity, and hypertension (WHO criteria) was present in 26.2 % of Mexican Americans and 7 % of Nauruans[10,25]. In Hong Kong Chinese subjects, serum triglyceride concentrations and waist:hip ratios were significantly increased amongst those women with albumin:creatinine ratios > 90th centile (2.1 mg/mmol), but these appeared less important than fasting serum insulin, which was an independent predictor of albumin:creatinine ratios, and HDL cholesterol was not related to microalbuminuria[12]. Thus, even in populations with a low prevalence of hyperlipidaemia such as the Chinese, central adiposity, insulin insensitivity and blood pressure are clearer correlates of microalbuminuria than dyslipoproteinaemia.

The broad consensus would be that in the absence of diabetes, at the most, modest differences in lipids are present in association with microalbuminuria. The fact that these may be more evident in obese populations might suggest that the dyslipidaemia may in fact reflect the underlying insulin insensitivity, which is well recognised to be associated with hypertriglyceridaemia. The close (patho)physiological correlation with HDL limits attempts by simple multivariate analysis to distinguish the contribution of triglycerides and HDL. Insulin insensitivity is a plausible explanation for these observations, as a common finding in both obesity and essential hypertension, with the potential through disinhibition to facilitate hepatic secretion of triglyceride-rich lipoproteins.

Other mechanisms may explain the findings. In particular, urinary loss of HDL apolipoprotein constituents and lipolytic enzymes could in theory accompany microalbuminuria. These abnormalities have been demonstrated in overt (often nephrotic range) proteinuria. If microalbuminuria was a surrogate for endothelial damage, one such effect could be reduced lipase activity. These considerations are more likely to explain changes in triglycerides and HDL; increases in LDL cholesterol, or suggestions of a change in its composition, are less easily explained. In particular, the molecular size of the major protein component of LDL (apoB) is much greater than that of apoA in HDL, and it would not be excreted in the urine alongside albumin. It is possible however, that the suggested altered LDL composition could reflect altered catabolism of triglyceride-rich lipoproteins, with a contribution to LDL from intermediate density lipoprotein (IDL). IDL is more triglyceride-rich than LDL, and is effectively incorporated in 'LDL' estimated by the Friedewald formula. This formula is a convenient method for estimating LDL, without the need for time-consuming preparative ultracentrifugation, where:

$$\text{LDL cholesterol} = \text{total serum cholesterol} - \text{HDL cholesterol} - (\text{total serum triglycerides} / 2.2) \text{ mmol/l}$$

The formula is based on the assumption that the ratio of triglyceride to cholesterol within very low density lipoprotein (VLDL) is 2.2 , and is unsuitable for lipaemic samples where total triglycerides are > 4.5 mmol/l. It is not clear currently whether the formula is perhaps also less secure in the presence of microalbuminuria. Thus our own suggestions of altered LDL composition in microalbuminuric non-diabetic subjects[87] should be confirmed in other studies where LDL is fully isolated and characterised.

Other methodological aspects require consideration. Discrepant alterations in high density lipoprotein need to take account of two factors. The first is the means by which HDL is isolated. This may be by precipitation methods which rely on the chemical properties of HDL, using either heparin–manganese or sodium phosphotungstate in the presence of magnesium chloride to remove VLDL and LDL, or by ultracentrifugation, which relies on the physical properties of HDL. HDL is often indirectly determined by ultracentrifugation, in that the lower density VLDL and LDL molecules are spun up and HDL is derived by subtraction of the cholesterol content of VLDL and LDL from total cholesterol. More sophisticated discontinuous gradient or single vertical spin ultracentrifuges can isolate HDL directly but these are not employed in many laboratories. The physical and chemical characteristics of

HDL are by no means analogous, thus it is perhaps not surprising that studies isolating HDL by different methods do not always produce comparable results. For example, it is known that the hydrated density of lipoprotein (a) (Lp(a)) is similar to HDL such that it is measured in ultracentrifuged 'HDL', whereas Lp(a) is precipitated out by sodium phosphotungstate and magnesium chloride alongside VLDL and LDL, and thus would not be incorporated in the 'HDL' isolated by this latter method.

The other point of importance is the gender-specific difference in patterns of HDL isolated by whatever means. HDL cholesterol is generally higher in women, thus reductions associated with microalbuminuria might be more apparent in those studies where women predominated, or there was lack of matching for gender between the normoalbuminuric and microalbuminuric groups.

Dyslipoproteinaemia and microalbuminuria in IDDM

In discussion of the impact of microalbuminuria in IDDM, consideration needs to be given to the complexities of lipoprotein metabolism in diabetes. As in the non-diabetic population, age, gender, body mass index and body fat distribution, tobacco and alcohol intake, and patterns of diet and exercise all exert an influence on lipoprotein concentrations in IDDM. An ostensibly more atherogenic profile with increased total and LDL cholesterol and total serum triglycerides, and reduced HDL cholesterol, accompanies ageing (except in women where HDL increases), and is more apparent in men than in women[89], and in smokers, obese individuals (body mass index $> 30 \text{ kg/m}^2$, particularly where fat is centrally distributed), sedentary individuals, and those whose diet is rich in saturated fat, calories and refined carbohydrate. Moderate to excessive alcohol consumption can produce apparently paradoxical increases in both triglycerides and HDL cholesterol, although in practice the rise in HDL cholesterol is usually attenuated. Consideration needs also to be given to the adverse effects of co-existent drug ingestion on lipoprotein metabolism, particularly with high doses of thiazide diuretics, non-cardioselective beta-blockers and corticosteroids.

More specific to IDDM is the influence of variable blood glucose control, non-enzymatic glycation and genetic polymorphism of lipoproteins[90,91], and insulin insensitivity on lipoprotein metabolism[92–94], all of which may further accentuate the atherogenic dyslipidaemic profile, although it has been suggested that the impact of hyperglycaemia may be less apparent amongst black women[95]. The impact of microalbuminuria must take account of the independent influence of these other factors on lipoprotein metabolism, and usually itself only exerts a modest impact by comparison. Insulin insensitivity assessed during a euglycaemic hyperinsulinaemic clamp has recently been independently related to both microalbuminuria and dyslipidaemia in IDDM[58].

Although quantitative lipid abnormalities are widely recognised to have prognostic importance in IDDM, there is increasing recognition of more subtle qualitative alterations in lipoprotein composition[96], which may be atherogenic in their own right, at least in normoglycaemic individuals[97]. Currently, relatively little is known about the impact of microalbuminuria on these features.

The definition of hypercholesterolaemia in IDDM is arbitrarily defined as ≥ 6.5 mmol/l, based on an associated significantly increased attributable cardiovascular risk in non-diabetic populations, and the understanding that this is at least doubled in IDDM. The prevalence of hypercholesterolaemia in IDDM has been reported to vary between 10 %[98] and 25 %[99], in part reflecting the different ages and other clinical characteristics of the study groups. It is approximately equivalent to that of an age- and gender-matched non-diabetic population. What seems clear however is that the prevalence varies according to the degree of albuminuria, increased by 5 % in those with microalbuminuria, and by 15 % in those with clinical proteinuria[98]. Multivariate analyses suggest that hypercholesterolaemia is independently predicted by, in order of importance, age, body mass index, glycated haemoglobin and albuminuria, with albuminuria assuming greater significance when the prevalence of clinical nephropathy was higher[98,99]. The influence of non-albuminuric factors and methodology of lipoprotein isolation has a bearing on the strength of the observations from the case-control studies which will be discussed.

With regard to hypertriglyceridaemia, this is best judged on fasting concentrations outside the 95th centile, estimated to be > 2.0 mmol/l[100]. The independent prognostic value of serum triglycerides in non-diabetic subjects is still viewed as contentious by some[101], despite observations to the contrary[102]. This in part reflects limitations of standard statistical methods, and ignorance of the fact that triglyceride and HDL cholesterol metabolism are intimately linked and that separate statistical analysis is inappropriate because of the much reduced biological variability of HDL cholesterol in comparison with triglycerides. In IDDM the independent prognostic value of serum triglycerides for cardiovascular disease appears more clear-cut. In contrast to serum cholesterol, the prevalence of fasting hypertriglyceridaemia appears to be greater in IDDM in comparison with the general population, and may be at least 30 %[99]. In this study, the independent influence of albuminuria was less apparent than was the case for cholesterol, and the key predictors (in order of importance) were the daily insulin requirement (a surrogate for insulin sensitivity), age, glycated haemoglobin and body mass index.

Estimates of HDL cholesterol in uncomplicated IDDM patients usually demonstrate concentrations higher than in non-diabetic age- and gender-matched control subjects[103].

At least ten cross-sectional case-control studies have examined the influence of microalbuminuria on lipids and lipoprotein concentrations in IDDM (Tables 6.1 and 6.2). The broad consensus which emerges is that quantitative differences in serum lipids are fairly subtle, and intermediate between those observed in normoalbuminuric and macroalbuminuric IDDM groups, with clear differences most evident amongst those with clinical nephropathy. Total and LDL cholesterol concentrations were comparable in virtually every study, with the exception of two[104,105]. The findings of Jay and colleagues[105] may be explained by the poorer blood glucose control in the microalbuminuric group accounting for increases in cholesterol. The absolute difference recorded by Jones and coworkers[104] was of the order of 0.5 mmol/l, a difference noted to be non-significant in other studies[106–108] raising the possibility that the difference arose by chance as the result of a small sample size and a type 2 statistical error. No doubt a meta-analysis would demonstrate that the difference did attain significance, but the clinical importance would remain uncertain.

The other point to bear in mind is that, in virtually all studies, LDL cholesterol was assessed by the Friedewald formula, thereby incorporating IDL and chylomicron remnants in its estimation. When LDL was definitively isolated by discontinuous gradient ultracentrifugation[87] and normoalbuminuric and microalbuminuric subjects were matched for total lipid concentrations, blood glucose control and other confounding factors, LDL concentration and composition were no different, although the (free) cholesterol concentration of the larger IDL_1 particle (flotation density 20–60 Svedberg units (Sf)) was increased. Thus the surface lipoproteins of molecules which are smaller and denser than the major LDL fraction (1.021–1.034 g/ml) may in fact account for the discrepant findings of Jones and coworkers[104].

A more recent report specifically examined LDL subclasses in normoalbuminuric, microalbuminuric and macroalbuminuric IDDM patients, and also found no major changes in density distribution or composition according to urinary albumin excretion, although differences emerged in comparison with non-diabetic subjects for all groups, most notably increased triglyceride

Table 6.1 *HDL cholesterol and fasting total serum triglycerides in published reports of microalbuminuric, compared with normoalbuminuric, IDDM patients*

Study	HDL cholesterol		Serum triglycerides	
	Normo	Micro	Normo	Micro
Vannini[117]	1.51[a]	1.46[e]	0.95[a]	0.99
Watts[107]	1.41[c]	1.11[f]	1.41[a]	1.52
Jensen[106]	1.42[a]	1.48[g]	0.98[a]	0.95
Jones[104]	1.24[b]	1.07[h]	0.68[d]	1.11
Dullart[114]	1.27[a]	1.15[e]	0.75[b]	0.92
Winocour[87]	1.38[b]	1.27[g]	1.57[a]	2.20
Jenkins[119]	1.40[a]	1.40[i]	nm	nm
Kapelrud[108]	1.18[a]	1.20[i]	0.88[b]	1.15
Winocour[116]	1.43[a]	1.40[g]	1.70[a]	1.60
	1.41[b]	1.32[e]		
Jay[105]	1.41[b]	1.71[f]	1.00[a]	1.14
Kahri[111]	1.64[c]	1.45[g]	0.83[b]	1.03

Normo: normoalbuminuria. Micro: microalbuminuria; nm: not measured.
Concentrations expressed in mmol/l.
[a] p ns, [b] $p < 0.05$, [c] $p < 0.01$, [d] $p < 0.001$, compared with microalbuminuric subjects. HDL isolated by [e] precipitation with sodium phosphotungstate and magnesium chloride, [f] precipitation with heparin and manganese chloride, [g] ultracentrifugation, by [h] precipitation with dextran and magnesium chloride, or [i] methodology not stated.

Table 6.2 *Lipoprotein Lp(a) concentrations in normoalbuminuric and microalbuminuric IDDM patients*

Study	APO (a) (U/I)		Methodology
	Normo	Micro	
Jenkins[119a]	86[e]	245	IRMA
Kapelrud[108b]	49[e]	100	ImmElec
Winocour[116b]	90[d]	137	IRMA
Jay[105b]	72[c]	105	ELISA

Normo: normoalbuminuria; Micro: microalbuminuria.
Figures are [a] geometric mean, or [b] median.
[c] p ns, [d] $p < 0.05$, [e] $p < 0.01$ compared with microalbuminuric patients.
Methodology: IRMA: immunoradiometric assay (Pharmacia).
            ImmElec: in house electrophoresis.
            ELISA: Enzyme-linked Immunosorbent assay (Immuno).

content of LDL[109]. In this study concentrations of isolated 'light' LDL (density 1.021–1.034 g/ml) were increased in microalbuminuric and macroalbuminuric compared with normoalbuminuric IDDM patients, and the increased concentrations of both cholesterol and apoB in this fraction confirmed an increased number of these particles. This contrasts with our earlier report[87], but the major difference was that we specifically matched patients for total lipid concentrations, whereas total cholesterol concentrations were clearly different in the study of Lahdenpera and colleagues[109]. As total cholesterol concentrations are usually comparable in microalbuminuric and normoalbuminuric IDDM subjects, the findings from the sample of the later study are not necessarily representative.

In a study comparing normoalbuminuric, microalbuminuric and proteinuric IDDM patients with non-diabetic control subjects matched for age and body weight, increased mass concentrations of IDL were found in the microalbuminuric and proteinuric as compared with the normoalbuminuric patients[110]. Triglyceride, free cholesterol, cholesterol ester and phospholipid concentrations in VLDL, IDL and LDL were also higher in the microalbuminuric and proteinuric groups, as were total cholesterol, total triglyceride and apo B concentrations. Heparin-stimulated lipoprotein lipase activity was similar in the three diabetic groups, whereas hepatic lipase activities were higher in the microalbuminuric and proteinuric groups. The interesting finding in this study was how marginal the differences were between non-diabetic and albuminuric IDDM subjects. The most important observation is that the superficially anti-atherogenic lipoprotein composition in normoalbuminuric IDDM patients was modified by the development of albuminuria, perhaps due to peripheral hyperinsulinaemia and the influence of hepatic lipase.

With regard to the effect of microalbuminuria on serum total triglycerides, slight increases are noted in some studies, but not in others, reflecting the skewed normal distribution of triglycerides and the need for non-parametric statistical analyses, as well as possible 'swamping' of the influence of microalbuminuria by poor blood glucose control. Jensen and colleagues[106] demonstrated a similar phenomenon for HDL cholesterol, where poor blood glucose control was a stronger factor than microalbuminuria in accounting for reduced HDL cholesterol.

Several studies have demonstrated, however, that HDL cholesterol is reduced in microalbuminuric IDDM patients[87,104,107,111], and it has been suggested that it is the potentially more cardioprotective HDL_2 cholesterol subfraction which is specifically reduced[87,111].

High density lipoprotein has also been subfractionated according to varying apolipoprotein content, LpA-I particles containing only apoA-I, and

LpA-I:A-II particles containing both apoA-I and apoA-II. The concentrations of these two particles were not altered by microalbuminuria, although HDL cholesterol:apoA-I + apoA-II ratios were significantly reduced in comparison to normoalbuminuric IDDM patients[111,112].

One purported mechanism to explain these quantitative and qualitative alterations is that HDL catabolism and urinary loss may be accelerated, leading to loss of the smaller HDL_3 cholesterol subfraction before it could be converted to HDL_2, thereby leading to a relative reduction of HDL_2 cholesterol[87]. Kahri and colleagues[111] have examined other possible factors which might explain the changes in HDL. Cholesteryl ester transfer protein (CETP) activity was not altered in microalbuminuria, and thus appears not to be implicated in the alterations in HDL, although the ratio of lipoprotein lipase:hepatic lipase was reduced, and correlated with HDL components. Urinary loss of HDL constituents, and enzymes involved in the lipolytic cascade have been implicated previously[113], as has the suggestion that endothelial control of lipopotein metabolism may be compromised. Urinary HDL cholesterol loss is only evident, however, at the stage of clinical proteinuria[113]. In addition, enhanced movement of cholesterol from HDL to triglyceride-rich lipoproteins may take place as a result of the increased activity of lecithin:cholesterol acyl transferase reported in diabetic nephropathy[114], but alterations in CETP activity are not apparent at the stage of microalbuminuria.

The method of isolation of HDL cholesterol could also be important, with the clearest reduction apparent when HDL is precipitated out by sodium phosphotungstate in the presence of magnesium chloride, or by heparin and manganese chloride. A rather surprising and unexplained increase in HDL and HDL_2 cholesterol isolated by the latter method has been reported in one study of microalbuminuric IDDM patients[105]. It is recognised that HDL cholesterol concentrations isolated by ultracentifugation in IDDM are higher than when isolated by precipitation[115], and this may be because Lp(a) cholesterol (*vide infra*) is incorporated in this particular 'HDL cholesterol' measurement.

This is supported by a significant correlation between Lp(a) and HDL only appparent in IDDM when HDL was isolated by ultracentrifugation[116].

Other components of the apolipoproteins have been studied in microalbuminuria. Increased serum concentrations of apoB, the major protein component of LDL, have been recorded[104,114,117], but are not apparent in other studies[87,107,109], again perhaps because of inappropriate matching for serum lipids, and because poorer blood glucose control in these latter studies could have obscured the effect of microalbuminuria. The study of Lahdenpera and coworkers[109] suggests that apoB concentrations may only be increased in the lighter density LDL fraction. As alluded to earlier, reductions in apoA (the major protein of HDL) concentrations have not been recorded.

The phospholipid and total protein concentrations, and composition of VLDL, IDL and LDL isolated by ultracentrifugation, are not intrinsically altered as a result of microalbuminuria[87,109]. A preliminary report has raised the possibilty that polymorphism in the apoE phenotype may be important in modifying the lipoprotein response to microalbuminuria, with possession of the ε2 allele reflected by less change in LDL and HDL cholesterol, and in apoB[118].

Quite apart from the possibility that Lp(a) may be measured in ultracentrifuged HDL, interest has focused on the possibility that, as in more advanced (diabetic and non-diabetic) nephropathy, Lp(a) concentrations could be increased in microalbuminuric IDDM patients[108,116,119]. Although there is presently no laboratory standardisation for the measurement of this molecule, it has been suggested to be an independent predictor of coronary heart disease in the non-diabetic population[120].

Lp(a) is composed of lipid and the apolipoproteins (a) and B, and apo(a) has structural (and possibly functional) homology with plasminogen, from which it appears to have arisen as a genetic mutant. The physiological role of Lp(a) is unknown, but it is an acute phase reactant and may interfere *in vitro* with plasminogen activation and thus fibrinolysis. Concentrations are predominantly genetically determined, in the main the consequence of expression of several different isoforms. Post-translational modification of apo(a) leading to altered concentrations is recognised increasingly, although the impact of poor blood glucose control and insulin insensitivity on increasing Lp(a) concentrations remains controversial[119,121,122]. Regardless of such possibilities, it is clearly recognised that the distribution of Lp(a) is markedly skewed, to the extent that unlike any other circulating biological constituent, physiological concentrations can vary from 0 to greater than 3000 mU/l.

The implication of this is that in order to examine critically the importance of post-translation modification on Lp(a) concentrations, for example, in microalbuminuric IDDM patients, Lp(a) quantitation with phenotyping in a large sample size of at least 200 would be required. As yet this has not been done, which may in part explain why despite evidence of greater Lp(a) concentrations in microalbuminuric IDDM patients in several studies[105,108,116,119] (Table 6.2), the difference did not always achieve significance[105]. A meta analysis in this instance would almost certainly confirm the impression of increased concentrations, but the possible mechanism remains speculative. Lp(a) may be a permissive factor in the progression of early diabetic nephropathy, or may rise as a consequence of reduced renal elimination. An alternative explanation to account for the observation that Lp(a) concentrations appeared no higher in macroalbuminuric in comparison with microalbuminuric IDDM patients[116,119] could be that both states reflect chronic endothelial damage, with a consequent increase in plasminogen activator, and compensatory increased endothelial synthesis of all acute phase reactants, in order to inhibit fibrinolysis.

The prognostic significance of the increased Lp(a) concentrations on coronary heart disease in microalbuminuric IDDM patients can only be resolved fully by large prospective studies, but at least two cross-sectional reports have not found Lp(a) to be a major determinant of coronary heart disease in IDDM[121,123].

Dyslipoproteinaemia and microalbuminuria in NIDDM

The impact of microalbuminuria on dyslipoproteinaemia in NIDDM appears to be less marked than in IDDM. This is partly because NIDDM is already characterised by reduced HDL cholesterol and increased serum triglyceride concentrations, fundamentally the consequence (and also possibly a determinant) of insulin insensitivity. It has also been suggested that insulin insensitivity may be intrinsic to microalbuminuria in NIDDM[77], although this has not been supported by the observations of Niskanen and colleagues[74], where fasting hypcrinsulinanemia (a surrogate for insulin insensitivity) was similar in microalbuminuric and normoalbuminuric patients at inception of a cross-sectional study, although interestingly somewhat higher in those with microalbuminuria after five years' observation (31 versus 21 mU/l, *p* ns).

Lipoprotein metabolism is fundamentally different in the two broad classifications of diabetes, particularly with regard to HDL cholesterol concentrations, which, if anything are greater in IDDM than in the general population. One point worthy of discussion is that the mechanism of microalbuminuria and dyslipoproteinaemia may be quite different in NIDDM, and is certainly more likely to be multifactorial.

The one microalbuminuric group with NIDDM where dyslipoproteinaemia might be expected to be most apparent are women with central adiposity, but lipoprotein patterns in this group have not been studied specifically. Consequently, the majority of studies is cross-sectional comparisons of microalbuminuric and normoalbuminuric men and women, with men predominating. Trends toward reduced HDL cholesterol and increased serum triglycerides only reached statistical significance in the minority of studies

(Table 6.3), with more clear-cut differences most evident in macroalbuminuria[70,112,124–126].

One interesting exception to this was in the study of Niskanen and co-workers[74], where differences emerged after a follow-up period of five years, implying that persistent microalbuminuria is associated with factors involved in lipoprotein metabolism which further aggravate pre-existing dyslipoproteinaemia. These changes could not be explained by age, sex, body mass index or estimates of blood glucose control, and altered intravascular and renal catabolism of triglyceride-rich lipoproteins seems the likeliest explanation. This would account for the further observation of modifed lipoprotein composition, with triglyceride saturation of LDL also evident after five years. Such changes are known to predict atherosclerotic disease in NIDDM and the general population[127–129].

Compositional lipoprotein analysis has also suggested increased cholesterol concentrations in remnant-like particles in a small cross-sectional study of Japanese microalbuminuric NIDDM subjects[130], but this was not confirmed in a study from Spain[131], where lipoprotein composition was more fully analysed by sequential ultracentrifugation, and microalbuminuric and normoalbuminuric NIDDM subjects had comparable cholesterol, triglyceride and protein concentrations in VLDL, IDL, LDL and HDL. A more recent Japanese study has reported a high prevalence of smaller, dense LDL particles in microalbuminuric NIDDM patients, with an increase in the post-prandial increment in triglyceride-rich lipoproteins following fat loading[132].

The majority of studies demonstrated not only no effect of microalbuminuria on total and estimated LDL cholesterol, but also a lack of change in concentrations of apoB, apoE, apoA, or the distribution of LpAI and LpAI:AII particles of HDL[68,70,71,74,112,124,126,131,133,134], although Seghieri and colleagues[131] suggested that NIDDM of less than five years' duration was exceptional to this, where increases in LDL cholesterol and apoB, and reductions in the apoA:apoB ratio were the rule. The likeliest explanation for such an observation is that the subgroup in whom dyslipoproteinaemia and microalbuminuria cluster were coincident with the group of shorter duration, the consequence of selection bias.

Previous observations in non-diabetic subjects might have led one to anticipate that microalbuminuria would be more clearly associated with dyslipoproteinaemic NIDDM patients in non-Europid ethnic groups, but this was apparently not the case in Mexican Americans, perhaps again because the underlying insulin insensitivity in this obese NIDDM cohort overshadowed the influence of microalbuminuria on lipoprotein metabolism[133].

Table 6.3 *HDL cholesterol and fasting total serum triglycerides in published reports of microalbuminuric and normoalbuminuric NIDDM patients*

Study	HDL cholesterol		Serum triglycerides	
	Normo	Micro	Normo	Micro
Seghieri[131]				
DDM >5 years	1.30[a]	1.20[d]	1.80[a]	2.00
DDM <5 years	1.30[a]	1.10	1.70[b]	2.10
Allawi[71]	1.22[a]	1.09[d]	1.84[a]	1.98
Niskanen[74]				
Basal	1.07[a]	1.07[e]	2.39[a]	2.45
+5 years	1.07[b]	0.92	2.38[b]	4.24
Tkac[70]	1.04[a]	1.13[f]	3.97[a]	3.15
Mattock[61]				
Males	NS[a]	NS	1.99[b]	2.66
Females	NS[a]	NS	1.85[b]	2.80
Stiegler[68]	1.30[a]	1.10[f]	1.80[a]	2.50
Stehouwer[197]				
Basal	1.20[a]	1.00[d]	2.40[a]	2.20
+5 years	1.20[a]	1.00	2.10[a]	1.90
Haffner[133]	1.04[a]	0.98[f]	1.95[a]	2.21
Jenkins[119]	1.10[a]	1.00[f]	2.00[a]	2.10
Nielsen[124]	1.23[a]	1.12[d]	1.30[a]	1.82
Groop[77]				
NBP	1.37[a]	1.21[f]	1.49[b]	2.17
HBP	1.20[a]	1.00[c]	2.81[a]	3.07[c]
Reverter[125]	1.28[a]	1.05[c]	1.37[a]	1.48
Peynet[112]	1.29[a]	1.36[d]	1.39[a]	1.79

Normo: normoalbuminuria; Micro: microalbuminuria. DDM: known duration of diabetes mellitus. NBP: normotensive; HBP: hypertensive. NS: concentrations not stated but comparable. Concentrations expressed in mmol/l.
[a] p ns, [b] $p < 0.05$, between groups; [c] $p < 0.05$ in comparison with NBP Normo group HDL isolated by [d] precipitation with sodium phosphotungstate and magnesium chloride, [e] precipitation with dextran and magnesium chloride, or [f] methodology not stated.

The role of apolipoprotein (a) in microalbuminuric NIDDM patients has been studied. Increased concentrations were demonstrated in contrast to normoalbuminuric subjects, the levels being comparable to those observed in non-diabetic individuals undergoing coronary artery bypass grafting[126]. These findings were not confirmed in other studies of Europids[124,134], or by Haffner and coworkers[133] in Mexican Americans. Part of the explanation for the discrepancy may be genetic differences between ethnic groups, as well as the relatively small numbers studied, bearing in mind the distribution of

Lp(a). These suggestions may also explain why higher apolipoprotein (a) concentrations amongst those NIDDM subjects with coronary heart disease have only been recorded inconsistently in Europids[126,135–137], as has been noted in prospective studies of non-diabetic subjects[120]. Alternatively, the influence of Lp(a) in coronary heart disease associated with NIDDM may be less important than in the general population, as has been suggested in IDDM[121,123,138].

Microalbuminuria, haemostasis and fibrinolysis

This discussion of the impact of microalbuminuria on thrombotic and antithrombotic factors will be prefaced by a brief outline of the physiology of haemostasis, whereby the fluidity of circulating blood is maintained. This is essentially achieved by the interaction of the endothelium with clotting and fibrinolytic factors, and with platelet function. Homeostasis is maintained in health by balance of all these factors; thus, it may be inappropriate to assess markers of thrombosis without reference to estimates of platelet function and fibrinolysis.

The key to integration of this complex balance is the vascular endothelium, which has both natural pro- and anticoagulant modulating properties. Endothelial function will be referred to briefly as it is covered in more detail elsewhere (Chapter 5), but it appears that endothelial trauma is the initiating factor which thereby leads to platelet adhesion, aggregation and degranulation, followed thereafter by activation of the intrinsic and/or extrinsic coagulation cascade, and the production of thrombin and fibrin clot.

The fibrinolytic system acts to restore normal tissue function and is activated after conversion of plasminogen to plasmin by the action of plasminogen activators, which themselves are physiologically under inhibitory control by tissue plasminogen activator-1 (PAI-1). Antithrombotic factors such as proteins C and S, and antithrombin III conserve the consumption of haemostatic factors, thereby also reducing the tendency to thrombosis. Activity of several of these factors is genetically determined, and also appears to be influenced by hyperglycaemia and acute inflammation.

It will be understood that such a complex system is finely balanced, such that minor alterations may accelerate either thrombosis or haemorrhage. Furthermore, it operates in such a way that geographically discrete endothelial sites may promote changes localised to the microenvironment, but not apparent systemically. A good example would be the retinal microvasculature in diabetes. In practice this means that efforts to assess coagulation by peripheral venous sampling may not reflect localised arterial pathology.

Furthermore there is inherent difficulty in assessing *in vivo* haemostatic function, particularly platelet behaviour. Laboratory *in vitro* tests of platelet function and clotting factors will not always mimic *in vivo* behaviour, and are very susceptible to activation during venepuncture. Finally, there are ongoing methodological difficulties and a lack of standardisation as to how clotting factors such as fibrinogen should best be measured.

It may be in part recognition of these difficulties that scarcely any reports at present have evaluated haemostasis and fibrinolysis in microalbuminuric non-diabetic patients, despite the suggestion of alterations in some studies in diabetes. We estimated fibrinogen concentrations by the Clauss technique and found microalbuminuria was associated with a non-significant increase (mean 0.4 g/l), and both urine albumin concentration and albumin:creatinine ratio correlated (albeit weakly) with fibrinogen ($r_s = 0.25$)[2]. At the time of writing, there were no other reports for comparison.

Microalbuminuria, haemostasis, fibrinolysis and platelet function in diabetes mellitus

Reviews of coagulation and fibrinolysis in diabetes are legion, and on balance there is a clear impression of a prothrombotic tendency. However, quite apart from the methodological difficulties alluded to earlier, the impact of diabetes itself needs to be taken into account, and in this respect is similar to the influence on lipoprotein metabolism of insulin insensitivity, hyperglycaemia and non-enzymatic glycation. The multiplicity of methods whereby platelet, haemostatic, anti-thrombotic and fibrinolytic function are measured means that there is no consensus on how they might be modified by the aforementioned metabolic alterations.

With regard to platelet function, hyperglycaemia appears at best to exert a modest influence on adhesion, aggregation and degranulation, with co-existent vascular disease a more potent indicator of abnormalities[139]. The *in vivo* role of insulin insensitivity and glycation is not clear.

Increased fibrinogen concentrations and clotting and antithrombotic factor activity are more clearly related to hyperglycaemia and insulin insensitivity, although the presence of established vascular disease is a more consistent correlate. Non-enzymatic glycation of anti-thrombin III has been noted to reduce its activity. Hypofibrinolysis and increased plasminogen activator inhibitor-1 (PAI-1) have been recorded in association with poorly controlled and complicated diabetes, and also with insulin insensitivity (in the shape of obesity).

The majority of studies of haemostatic factors in microalbuminuric diabetic patients has focused on IDDM. Fibrinogen has usually been measured by clotting methods, although turbidimetry has also been utilised. Of those studies reported to date, elevated fibrinogen concentrations have been clearly demonstrated in both IDDM and in NIDDM, when a group with overt macroalbuminuria was included[69,106,140,141]. Microalbuminuria was less consistently associated with hyperfibrinogenaemia, with significant differences of 0.3 or 0.7 g/l recorded in IDDM in three reports[104,140,142], and with a significant 0.5 g/l difference in microalbuminuric Japanese NIDDM[143], in contrast to non-significant trends in the other reports in IDDM[106,141,144] and NIDDM[69,141,145,146]. This suggests that larger numbers would be required to demonstrate clearly a significant difference, but also the fact that the absolute order of the difference would be small. It is important to note that blood glucose control was particularly poor in one study[140] (mean HbA_{1c} 9.1 %), and multivariate analysis demonstrated this to be a more potent indicator of fibrinogen than microalbuminuria.

It seems reasonable to conclude that microalbuminuria and hyperglycaemia exert a cumulative impact on plasma fibrinogen. This may reflect underlying endothelial damage (*vide infra*), altered synthetic rates of fibrinogen associated with microalbuminuria, and subsequent delayed catabolism of glycated fibrinogen[147]. The reported increased partial thromboplastin time in microalbuminuric IDDM[140] was attributed to the increased fibrinogen.

Clotting factor concentration and (*in vitro*) activity are not necessarily synonymous, which may in part explain the discrepant findings of increased factor VIIc activity[140,142], without an apparent increase in factor VII concentration in either IDDM[104,141] or NIDDM[71,141,146]. The accentuated activity could have contributed to the reduced prothrombin ratio, and might be explained on the basis of an associated increase in circulating triglyceride-rich IDL and LDL, which are known templates for activation of factor VII. This is supported to some extent by the observation that serum cholesterol and triglycerides are independent predictors of factor VIIc activity[140,142]. By contrast, factor VIIIc appears to be less susceptible to activation[144,146], with increased concentrations only recorded in established nephropathy (> 140 µg/min)[148]. Factor VIII concentration was not significantly different in normoalbuminuric and microalbuminuric NIDDM patients[69,71]. As with fibrinogen and factor VII[141], increased factor VIII is present in those with frank proteinuria[69].

Antithrombin III activity is not reduced in microalbuminuric IDDM[140,144] or NIDDM patients[146], and indeed there is a suggestion that it may be increased in overt nephopathy[140], despite no apparent increase in the *ex vivo* rate of thrombin generation[148]. This is at odds with an earlier report suggesting that thrombogenesis via the intrinsic pathway could indeed be accelerated[149]. Lee and colleagues[140] suggested that levels of the other antithrombotic factors S and C were also increased in IDDM, although this was not confirmed by Knobl and coworkers[141] in either IDDM or NIDDM, but Lee[140] suggested that this could arise as part of a homeostatic compensatory response. Blood glucose control and serum cholesterol again seemed to be more important determinants of these factors than albuminuria, and although total protein S was predicted by albuminuria on multiple regression analysis, activity of factor S is reflected more by 'free' levels[140].

Global tests of fibrinolysis do not appear to be altered in microalbuminuric IDDM patients[140], although a marked increase in PAI was noted, but this probably reflects endothelial dysfunction, as (presumed compensatory) activation has been noted in established nephropathy[150]. No significant alteration in PAI-1 or plasmin activity was noted in microalbuminuric NIDDM patients[145,146], although others have recorded a correlation between microalbuminuria and PAI-1 in both NIDDM and IDDM patients[142,151,152]. A stronger association between insulin resistance and the other two variables probably accounts for the univariate association. Extensive assessment of rheological function has also established that plasma and whole blood viscosity at low and high shear rates are not altered by microalbuminuria, and neither are indices of erythrocyte aggregation and deformability[105].

Platelet function studies are particularly difficult to carry out *ex vivo*, without running the risk of platelet activation. Spontaneous platelet hyperaggregation has been reported in uncomplicated diabetes[153], but estimates of microalbuminuria were not made in this study. *In vitro* aggregation in response to adrenaline and ADP appears to be unaffected by either microalbuminuria or macroalbuminuria in IDDM[144]. The observation that collagen-induced aggregation was increased in those with microalbuminuria, in comparison with both normoalbuminuric and macroalbuminuric groups is not easily explained. More evident *in vivo* platelet hyperactivity was suggested by increased concentrations of both platelet factor IV and β-thromboglobulin in microalbuminuric as well as macroalbuminuric IDDM patients[144]. These proaggregatory substances are normally resident in granules within platelets, and increased activity is compatible with platelet activation and degranulation. In contrast to IDDM, platelet aggregation to both collagen and ADP was unaltered in Japanese NIDDM subjects[143]; thus, it appears likely that microalbuminuria *per se* does not primarily affect platelet function.

These alterations in clotting factors, fibrinolysis and platelet function are summarised in Table 6.4.

Free radical activity and microalbuminuria in diabetes

Free radicals are highly unstable reactive oxygen species which are capable of inducing peroxidation of lipids and proteins. Whilst primarily an intracellular defence mechanism, free radical activity also takes place systemically and in certain circumstances may lead to tissue damage. In particular, free-radical-mediated lipid and lipoprotein peroxidation has been implicated in atherosclerosis and in diabetic microvascular disease. *In vivo* measurement of free radical activity has serious methodological limitations and indeed it is uncertain whether circulating measures have any bearing on free-radical-mediated tissue damage at the local microenvironmental level.

The activity of free radicals is physiologically controlled by the presence of circulating antioxidants such as superoxide dismutase, caeruloplasmin, ascorbic acid, glutathione, vitamin E (α-tocopherol) and plasma and lysate thiols. High-density lipoprotein is also now recognised as possessing antioxidant activity.

Consequently, indirect methods are employed to assess free-radical-mediated lipid and protein peroxidation. Thus oxidation of polyunsaturated fatty acids or of LDL cholesterol can be estimated by respective measurement of the diene-conjugated isomer of linoleic acid or of the lipid peroxide malondialdehyde. Fluorescence of serum proteins occurs after peroxidation and can also indicate free radical effects. The problem with all these estimates is that they are non-specific, poorly reproducible and, in the context of diabetes, susceptible to the impact of non-enzymatic glycation. *In vitro* assessment of the susceptibilty of LDL to oxidation in the presence of copper ions has also been utilised, but again may have little bearing on the *in vivo* situation, and the measurement of antioxidant activity is probably only of value when examined in relation to a reliable marker of lipid or protein peroxidation. The recent use of direct measurement of oxidised cholesterol byproducts, such as ketocholesterol, may enable further progress in this area.

Having said that, it will become clear that it is uncertain whether present methodology is sufficiently sophisticated to enable a valid discussion of the impact of free radicals in microalbuminuria, and to date this has only been addressed in diabetes. It has been claimed that diabetes is a state of heightened free radical activity and reduced activity of certain antioxidants, in part due to the capacity of non-enzymatically glycated proteins to induce peroxidation[154,155]. A preliminary report, however, has found no evidence of

Table 6.4. *Summary of the abnormalities in clotting factors, fibrinolysis and platelet function in IDDM and NIDDM patients with microalbuminuria compared with normoalbuminuric patients*

	IDDM	NIDDM
Clotting factors		
Fibrinogen	N-↑	N-↑
Factor VIIc concentration	N	N
Factor VIIc activity	↑	↑
Factor VII concentration	N	N
Antithrombin III activity	N	N
Fibrinolysis		
Global fibrinolysis	N	?
PAI	↑	?
PAI-1	?	N
Plasmin activity	?	N
Viscosity	N	?
Erythrocyte aggregation and deformability	N	?
Platelet function		
In vitro aggregation to		
ADP/adrenaline	N	N
collagen	↑	N
Factor IV	↑	?
β-thromboglobulin	↑	?

N: similar to values in normoalbuminuric patients.
↑: increased compared with values in normoalbuminuric patients.
?: unknown.

increased ketocholesterol concentrations (the major oxidised cholesterol byproduct) in uncomplicated NIDDM patients in comparison with age-matched controls[156].

In Albustix-negative IDDM patients with retinopathy, there was no evidence of enhanced free-radical-mediated peroxidation of proteins or lipids in two reports[157,158]. Although not stated explicitly, at least a proportion of the sample would have been expected to have microalbuminuria, in view of the close association between retinopathy and early nephropathy. A similar lack of alteration in lipid peroxides in microalbuminuric IDDM and NIDDM patients was noted by Knobl and colleagues[141] but, in contrast, increased diene conjugates were recorded by Jennings and coworkers[155] in IDDM complicated by microangiopathy, and one sole study in NIDDM has demonstrated increased concentrations of both diene conjugates and malondialdehyde in association with microalbuminuria[145]. This apparent discrepancy could be explained by the different mechanisms accounting for albuminuria. In the study of Collier and colleagues[157] it was stated that there was no clinical or electrocardiographic evidence of ischaemic or peripheral vascular disease, but the presence of subclinical cardiovascular disease in a population at high risk was not excluded.

The younger age group in the IDDM studies would make this much less likely, and indeed microalbuminuria may be a marker of established athero-sclerotic disease in NIDDM (see later). Recent studies have demonstrated that diene conjugates, lipid peroxides and antioxidant activity are increased in atherosclerotic disease, but no more so in diabetes in comparison with a non-diabetic group[159,160]. The overall impression is therefore that established cardiovascular disease *per se* can itself lead to increased free radical damage and microalbuminuria, thereby explaining the association between these latter two variables. Free radical damage and increased lipid peroxides are more evident, however, in established nephropathy[141].

Microalbuminuria and smoking

Although the evidence that smoking is a major cardiovascular risk factor is incontrovertible, an independent effect on microalbuminuria is less certain.

In non-diabetic subjects there has been a suggestion that a marginally significant increase in albuminuria is apparent when more than ten cigarettes a day are smoked[88], although a smaller study did not confirm this in IDDM or healthy control subjects[161]. A putative mechanism is that smoking could itself chronically alter glomerular and tubular function, thereby being associated with both microalbuminuria and cardiovascular disease, but through quite different mechanisms. Cross-sectional studies in IDDM have examined the impact of smoking on microalbuminuria with contrasting findings. Smoking does not appear to be associated with microalbuminuria if the duration of IDDM is less than ten years[161,162], but is clearly related to albuminuria where the average duration of IDDM is of the order of 14-15 years[162,163], in keeping with the observation from both cross-sectional and longitudinal studies that even if smoking does not necessarily initiate albuminuria, it is an important factor in the progression towards Albustix-positive clinical nephropathy[163,164]. A recent intriguing report suggested that chronic smoking could attenuate the exaggerated vasoconstrictor response to noradrenaline previously decribed in microalbuminuric IDDM patients. It was speculated that this could represent down-regulation of α-adrenorecep-tors if smokers temporarily ceased smoking during acute experimentation[165].

Future research in this area may require protocols to be modified to take account of such a possibility. The impact of smoking on microalbuminuria in NIDDM is at present even less certain.

Microalbuminuria and insulin resistance

It is clear that microalbuminuria is associated with a number of clinical abnormalities, all of which are recognised to be insulin-resistant states, such as hypertension, obesity and dyslipidaemias. It is thus not surprising that non-diabetic and diabetic microalbuminuric subjects are more insulin resistant than their normoalbuminuric peers. However, several lines of evidence suggest that the association with other insulin-resistant states does not fully explain the degree of insulin resistance seen in microalbuminuria.

In elderly non-diabetic subjects followed for a mean of 3.5 years, those with microalbuminuria (albumin:creatinine ratio in an early morning urine sample ≥3.22 mg/mmol) plus hyperinsulinaemia (fasting serum insulin ≥114.0 pmol/l) had the highest rate of coronary heart disease mortality and coronary heart disease events[166]. In patients with essential hypertension, plasma glucose and insulin levels during a 75 g oral glucose tolerance test were both significantly higher in microalbuminuric compared to normoalbuminuric individuals, suggesting that those with microalbuminuria were more insulin resistant than those with normal albumin excretion[167]. A significant correlation was present between the area under the insulin curve and the albumin excretion rate.

In IDDM, in one study using the hyperinsulinaemic, euglycaemic clamp technique, glucose disposal rates were lower in microalbuminuric compared with normoalbuminuric patients[168]. Microalbuminuric patients had higher mean 24-h systolic blood pressure, blood pressure load and a more atherogenic lipid profile than normoalbuminuric subjects. However, on linear regression analysis, glucose disposal rate was inversely correlated with albumin excretion rate in the microalbuminuric group, and with body mass index in both groups. Total glucose disposal rate remained lower in the microalbuminuric group after adjustment for body mass index.

In NIDDM, again using the hyperinsulinaemic euglycaemic clamp technique, microalbuminuric patients have been demonstrated to have lower total glucose disposal rates compared with normoalbuminuric subjects[169]. Differences in glucose disposal persisted even after exclusion of hypertensive microalbuminuric subjects. Two groups have performed detailed metabolic studies of non-diabetic control subjects, normotensive normoalbuminuric NIDDM, microalbuminuric normotensive NIDDM, normoalbuminuric hypertensive NIDDM and microalbuminuric hypertensive NIDDM patients[170,171]. Total glucose disposal rates during a hyperinsulinaemic euglycaemic clamp were similar in non-diabetic and uncomplicated NIDDM subjects and reduced to a similar degree in microalbuminuric normotensive and normoalbuminuric hypertensive subjects (Fig. 6.3). The most profound reduction in glucose disposal was seen in the group with both microalbuminuria and hypertension. The reduction in total glucose disposal was almost completely accounted for by a reduction in non-oxidative glucose metabolism, i.e. in glycogen storage in skeletal muscle.

Intriguingly, Forsblom and colleagues[172] studied non-diabetic relatives of patients with NIDDM. In relatives with microalbuminuria, systolic blood pressure and fasting glucose concentrations were higher and HDL-cholesterol and apolipoprotein A-I lower than in normoalbuminuric relatives. In hyperinsulinaemic, euglycaemic clamps, total glucose disposal rates were

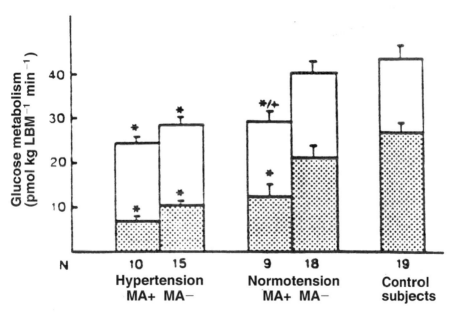

Fig. 6.3. Rates of insulin-stimulated total glucose metabolism (shown by the height of the total bars), glucose oxidation (open bars) and non-oxidative glucose metabolism (hatched bars) in normotensive and hypertensive NIDDM patients with (MA +) and without (MA-) microalbuminuria. Values are mean ± SEM. *: $p < 0.05$ compared with non-diabetic control subjects; +: $p < 0.05$ compared with NIDDM patients with normal blood pressure and normal albumin excretion rate; LBM: lean body mass. Reproduced from reference 77 with permission (copyright Springer-Verlag).

lower in the microalbuminuric subjects, and once again this difference was almost completely explained by lower non-oxidative glucose disposal rates.

This work suggests that insulin resistance in microalbuminuria is greater than can be explained by the contributions from the features which are associated with abnormal albumin excretion. From the family studies it would appear that there may be a hereditary element contributing to the appearance of the clinical phenotype of microalbuminuria, hypertension, obesity and dyslipidaemia.

Microalbuminuria, coronary heart disease and the role of immune complexes–complement system

There is a body of evidence suggesting an immunological basis for both diabetic microvascular disease[173] and for coronary heart disease[174], raising the possibility that the association between microalbuminuria and coronary heart disease could be indirect and immunologically mediated. The relationship between microalbuminuria and reduced complement C_4 concentrations in IDDM[173] could either reflect increased consumption by immune complex formation, or alternatively lead to failure of clearance of immune complexes. Either scenario could result in damage to both large vessels and the microvasculature.

More recent evidence has demonstrated that NIDDM and coronary heart disease are both independently associated with activation of the complement system, either by a classical (immune complex mediated) or alternative pathway[175]. The co-existence of microalbuminuria made little difference, although macroalbuminuria was associated with raised plasma concentrations of C3d, a split product arising following activation of the classical complement pathway.

However, the demonstration that glycated lipoproteins were immunogenic[176] could be relevant to the impact of diabetes on atherosclerosis, and simply be an additional additive mechanism which operated to a similar extent in normoalbuminuric and microalbuminuric subjects, and was exaggerated once macroalbuminuria and hyperlipidaemia were present.

Microalbuminuria and non-atherosclerotic cardiovascular disease

Systemic haemodynamics are an important determinant of glomerular albumin handling, and this has led to the realisation that microalbuminuria may be a secondary non-specific feature of all significant cardiovascular disease, regardless of the primary pathology. This is most clearly illustrated in subjects with congestive cardiac failure where microalbuminuria is thought to reflect altered glomerular capillary haemodynamics to a greater extent than altered permeability, although there is some evidence to suggest that the fractional clearance of albumin could be preferentially enhanced when glomerular plasma flow is reduced[177], and tubular dysfunction may also be involved in the proteinuria of cardiac failure[178]. Hypertensive cardiac disease is another situation described previously where there is a logical basis for associated microalbuminuria.

The role of other forms of cardiovascular disease such as cardiovascular autonomic neuropathy and cardiomyopathy has to date only been studied in diabetes. Subclinical alteration of parasympathetic vagal control of heart rate responses has been noted in association with microalbuminuria in IDDM[54,179]. This is particularly apparent at night when additional alterations in sympathetic activity could be implicated in the process by altering nocturnal systemic and renal haemodynamics.

Support for this comes from 24-h blood pressure monitoring in subjects with microalbuminuria, where absence of the physiological fall in nocturnal blood pressure has been related to other features of autonomic dysfunction[49–51,55]. It is also possible, of course, that both autonomic dysfunction and microalbuminuria in IDDM have a common pathogenesis, or that early nephropathy may itself lead to autonomic neuropathy. This can only be resolved by prospective studies early in the natural history of IDDM, but it has been shown that early autonomic dysfunction predicts a decline in glomerular filtration in established nephropathy, whilst at the same time progressing itself[180]. Cardiovascular autonomic neuropathy may be implicated in subsequent mortality, perhaps by sudden death due to ventricular dysrhythmia, and this is supported by prospective studies where symptomatic autonomic neuropathy is associated with a > 50 % mortality rate over the subsequent ten years, often due to cardiovascular or unexplained causes[181]. Where (as is commonly the case) there is coexistent coronary atherosclerosis, alterations in heart rhythms and cardiovascular tone could tip the balance in individuals with critical coronary ischaemia.

It has been suggested that diabetes may be complicated by a specific diabetic cardiomyopathy due to microvascular disease[182]. Thus, diabetic microangiopathy affecting both the myocardium and the kidney could theoretically account for features of cardiac dysfunction in association with microalbuminuria in subjects without coronary atherosclerosis. There are several studies in microalbuminuric IDDM patients with normal autonomic tone demonstrating intraventricular septal hypertrophy and left ventricular diastolic impairment[183–185], which complement earlier reports of histological endomyocardial abnormalities in IDDM complicated by diabetic retinopathy and nephropathy, but with patent coronary arteries[182]. Sampson and colleagues[183,184] have attributed these abnormalities to minor increases in blood pressure, and suggested that the findings are the earliest reflection of hypertensive heart disease. Similar observations have been made in non-diabetic atherosclerotic patients[18]. Others have noted such abnormalities in the absence of subtle differences in blood pressure in IDDM[185].

Microalbuminuria and atherosclerotic cardiovascular disease in non-diabetic subjects

The predominant area of interest has focused on the relationship between coronary heart disease and microalbuminuria. The method by which coronary heart disease is defined may be relevant. Thus, the association with morbidity measures (angina, previous myocardial infarction, angiographically defined disease) may not necessarily be paralleled by the relationship with coronary heart disease mortality, or with peripheral or cerebrovascular disease.

Several cross-sectional studies have documented features of coronary heart disease in association with microalbuminuria. Yudkin and colleagues[24] examined 187 subjects averaging 60 years of age, with a high prevalence of diabetes (7 %), hypertension (50 %), microalbuminuria (10.2 %), and coronary heart disease (37 %, based on Minnesota coded ECGs, or a history of angina or myocardial infarction). Microalbuminuria was present in 20.6 % with coronary heart disease, as opposed to 4.3 % without ($p = 0.001$). The corollary was that coronary heart disease was present in 74 % of microalbuminuric subjects, but in only 32.9 % of those with albumin excretion rate < 20 µg/min ($p = 0.001$). These findings were independent of the influence of altered glucose tolerance, hypertension, smoking, gender, age, ethnic origin or body mass. The population surveyed was not broadly representative in that they were selected with an anticipated high yield of glucose intolerance.

In our own study of 447 Caucasian men and women (average age 48 years), coronary heart disease was defined by similar criteria to those of Yudkin and coworkers[24], but the prevalence of coronary heart disease (< 10 %), microalbuminuria (6.3 %), diabetes (1.3 %) and hypertension (10.3 %) was lower[2]. Although the prevalence of ischaemia on resting ECG was more common amongst those with microalbuminuria (17.9 versus 2.7 %, $p < 0.05$), there was no significant difference in the prevalence of angina (3.6 versus 4.1 %) or of previous myocardial infarction (3.6 versus 1.0 %). Using the presence of abnormal ECGs as the most sensitive criterion of coronary heart disease, 33 % had concomitant microalbuminuria.

Agewall and coworkers[4] examined 331 non-diabetic hypertensive men whose age averaged 67 years, and also assessed coronary heart disease using Minnesota coded ECGs (abnormal in 18.7 %), angina (in 12.6 %) or past myocardial infarction (6.3 %) criteria. Microalbuminuria was present in 25 % of cases, but had a low sensitivity as a marker of concomitant coronary heart disease however assessed. The prevalence of microalbuminuria was significantly higher amongst those with ECG or historical evidence of cardiovascular damage (34.2 %) in comparison with those without (20.4 %).

Haffner and colleagues[25] examined 316 Mexican Americans whose mean age was 50 years. Coronary heart disease was based on self reporting of previous myocardial infarction, which was apparently more common amongst those with microalbuminuria (7.1 versus 1.7 %, p < 0.05), although with exclusion of hypertensive subjects, the difference was no longer significant (3.6 versus 0.8 %).

There is thus a distinct impression that microalbuminuria may more commonly be a marker of coronary heart disease in the presence of co-existent hypertension, where potentially similar mechanisms may be implicated in the sequelae of glomerular and coronary artery vasculopathy. The fact that microalbuminuria and coronary heart disease do not always accompany one another suggests that additional common predisposing factors are operative, and also highlights the non-specific nature of microalbuminuria. In addition to cardiac failure[177,178] it is now widely recognised that microalbuminuria is an acute phase response following myocardial infarction[178,186,187]. It has been suggested that this reflects transitory glomerulotubular dysfunction secondary to neurohormonal activation of the adrenergic system and renin–angiotensin–aldosterone axis. The possibility that thrombolytic therapy with streptokinase could also be implicated in microalbuminuria has been effectively excluded[188]. It is important, however, to ensure that estimation of microalbuminuria in coronary heart disease takes account of these acute reversible phenomena.

Despite such caveats, the detection of microalbuminuria can predict subsequent cardiovascular morbidity and mortality. The studies of Yudkin and colleagues[24] and Damsgaard and coworkers[189] focused on a group where coronary heart disease was initially present in 30–40 % of the cohort, and there was a high prevalence of accompanying hypertension. The mortality rate in both studies was considerably magnified by the presence of microalbuminuria: in elderly people in Denmark this was three-fold (14 % over a six-year follow-up period)[189], and in England sixteen-fold (33 % over a 3.6-year follow-up period)[24]. Damsgaard and colleagues[189] found that microalbuminuria interacted with the presence of hypertension, male gender and serum creatinine, all of which were independent predictors of mortality. Mortality in 50 % of cases could be attributed to cardiovascular disease (mainly coronary heart disease), but 30 % had cancer, usually of the genito-urinary tract (*vide infra*), and 13 % who subsequently died from cardiovascular disease were normoalbuminuric.

In summary, microalbuminuria is closely related to coronary heart disease, particularly in the presence of other coronary heart disease risk factors. Its detection in patients with overt coronary heart disease or at high risk of coronary heart disease should suggest the need for more active management of modifiable cardiovascular risk factors, because of the anticipated increased mortality risk. Definitive proof to justify such a policy would only come from a longitudinal intervention study of management of risk factors in patients with and without microalbuminuria, with coronary heart disease morbidity and mortality as the outcome measures.

The relationship between microalbuminuria and peripheral and/or cerebrovascular disease in comparison with coronary heart disease is not necessarily synonomous. Yudkin and colleagues[24] classified peripheral vascular disease (PVD) as an ankle to brachial systolic pressure ratio of < 0.90 in either leg, and recorded a prevalence of PVD of 13.1 %, in whom microalbuminuria was present in 33.3 %, in comparison with 6.3 % without PVD ($p < 0.001$). The corollary was that PVD was present in 9.7 % of normoalbuminuric subjects compared with 44 % with microalbuminuria ($p < 0.001$). There is thus an impression that in the general population, PVD may be a less frequent accompaniment of microalbuminuria than coronary heart disease. Hickey and colleagues[190] assessed PVD more stringently by symptoms of claudication accompanied by an ankle–brachial pressure index of less than 0.80, and found that resting albumin:creatinine ratios were higher than in controls, but that exercise-induced microalbuminuria was a clearer discriminator from healthy controls. Furthermore, the degree of exercise-induced microalbuminuria appeared to be related to the severity of the claudication; thus, its reduction following surgery was of value in assessing outcome.

The relationship between microalbuminuria and cerebrovascular disease is even less clear, although it may predict hypertensive haemorrhagic cerebrovascular episodes in the elderly[189].

Microalbuminuria and atherosclerotic cardiovascular disease in diabetic subjects

The association in diabetes was first hinted at by retrospective case control studies in NIDDM which demonstrated an increased mortality, predominantly from cardiovascular disease[191-193]. The predictive cut-off point in these studies was > 15 mg/l, or > 10 µg/min in an overnight collection. These studies were of course unable to elaborate what factors in the intervening period may have been of prognostic importance, nor were attempts made to establish whether the impact of microalbuminuria was not only independent of blood pressure, age and serum creatinine, but also took no regard of serum lipids.

Cross-sectional studies have thus attempted to confirm the higher prevalence of cardiovascular disease associated with microalbuminuria, and to clarify whether the relationship is independent of other vascular risk factors. It is useful to examine carefully the patient characteristics in these reports. Mattock and colleagues[61] examined 141 Europid men and women with NIDDM, of whom one third had electrocardiographic and clinical features of coronary heart disease, and almost 50 % had hypertension. Albumin excretion rates (AER) amongst those with coronary heart disease were more than double those without coronary heart disease, and multiple logistic regression showed that AER was the strongest independent predictor of coronary heart disease.

Marshall and Alberti[32] examined 524 men and women with NIDDM, of whom only 18 % had treated hypertension, 23.4 % had symptomatic coronary heart disease, and 7 % had microalbuminuria. The prevalence of coronary heart disease was greater amongst those with microalbuminuria, particularly if AER was > 30 µg/min (38 versus 19 % with normoalbuminuria). Although a univariate association between albuminuria and coronary heart disease was noted, a much clearer relationship was noted in patients with clinical or symptomatic peripheral vascular disease, in whom AER was > 10 µg/min in 40 % of cases. Alternatively, the prevalence of PVD increased three-fold when AER was > 30 µg/min (29 versus 10 % with normoalbuminuria).

The suggestion that microalbuminuria was more closely associated with PVD than coronary heart disease in NIDDM was supported by Patrick and colleagues[63] who studied 149 newly diagnosed cases, of whom 26 % had microalbuminuria and approximately 16 % received treatment for hypertension. Whilst the overall prevalence of CVD was greater amongst those with microalbuminuria (47 versus 23 %, $p \leqslant 0.01$), this was exclusively

due to PVD (34 versus 9 %), but the significance of this was only modest
(*p* < 0.05) after correcting for the age difference. There was a notable lack
of difference in clinically documented cerebrovascular disease or coronary
heart disease amongst those with or without microalbuminuria, and the
difference in PVD prevalence was in fact no longer significant after 12
months' follow-up.

With the exception of a greater prevalence of self-reported angina in comparison with those who were normoalbuminuric, only non-significant
increases in the prevalence in all other measures of vascular disease were
noted by Nielsen and colleagues[124] although clear increases were more apparent in macroalbuminuric subjects.

Penno and coworkers[194] reported on 318 subjects with NIDDM, of whom
42.5 % were microalbuminuric, over 50 % hypertensive, and of whom 23 %
had coronary heart disease. The prevalence of coronary heart disease and
PVD was twice as great amongst those with microalbuminuria, and in this
study it was suggested that the association was independent of other established vascular risk factors.

A small study in 234 Mexican American NIDDM subjects with a high
prevalence of microalbuminuria (30.8 %) but less hypertension (26.2 %),
also found no excess of coronary heart disease, but this was based purely
on self-reporting of previous myocardial infarction, clearly a particularly
crude marker of coronary heart disease[133].

In the largest study by Gall and coworkers[60] of 557 NIDDM patients, 58
% were hypertensive, 27 % had microalbuminuria, and ECG features of
coronary heart disease were evident in 24 % of cases. This report may be
more representative than others, and is of interest since the prevalence of
several measures of CVD was not significantly greater amongst those with
microalbuminuria (abnormal ECG 26 versus 22 %, angina 9 versus 10 %,
intermittent claudication 9 versus 7 %, cerebrovascular events 8 versus 4 %,
and transient cerebral ischaemia 3 versus 2 %). The odds ratio of microalbuminuria for coronary heart disease was only 1.06 (NS), and microalbuminuria was thus a weak determinant of coronary heart disease. The situation
was quite different for macroalbuminuria when coronary heart disease was
clearly more prevalent and directly related to the degree of albuminuria. It is
important to note that documentation of coronary heart disease in this study
gave a greater yield when ECG rather than only clinical evidence of coronary
heart disease, was sought. This could partly reflect cardiac autonomic dysfunction leading to silent myocardial ischaemia.

Thus, whilst microalbuminuria is related to vascular disease in NIDDM,
this is most notable when there is coexisting hypertension. However, even

under these circumstances, it is not a specific and consistent marker of cardiovascular disease, although it could in theory reflect the severity of disease, particularly coronary heart disease and PVD. This latter hypothesis would be supported if microalbuminuria in NIDDM patients with coronary heart disease and PVD was associated with a poorer prognosis than those who were initially normoalbuminuric.

Longitudinal studies have given support to this possibility. Mattock and colleagues[62] prospectively followed up a cohort (33 % with coronary heart disease and 25 % with microalbuminuria at baseline) for a period of 3.4 years, during which time the cumulative mortality was 10 %. The mortality was seven-fold greater (28 versus 4 %) amongst those who were initially microalbuminuric, and most importantly, microalbuminuria remained an independent predictor after adjustment for blood pressure, lipids, and pre-existing coronary heart disease. Coronary heart disease accounted for 50 % of mortality, but an important point corroborated elsewhere[189,191,195] was that microalbuminuria was also more apparent amongst the 15–20 % who died from cancer. The role of proteinuria in cancer will be discussed in more detail in Chapter 7.

These findings concur with a population-based study of 236 subjects with NIDDM who were followed up for 6.1 years, during which a 39.4 % cumulative mortality was noted[195]. At baseline there was a significant proportion with microalbuminuria (34.3 %), hypertension (48.3 %), and pre-existing coronary heart disease (14.2 % with symptoms on a questionnaire). The standardised mortality rate (SMR) for the cohort was only significantly increased in women, although a less marked increase was noted in men, but this to some extent reflects the high incidence of all-cause and coronary heart disease mortality in men whose average age was 68 years. A larger sample size would be required to demonstrate a relative increase in SMR. However, as in Mattock's study[62], microalbuminuria (> 40 mg/l) in men and women was an independent predictor of all-cause mortality, in addition to age and the severity of diabetic retinopathy. Over 40 % of mortality was due to cardiovascular disease, and 19 % to cancer-related deaths.

In a three-year prospective study in 290 NIDDM subjects with a high prevalence of microalbuminuria (> 40 %), hypertension (50 %), PVD (40 %) and coronary heart disease (> 50 %), only macroalbuminuria was a clear marker of vascular mortality, and progression of PVD and carotid stenosis[68]. A recent follow-up study in Newcastle confirms that microalbuminuric NIDDM patients have a greater all-cause total mortality rate, with a high proportion with vascular deaths in microalbuminuric compared with normoalbuminuric, subjects[196]. This could suggest that microalbuminuria may therefore be a marker of subsequent mortality from causes such as cancer in NIDDM, as in the non-diabetic elderly population[189], in addition to cardiovascular disease. The non-specific nature of microalbuminuria is again highlighted, although when there is additional evidence of vascular dysfunction such as increased circulating endothelial constituents[197], microalbuminuria then seems a more precise marker of subsequent coronary heart disease in NIDDM.

The importance of microalbuminuria to coronary heart disease in IDDM is less clear, mainly because of the low cardiovascular morbidity and mortality amongst this relatively young population[198]. The situation is much clearer when the duration of diabetes exceeds 20 years, and once established nephropathy and macroalbuminuria supervene (*vide infra*). However, several longitudinal studies suggest that microalbuminuria in IDDM is associated with a greater chance of dying from cardiovascular disease, although the increase in relative risk is small and the effect only becomes apparent once clinical proteinuria is present[199–201]. This is logical given the clear evidence that microalbuminuria is a precursor of clinical nephropathy in IDDM, at which stage the risk of coronary heart disease mortality is considerable.

Proteinuria, macroalbuminuria and cardiovascular disease

Virtually all of the previously noted associations with microalbuminuria are even more evident in diabetic and non-diabetic subjects with overt proteinuria, which is a clear and independent predictor of a greatly enhanced risk of coronary heart disease mortality in diabetic, hypertensive and general populations[202–206]. Proteinuria in hypertensive populations probably reflects the severity of the hypertensive process[202] but of course also will result in adverse changes in lipoporoteins and coagulation which will compound the cardiovascular risk[84–85].

The impact of proteinuria on total and cardiovascular mortality in diabetes is particularly dramatic. Longitudinal studies in Denmark and the United States into IDDM have shown that the relative mortality rate is on average magnified ten-fold, in comparison with non-proteinuric IDDM patients of similar age, where the relative mortality rate is still twice that of the age- and sex-matched non-diabetic population [205,207]. The relative magnification of mortality rates is as high as 100-fold in proteinuric women with IDDM in comparison with non-diabetic women of similar age[205]. Whereas a significant cause of death in these earlier studies was uraemia, there are now greater facilities for support of end-stage renal disease, and indeed the long-term prognosis of diabetic nephropathy appears to have improved[208,209]. Consequently an increasing proportion of deaths will be attributed to a cardiovascular cause. Account should also be taken of the fact that the incidence of persistent proteinuria and diabetic nephropathy may be declining[210], in part the result of improvements in diabetes care. This raises the as yet unanswered question as to whether the incidence of microalbuminuria has also changed, in which case the longer-term cardiovascular prognosis in IDDM might also be expected to improve in time.

Whilst proteinuria in NIDDM magnifies 3.5-fold the relative mortality rate[206] this is more clearly from an excess of cardiovascular as opposed to renal causes. The pathogenesis of albuminuria in IDDM and NIDDM is not identical and in NIDDM is more closely linked to established coronary heart disease. However, as in IDDM, the coexistence of hypertension and proteinuria act synergistically to magnify mortality risk.

The mechanism whereby proteinuria amplifies coronary heart disease risk so profoundly in comparison with microalbuminuria must in part reflect the more consistent aggregation of clear disturbances in established cardiovascular risk factors, although these factors can only be considered contributory.

Influences specific to diabetes such as the impact of non-enzymatic glycation on immune function and vascular structure and function are presumably also implicated, but the Steno hypothesis (Chapter 5), whereby albuminuria reflects a generalised angiopathy of the micro- and macrovasculature, offers the best explanation for the greatly enhanced risk of cardiovascular mortality.

The importance of proteinuria to coronary heart disease morbidity and mortality in diabetes needs to be put in context. In IDDM its detection in younger patients with a duration of diabetes of 15 years or more magnifies considerably the relative risk of coronary heart disease in comparison, for example, with a 30-year-old without IDDM or in an individual with IDDM uncomplicated by nephropathy. However in absolute terms, the incidence of coronary heart disease in 30-year-old patients is relatively small, and coronary heart disease is most prevalent after the age of 50. In such circumstances the impact of proteinuria will be less apparent, and indeed proteinuria may be recorded in less than 50 % of IDDM patients with established coronary heart disease[198]. Our own cross-sectional study confirms this, in that although albumin excretion rates are clearly greater amongst IDDM patients with coronary heart disease as opposed to those without, albuminuria is not an independent predictor of coronary heart disease, and the major determinants are age, blood pressure and serum lipids[123].

Conclusion

Thus, in both insulin-dependent and non-insulin-dependent diabetes, micro-albuminuria is associated with a collection of other abnormalities, depicted in Fig. 6.4. Whether the central factor in this clustering is microalbuminuria itself or another fundamental disease process is not yet clear, but many of the abnormalities are obviously closely inter-related, so that it is difficult to determine cause and effect.

The relationship between cardiovascular disease and both micro- and macroalbuminuria is clearly complex, partly because of the nature of the association. It seems likeliest that micro- or macroalbuminuria is directly implicated in a build-up of factors involved in the pathogenesis of cardio-vascular disease, and that in turn some of these factors, such as hyperten-sion, perpetuate and aggravate the albuminuria. In addition albuminuria may be a manifestation of various forms of established cardiovascular dis-ease and endothelial dysfunction, and a marker of other phenomena, such as immunological changes, which are relevant to the pathogenesis and progression of atherosclerosis. The impact of any genetic component is presently speculative. A schematic outline is presented in Fig. 6.5.

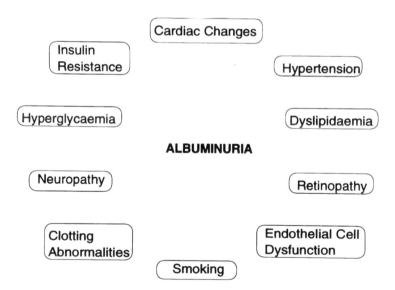

Fig. 6.4. Clinical abnormalities which tend to cluster with microalbuminuria in insulin-dependent, non-insulin-dependent diabetic and non-dia-betic subjects. Reproduced from reference 211 with permission (copyright John Wiley & Sons Limited).

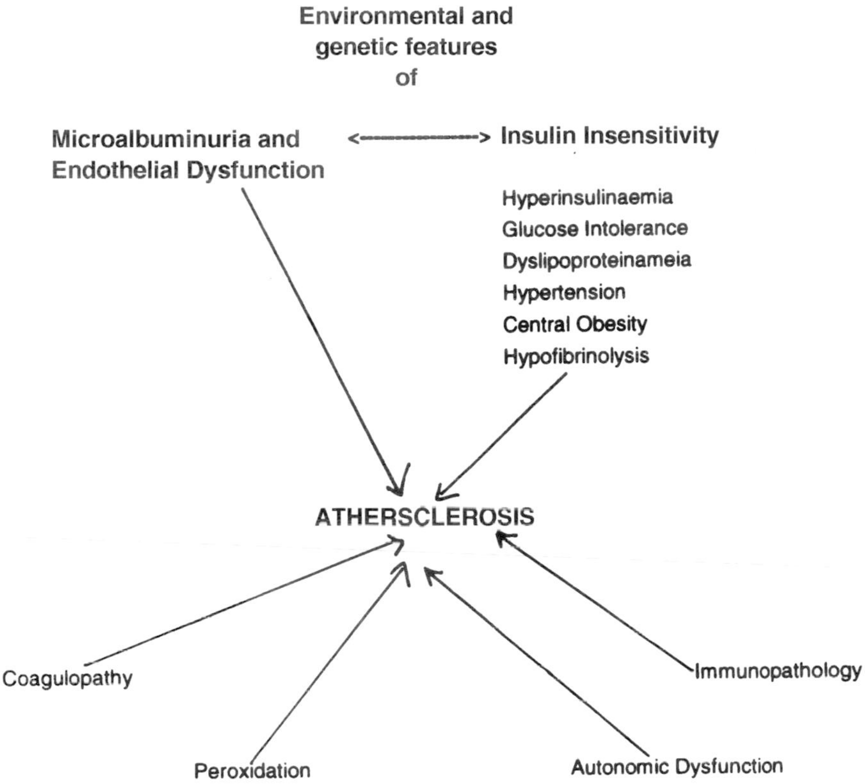

Environmental and
genetic features
of

Microalbuminuria and   <------------> Insulin Insensitivity
Endothelial Dysfunction

                            Hyperinsulinaemia
                            Glucose Intolerance
                            Dyslipoproteinameia
                            Hypertension
                            Central Obesity
                            Hypofibrinolysis

ATHERSCLEROSIS

Coagulopathy   Immunopathology

            Peroxidation   Autonomic Dysfunction

Fig. 6.5. Schematic diagram of the factors important in the development of atherosclerosis.

References

1. Parving H-H, Jensen H, Mogensen CE, Evrin PE. Increased urinary albumin excretion rate in benign essential hypertension. *Lancet* 1974; **1**:1190–1192.
2. Winocour PH, Harland JOE, Millar JP, Laker MF, Alberti KGMM. Microalbuminuria and associated risk factors in the community. *Atherosclerosis* 1992; **93**:71–81.
3. Metcalf P, Baker J, Scott A, Wild C, Scragg R, Dryson E. Albuminuria in people at least 40 years old: effect of obesity, hypertension, and hyperlipidaemia. *Clin Chem* 1992; **38**:1802–1808.
4. Agewall S, Persson B, Samuelsson O, Ljungmann S, Herlitz H, Fagerberg B. Microalbuminuria in treated hypertensive men at high risk of coronary disease. *J Hypertension* 1993; **11**:461–469.
5. Bigazzi R, Bianchi S, Campese VM, Baldari G. Prevalence of microalbuminuria in a large population of patients with mild to moderate essential hypertension. *Nephron* 1992; **61**:94–97.
6. Gosling P, Beevers DG. Urinary albumin excretion and blood pressure in the general population. *Clin Sci* 1989; **76**:39–42.
7. Hoegholm A, Bang LE, Kristensen KS, Nielsen JW, Holm J. Microalbuminuria in 411 untreated individuals with established hypertension, white coat hypertension and normotension. *Hypertension* 1994; **24**:101–105.

8. Gould MM, Mohamed-Ali V, Goubet SA, Yudkin JS, Haines AP. Microalbuminuria: associations with height and sex in non-diabetic subjects. *Br Med J* 1993; **306**:240–306.

9. Giaconi S, Levanti C, Fommei E, Innocenti F, Seghieri G, Palla L *et al.* Microalbuminuria and casual and ambulatory blood pressure monitoring in normotensives and in patients with borderline and mild essential hypertension. *Am J Hypert* 1989; **2**:259–261.

10. Collins VR, Dowse GK, Finch CF, Zimmet PZ, Linnane AW. Prevalence and risk factors for micro- and macroalbuminuria in diabetic subjects and entire population of Nauru. *Diabetes* 1989; **38**:1602–1610.

11. Gerber LM, Shmukler C, Alderman MH. Differences in urinary albumin excretion rate between normotensive and hypertensive, white and non-white subjects. *Arch Intern Med* 1992; **152**:373–377.

12. Woo J, Cockram CS, Swaminathan R, Lau E, Chan A, Cheung R. Microalbuminuria and other cardiovascular risk factors in nondiabetic subjects. *Int J Cardiol* 1992; **37**:345–350.

13. Lokkegaard N, Haupter I, Kristensen TB. Microalbuminuria in obesity. *Scand J Urol Nephrol* 1992; **26**:275–278.

14. Nosadini R, Semplicini A, Fioretto P, Lusiani L, Trevisan R, Donadon V *et al.* Sodium–lithium countertransport and cardiorenal abnormalities in essential hypertension. *Hypertension* 1991; **18**:191–198.

15. Winocour PH, Thomas TH, Brown L, Laker MF, Wilkinson R, Alberti KGMM. Serum insulin and triglyceride levels influence erythrocyte sodium–lithium countertransport activity in normoglycaemic individuals. *Clin Chim Acta* 1992; **208**:193–203.

16. Rutherford PA, Thomas TH, Carr SJ, Taylor R, Wilkinson R. Kinetics of sodium–lithium counter-transport activity in patients with uncomplicated type 1 diabetes. *Clin Sci* 1992; **82**:291–299.

17. Hasstedt SJ, Wu LL, Ash KO, Kuida H, Williams R. Hypertension and sodium–lithium countertransport in Utah pedigrees:evidence for major locus inheritance. *Am J Human Genet* 1988; **43**:14–22.

18. Pedrinelli R, Di Bello V, Catapano G, Talarico L, Materazzi F, Santoro G *et al.* Microalbuminuria is a marker of left ventricular hypertrophy but not hyperinsulinaemia in non-diabetic atherosclerotic patients. *Arteriosclerosis and Thrombosis* 1993; **13**:900–906.

19. Bigazzi R, Bianchi S, Baldari D, Sgherri G, Baldari G, Campese VM. Microalbuminuria in salt-sensitive patients. A marker for renal and cardiovascular risk factors. *Hypertension* 1994; **23**:195–199.

20. Fauvel JP, Hadj-Aissa A, Laville M, Fadat G, Labeeuw M, Zech P, Pozet N. Microalbuminuria in normotensives with genetic risk of hypertension. *Nephron* 1991; **57**:375–376.

21. Cottone S, Cerasola G. Microalbuminuria, fractional clearance and early renal permselectivity changes in essential hypertension. *Am J Nephrol* 1992; **12**:326–329.

22. Scarpelli PT, Chegai E, Castigli E, Livi R, Cagnoni M, Cappelli G. Renal handling of albumin and beta-2-microglobulin in human hypertension. *Nephron* 1985; **40**:122–123.

23. Ellekilde G, Von Eyben FE, Holm J, Hemmingsen L. Above-normal urinary excretion of retinol-binding protein and albumin in Albustix-negative hypertensive patients. *Clin Chem* 1991; **37**:1446–1447.

24. Yudkin JS, Forrest RD, Jackson CA. Microalbuminuria as predictor of vascular disease in non-diabetic subjects. Islington Diabetes Survey. *Lancet* 1988; **2**:530–533.

25. Haffner SM, Stern MP, Gruber MKK, Hazuda HP, Mitchell BD, Patterson JK. Microalbuminuria. Potential marker for increased cardiovascular risk factors in nondiabetic subjects? *Arteriosclerosis* 1990; **10**:727–731.

26. Hotz P, Pilliod J, Berode M, Rey F, Boillat M-A. Glycosaminoglycans, albuminuria and hydrocarbon exposure. *Nephron* 1991; **58**:184–191.

27. Yaqoob M, Bell GM, Stevenson A, Mason H, Percy DF. Renal impairment with chronic hydrocarbon exposure. *Q J Med* 1993; **86**:165–174.

28. Pedrinelli R, Giampietro O, Carmassi F, Melillo E, Dell'Ormo G, Catapano G et al. Microalbuminuria and endothelial dysfunction in essential hypertension. *Lancet* 1994; **344**:14–18.

29. Norgaard K, Feldt-Rasmussen B, Borch-Johnsen K, Saelen H, Deckert T. Prevalence of hypertension in type 1 (insulin-dependent) diabetes mellitus. *Diabetologia* 1990; **33**:407–410.

30. Ramirez L, Rosenstock J, Arauz C, Hellenbrand D, Raskin P. Low prevalence of microalbuminuria in normotensive patients with insulin-dependent diabetes mellitus. *Diabet Res Clin Pract* 1991; **12**:85–90.

31. Berglund J, Lins P-E, Adamson U, Lins L-E. Microalbuminuria in long-term insulin-dependent diabetes mellitus. *Acta Med Scand* 1987; **222**:333–338.

32. Marshall SM, Alberti KGMM. Comparison of the prevalence and associated features of abnormal albumin excretion in insulin-dependent and non-insulin-dependent diabetes. *Q J Med* 1989; **70**:61–71.

33. Drury P, Tarn AC. Are the WHO criteria for hypertension appropriate in young insulin-dependent diabetics? *Diabet Med* 1985; **2**:79–82.

34. Acheson RM. Blood pressure in a national sample of US adults: Percentile distribution by age, sex and race. *Int J Epidemiol* 1973; **2**:293–301.

35. Cowie CC, Port FK, Wolfe RA, Savage PJ, Moll PP, Hawthorne VM. Disparities in incidence of diabetic end-stage renal disease according to race and type of diabetes. *N Engl J Med* 1989; **321**:1074–1079.

36. Carr S, Mbanya JC, Thomas TH, Keavey P, Taylor R, Alberti KGMM, Wilkinson R. Increase in glomerular filtration rate in patients with insulin-dependent diabetes and elevated erythrocyte sodium–lithium countertransport. *N Engl J Med* 1990; **322**:500–505.

37. Microalbuminuria Collaborative Study Group, United Kingdom. Risk factors for development of microalbuminuria in insulin dependent diabetic patients:a cohort study. *Br Med J* 1993; **306**:1235–1239.

38. Viberti GC, Keen H, Wiseman MJ. Raised arterial pressure in parents of proteinuric insulin dependent diabetics. *Br Med J* 1987; **295**:515–517.

39. Krowlewski A, Canessa M, Warran JH, Laffel LMB, Christlieb AR, Knowler WC, Rond LI. Predisposition to hypertension and susceptibility to renal disease in insulin-dependent diabetes mellitus. *N Engl J Med* 1988; **318**:140–145.

40. Mangili R, Bending JJ, Scott G, Li LK, Gupta A, Viberti GC. Increased sodium-lithium countertransport in red cells of patients with insulin dependent diabetes and nephropathy. *N Engl J Med* 1988; **318**:146–150.

41. Walker JD, Tariq T, Viberti GC. Sodium–lithium countertransport activity in red cells of patients with insulin dependent diabetes and nephropathy and their parents. *Br Med J* 1990; **301**:635–638.

42. Jones SL, Trevisan R, Tariq T, Semplicini A, Mattock M, Walker JD *et al*. Sodium lithium countertransport activity is increased in microalbuminuric diabetics. *Hypertension* 1990; **19**:570–575.

43. Elving L, Wetzels JFM, de Nobel E, Berden JHM. Erythrocyte sodium–lithium counter-transport is not different in type 1 (insulin-dependent) diabetic patients with and without nephropathy. *Diabetologia* 1991; **34**: 126-128.

44. Jensen JS, Mathiesen ER, Norgaard K, Hommel E, Borch-Johnsen K, Funder J, *et al*. Increased blood pressure and erythrocyte sodium/lithium countertransport activity are not inherited in diabetic nephropathy. *Diabetologia* 1990; **33**:619–624.

45. Rutherford PA, Thomas TH, Carr SJ, Taylor R, Wilkinson R. Changes in erythrocyte sodium–lithium countertransport activity in diabetic nephropathy. *Clin Sci* 1992; **82**:301–307.

46. Winocour PH, Catalano C, Thomas TH, Wilkinson R, Alberti KGMM. Increased red cell sodium lithium countertransport activity, total exchangeable sodium, and hormonal control of sodium balance in normoalbuminuric type 1 diabetes. *Diabet Med* 1993; **10**:825–832.

47. Mathiesen ER, Oxenboll B, Johansen K, Svendsen PA, Deckert T. Incipient nephropathy in Type 1 (insulin dependent) diabetes. *Diabetologia* 1984; **26**:406–410.

48. Mathiesen ER, Ronn B, Jensen T, Storm B, Deckert T. Relationship between blood pressure and urinary albumin excretion in development of microalbuminuria. *Diabetes* 1990; **39**:245–249.

49. Benhamou P, Pitiot M, Halimi S, Siche JP, de Gaudemaris R, Bachelot I, Boizel R, Mallion JM. Early disturbances of ambulatory blood pressure load in normotensive type 1 diabetic patients with microalbuminuria. *Diabetes Care* 1992; **15**:1614–1619.

50. Moore WV, Donaldson DL, Chonko AM, Ideus P, Wiegmann TB. Ambulatory blood pressure in type 1 diabetes mellitus. Comparison to presence of incipient nephropathy in adolescents and young adults. *Diabetes* 1992; **41**:1035–1041.

51. Hornung RS, Mahler RF, Raftery EB. Ambulatory blood pressure and heart rate in diabetic patients:an assessment of autonomic function. *Diabet Med* 1989; **6**:579–585.

52. Germano G, Damiani S, Caparra A, Cassone-Faldetta M, Germano U, Coia F, *et al*. Ambulatory blood pressure recording in diabetic patients with abnormal responses to cardiovascular autonomic function tests. *Acta Diabetol* 1992; **28**:221–228.

53. Spallone V, Barini A, Gambardella S, Frontoni S, Maiello MR, Menzinger G. Relationship between autonomic neuropathy, 24-h blood pressure profile, and nephropathy in normotensive IDDM patients. *Diabetes Care* 1994; **17**: 578–584.

54. Winocour PH, Dhar H, Anderson DC. The relationship between autonomic neuropathy and urinary sodium and albumin excretion in insulin-treated diabetics. *Diabet Med* 1986; **3**:436–440.

55. Hansen KW, Christensen CK, Andersen PH, Pedersen MM, Christiansen JS, Mogensen CE. Ambulatory blood pressure in microalbuminuric type 1 diabetic patients. *Kidney Int* 1992; **41**:847–854.

56. Lurbe A, Redon J, Pascual J, Tacons J, Alvarez V, Batlle DC. Altered blood pressure during sleep in normotensive subjects with type 1 diabetes. *Hypertension* 1993; **21**:227–235.

57. Cohen DL, Close CF, Viberti GC. The variability of overnight urinary albumin excretion in insulin-dependent diabetic and normal control subjects. *Diabet Med* 1987; **4**:437–440.

58. Yip J, Mattock MB, Morocutti A, Sethi M, Trevisan R, Viberti GC. Insulin resistance in insulin-dependent diabetic patients with microalbuminuria. *Lancet* 1993; **342**:883–887.

59. Bengtsson C, Blohme G, Lapidus L, Lissner L, Lundgren H. Diabetes incidence in users and non-users of antihypertensive drugs in relation to serum insulin, glucose tolerance and degree of adiposity: a 12-year prospective population study of women in Gothenburg, Sweden. *J Intern Med* 1992; **231**:583–588.

60. Gall M-A, Rossing P, Skott P, Damsbo P, Vaag A, Bech A *et al.* Prevalence of micro- and macroalbuminuria, arterial hypertension, retinopathy and large vessel disease in European type 2 (non-insulin-dependent) diabetic patients. *Diabetologia* 1991; **34**:655–661.

61. Mattock MB, Keen H, Viberti GC, El-Gohari MR, Murrells TJ, Scott GS *et al.* Coronary heart disease and urinary albumin excretion rate in type 2 (non-insulin-dependent) diabetic patients. *Diabetologia* 1988; **31**:82–87.

62. Mattock MB, Morrish NJ, Viberti GC, Keen H, Fitzgerald AP, Jackson G. Prospective study of microalbuminuria as predictor of mortality in NIDDM. *Diabetes* 1992; **41**:736–741.

63. Patrick AW, Leslie PJ, Clarke BF, Frier BM. The natural history and associations of microalbuminuria in type 2 diabetes during the first year after diagnosis. *Diabet Med* 1990; **7**:902–908.

64. Keen H, Chlouverakis C, Fuller J, Jarrett RJ. The concomitants of raised blood sugar:studies in newly-detected hyperglycaemics. *Guy's Hosp Rep* 1969; **118**:247–254.

65. Haneda M, Kikkawa R, Togawa M, Koya D, Kajiwara N, Uzu T, Shigeta Y. High blood pressure is a risk factor for the development of microalbuminuria in Japanese subjects with non-insulin-dependent diabetes mellitus. *J Diabet Comp* 1992; **6**:181–185.

66. Nelson RG, Kunzelman CL, Pettitt DJ, Saad MF, Bennett PH, Knowler WC. Albuminuria in type 2 (non-insulin-dependent) diabetes mellitus and impaired glucose tolerance in Pima Indians. *Diabetologia* 1989; **32**:870–876.

67. Tai T-Y, Chuang L-M, Tseng T-H, Wu H-P, Chen M-S, Lin BJ. Microalbuminuria and diabetic complications in Chinese non-insulin-dependent diabetic patients: a prospective study. *Diabetes Res Clin Pract* 1990; **9**:59–63.

68. Stiegler H, Standl E, Schulz K, Roth R, Lehmacher W. Morbidity, mortality, and albuminuria in type 2 diabetic patients: a three-year prospective study of a random cohort in general practice. *Diabet Med* 1992; **9**:646–653.

69. Schmitz A, Ingerslev J. Haemostatic measures in type 2 diabetic patients with microalbuminuria. *Diabet Med* 1990; **7**:521–525.

70. Tkac I, Molcanyiova A, Tkacova R, Takac M. Levels of cardiovascular risk factors in type 2 diabetes are dependent on the stage of proteinuria. *J Intern Med* 1992; **231**:109–113.

71. Allawi J, Jarrett RJ. Microalbuminuria and cardiovascular risk factors in type 2 diabetes mellitus. *Diabet Med* 1990; **7**:115–118.
72. Schmitz A, Pedersen MM, Hansen KW. Blood pressure by 24 h ambulatory recordings in type 2 (non-insulin-dependent) diabetics. Relationship to urinary albumin excretion. *Diabete Metabolisme* 1991; **17**:301–307.
73. Gatling W, Knight C, Mullee MA, Hill RD. Microalbuminuria in diabetes: a population study of the prevalence and an assessment of three screening tests. *Diabet Med* 1988; **5**:343–347.
74. Niskanen L, Uusitupa M, Sarlund H, Siitonen O, Voutilainen E, Penttila J, Pyorala K. Microalbuminuria predicts the development of serum lipoprotein abnormalities favouring atherosclerosis in newly diagnosed Type 2 (non-insulin-dependent) diabetic patients. *Diabetologia* 1990; **33**:237–243.
75. Nakano S, Uchida K, Azukizawa S, Iwasaki R, Kaneko M, Morimoto S. Circadian rhythm of blood pressure in normotensive NIDDM subjects. Its relationship to microvascular complications. *Diabetes Care* 1991; **14**:8: 707–711.
76. Gall M-A, Rossing P, Jensen JS, Funder J, Parving H-H. Red cell Na^+/Li^+ countertransport in non-insulin-dependent diabetics with diabetic nephropathy. *Kidney Int* 1991; **39**:135–140.
77. Groop L, Ekstrand A, Forsblom C, Widen E, Groop P-H, Teppo A-M, Eriksson J. Insulin resistance, hypertension and microalbuminuria in patients with type 2 (non-insulin-dependent) diabetes mellitus. *Diabetologia* 1993; **36**:642–647.
78. Nosadini R, Solini A, Velussi M, Muollo B, Frigato F, Sambataro M, *et al.* Impaired insulin-induced glucose uptake by extrahepatic tissue is hallmark of NIDDM patients who have or will develop hypertension and microalbuminuria. *Diabetes* 1994; **43**:491–499.
79. Allawi J, Rao PV, Gilbert R, Scott G, Jarrett RJ, Keen H, *et al.* Microalbuminuria in non-insulin-dependent diabetes: its prevalence in Indian compared with Europid subjects. *Br Med J* 1988; **296**:462–464.
80. Cheung CK, Yeung YTF, Cockram CS, Swaminathan R. Urinary excretion of albumin and enzymes in non-insulin-dependent Chinese diabetics. *Clin Nephrol* 1990; **34**:125–130.
81. Lunt H, Lim CW, Crooke MJ, Smith RBW. Comparison of urinary albumin excretion between Maoris, Pacific Island Polynesians and Europeans with non-insulin-dependent diabetes. *Diabetes Res Clin Pract* 1990; **8**:45–50.
82. Erasmus RT, Oyeyinka G, Arije A. Microalbuminuria in non-insulin-dependent (type 2) Nigerian diabetics: relation to glycaemic control, blood pressure and retinopathy. *Postgrad Med J* 1992; **68**:638–642.
83. Alexander JH, Schapel GJ, Edwards KDG. Increased incidence of coronary heart disease associated with combined elevation of serum triglyceride and cholesterol concentrations in the nephrotic syndrome in man. *Med J Aust* 1974; **2**:119–122.
84. Cramp DG, Moorhead JF, Wills MR. Disorders of blood lipids in renal disease. *Lancet* 1975; **1**:672–673.
85. Mallick NP, Short CD. The nephrotic syndrome and ischaemic heart disease. *Nephron* 1981; **27**:54–57.
86. Smellie WSA, Warwick GL. Primary hyperlipidaemia is not associated with increased urinary albumin excretion. *Nephrol Dial Transplant* 1991; **6**: 398–401.

87. Winocour PH, Durrington PN, Bhatnagar D, Ishola M, Mackness M, Arrol S. Influence of early diabetic nephropathy on very low density lipoprotein (VLDL), intermediate density lipoprotein (IDL), and low density lipoprotein (LDL) composition. *Atherosclerosis* 1991; **89**:49–57.

88. Metcalf PA, Baker JR, Scragg RKR, Dryson E, Scott AR, Wild CJ. Albuminuria in people at least 40 years old: effect of alcohol consumption, regular exercise, and cigarette smoking. *Clin Chem* 1993; **39**:1793–1797.

89. Walden CE, Knopp RH, Wahl PW, Beach KW, Strandness E. Sex differences in the effect of diabetes mellitus on lipoprotein triglyceride and cholesterol concentrations. *N Engl J Med* 1984; **311**:953–959.

90. Curtiss LK, Witztum JL. Plasma apolipoproteins AI, AII, CI and E are glucosylated in hyperglycaemic diabetic subjects. *Diabetes* 1985; **34**:452–461.

91. Winocour PH, Tetlow L, Durrington PN, Ishola M, Hillier V, Anderson DC. Apolipoprotein E polymorphism and lipoproteins in insulin-treated diabetes mellitus. *Atherosclerosis* 1989; **75**:167–172.

92. Lopes-Virella MF, Sherer GK, Lees AM, Wohltmann H, Mayfield R, Sagel G, et al. Surface binding, internalization and degradation by cultured human fibroblasts of low density lipoproteins isolated from type 1 (insulin-dependent) diabetic patients: changes with metabolic control. *Diabetologia* 1982:22: 430–436.

93. Lopes-Virella MF, Wohltmann HJ, Mayfield RK, Loadholt CB, Colwell JA. Effect of metabolic control on lipid, lipoprotein and apolipoprotein levels in insulin-dependent diabetic patients:a longitudinal study. *Diabetes* 1983; **32**:20–25.

94. Gonen B, White N, Schonfeld G, Skor D, Miller P, Santiago J. Plasma levels of apoprotein B in patients with diabetes mellitus:the effect of glycemic control. *Metabolism* 1985; **34**:675–679.

95. Semenkovich CF, Ostlund RE, Schectman KB. Plasma lipids in patients with type 1 diabetes mellitus. Influence of race, gender, and plasma glucose control:lipids do not correlate with glucose control in black women. *Arch Intern Med* 1989; **149**:51–56.

96. Winocour PH, Durrington PN, Bhathagar D, Ishola M, Arrol S, Mackness M. Abnormalities of VLDL, IDL, and LDL characterize insulin-dependent diabetes mellitus. *Arteriosclerosis Thrombosis* 1992; **12**:920–928.

97. Kuksis A, Myher JJ, Geher K, Jones GJ, Breckenridge W, Feather T et al. Decreased phosphatidylcholine:free cholesterol ratio as an indicator of risk for ischaemic heart disease. *Arteriosclerosis* 1982; **2**:296–302.

98. Haaber AB, Kofoed-Enevoldsen A, Jensen T. The prevalence of hypercholesterolaemia and its relationship with albuminuria in insulin-dependent diabetic patients: an epidemiological study. *Diabet Med* 1992; **9**:557–561.

99. Winocour PH, Durrington PN, Ishola M, Hillier VF, Anderson DC. The prevalence of hyperlipidaemia and related clinical features in insulin-dependent diabetes mellitus. *Q J Med* 1989; **70**:265–276.

100. Lewis B, Chait A, Wootton IDP, Oakley CM, Krikler DM, Sigurdson G, et al. Frequency of risk factors for ischaemic heart disease in a healthy British population with particular reference to serum lipoprotein levels. *Lancet* 1974; **1**:141–146.

101. Hulley SB, Rosenman RH, Bawal RD, Brand RJ. Epidemiology as a guide to clinical decisions. The association between triglyceride and coronary heart diseases. *N Engl J Med* 1980; **302**:1383–1389.
102. Bainton D, Miller NE, Bolton CH, Yarnell JWG, Sweetman PM, Baker IA, *et al.* Plasma triglyceride and high density lipoprotein cholesterol as predictors of ischaemic heart disease in British men. The Caerphilly and Speedwell Collaborative Heart Disease Studies. *Br Heart J* 1992; **68**:60–66.
103. Winocour PH, Durrington PN, Ishola M, Anderson DC. Lipoprotein abnormalities in insulin-dependent diabetic patients. *Lancet* 1986; **1**: 1176–1178.
104. Jones SL, Close CF, Mattock MB, Jarrett RJ, Keen H, Viberti GC. Plasma lipid and coagulation factor concentrations in insulin dependent diabetics with microalbuminuria. *Br Med J* 1989; **298**:487–490.
105. Jay RH, Jones SL, Hill CE, Richmond W, Viberti GC, Rampling MW, Betteridge DJ. Blood rheology and cardiovascular risk factors in type 1 diabetes:relationship with microalbuminuria. *Diabet Med* 1991; **8**:662–667.
106. Jensen T, Stender S, Deckert T. Abnormalities in plasma concentrations of lipoproteins and fibrinogen in type 1 (insulin-dependent) diabetic patients with increased urinary albumin excretion. *Diabetologia* 1988; **31**:142–145.
107. Watts GF, Naumova R, Slavin BM, Morris RW, Houlston R, Kubal C, Shaw KM. Serum lipids and lipoproteins in insulin-dependent diabetic patients with persistent microalbuminuria. *Diabet Med* 1989; **6**:25–30.
108. Kapelrud H, Bangstad H-J, Dahl-Jorgensen K, Berg K, Hanssen KF. Serum Lp(a) lipoprotein concentrations in insulin dependent diabetic patients with microalbuminuria. *Br Med J* 1991; **303**:675–678.
109. Lahdenpera S, Groop P-H, Tilly-Kiesi M, Elliot TG, Viberti GC, Taskinen MR. LDL subclasses in IDDM patients: relation to diabetic nephropathy. *Diabetologia* 1994; **37**:681–688.
110. Groop PH, Elliott T, Ekstrand A, Franssila-Kallunki A, Friedman R, Viberti GC, Taskinen MR. Multiple lipoprotein abnormalities in Type 1 diabetic patients with renal disease. *Diabetes* 1996; **45**:974–979.
111. Kahri J, Groop P-H, Elliot T, Viberti GC, Taskinen MR. Plasma cholesteryl ester transfer protein and its relationship to plasma lipoproteins and apolipoprotein A-I- containing lipoproteins in IDDM patients with microalbuminuria and clinical nephropathy. *Diabetes Care* 1994; **17**:412–419.
112. Peynet J, Guillausseau PJ, Legrand A, Altman JJ, Flourie F, Chanson P, *et al.* Serum LpAI lipoprotein particles in diabetic patients with and without renal lesions of different grades. *Diabete Metabolisme* 1993; **19**:355–360.
113. Haaber AB, Deckert M, Stender S, Jensen T. Increased urinary loss of high density lipoproteins in albuminuric insulin-dependent diabetic patients. *Scand J Clin Lab Invest* 1993; **53**:191–196.
114. Dullaart RPF, Dikkeschei LD, Doorenbos H. Alterations in serum lipids and apolipoproteins in male type 1 (insulin-dependent) diabetic patients with microalbuminuria. *Diabetologia* 1989; **32**:685–689.
115. Durrington PN. A comparison of three methods of measuring high density lipoprotein cholesterol in diabetics and non-diabetics. *Ann Clin Biochem* 1980; **17**:199–204.
116. Winocour PH, Bhatnagar D, Ishola M, Arrol S, Durrington PN. Lipoprotein (a) and microvascular disease in type 1 (insulin-dependent) diabetes. *Diabet Med* 1991; **8**:922–927.

117. Vannini P, Ciavarella A, Flammini M, Bargossi A, Forlani G, Borgnino LC, Orsoni G. Lipid abnormalities in insulin-dependent diabetic patients with albuminuria. *Diabetes Care* 1984; **7**:151–154.

118. Groop PH, Elliot T, Friedman R, Viberti GC, Taskinen MR. The presence of the ε2 allele protects against dyslipidaemia in type 1 diabetic patients with renal disease (Abstract). *Diabetologia* 1993; **36**(Supp 1) A79.

119. Jenkins AJ, Steele JS, Janus ED, Best JD. Increased plasma apolipoprotein (a) levels in IDDM patients with microalbuminuria. *Diabetes* 1991; **40**:787–790.

120. Mbewu A, Durrington PN. Lipoprotein (a) : structure, properties and possible involvement in thrombogenesis and atherogenesis. *Atherosclerosis* 1990; **85**:1–4.

121. Maser RE, Drash AL, Usher D, Kuller LH, Beker DJ, Orchard TJ. Lipoprotein (a) concentration shows little relationship to IDDM complications in the Pittsburgh Epidemiology of Diabetes Complications Study Cohort. *Diabetes Care* 1993; **16**:755–758.

122. Haffner SM, Tuttle KR, Rainwater DL. Decrease of lipoprotein (a) with improved glycaemic control in IDDM subjects. *Diabetes Care* 1991; **14**: 302–307.

123. Winocour PH, Durrington PN, Bhatnagar D, Mbewu AD, Ishola M, Mackness M, Arrol S. A cross-sectional evaluation of cardiovascular risk factors in coronary heart disease associated with type 1 (insulin-dependent) diabetes mellitus. *Diabetes Res Clin Pract* 1992; **18**:173–184.

124. Nielsen FS, Voldsgaard AI, Gall MA, Rossing P, Hommel E, Andersen P, Dyerberg J, Parving HH. Apolipoprotein (a) and cardiovascular disease in Type 2 (non-insulin-dependent) diabetic patients with and without diabetic nephropathy. *Diabetologia* 1993; **36**:438–444.

125. Reverter JL, Senti M, Rubies-Prat J, Lucas A, Salinas I, Pizarro E, *et al.* Relationship between lipoprotein profile and urinary albumin excretion in Type II diabetic patients with stable metabolic control. *Diabetes Care* 1994; **17**:189–194.

126. Jenkins AJ, Steele JS, Janus ED, Santamaria JD, Best JD. Plasma apolipoprotein (a) is increased in Type 2 (non-insulin-dependent) diabetic patients with microalbuminuria. *Diabetologia* 1992; **35**:1055–1059.

127. Uusitupa M, Niskanen L, Siitonen O, Voutilainen E, Pyorala K. Five-year incidence of atherosclerotic vascular diseases in relation to general risk factors, insulin level and lipoprotein abnormalities in non-insulin-dependent diabetic and non-diabetic subjects. *Circulation* 1990; **82**:27–36.

128. Uusitupa MIJ, Niskanen LK, Siitonen O, Voutilainen E, Pyorala K. Ten-year cardiovascular mortality in relation to risk factors and abnormalities in lipoprotein composition in Type 2 (non-insulin-dependent) diabetic and non-diabetic subjects. *Diabetologia* 1993; **36**:1175–1184.

129. Austin MA, Breslow JL, Hennekens CH, Buring JE, Willett WC, Krauss RM. Low density lipoprotein subclass patterns and risk of myocardial infarction. *J Am Med Ass* 1988; **260**:1917–1921.

130. Shimizu H, Mori M, Saito T. An increase of serum remnant-like particles in non-insulin-dependent diabetic patients with microalbuminuria. *Clin Chim Acta* 1993; **221**:191–196.

131. Seghieri G, Alviggi L, Caselli P, De Giorgio LA, Breschi C, Gironi A, *et al.* Serum lipids and lipoproteins in type 2 diabetic patients with persistent microalbuminuria. *Diabet Med* 1990; **7**:810–814.

132. Hirano T, Naito H, Kurokawa M, Ebara T, Nagano S, Adachi M, Yoshino G. High prevalence of small LDL particles in non-insulin-dependent diabetic patients with nephropathy. *Atherosclerosis* 1996; **123**:57–72.

133. Haffner SM, Morales PA, Gruber K, Hazuda HP, Stern MP. Cardiovascular risk factors in non-insulin-dependent diabetic subjects with microalbuminuria. *Arteriosclerosis Thrombosis* 1993; **13**:205–210.

134. Schnack C, Pietschmann P, Knobl P, Schuller E, Prager R, Schernthaner G. Apolipoprotein (a) levels and atherogenic lipid fractions in relation to the degree of urinary albumin excretion in Type 2 Diabetes Mellitus. *Nephron* 1994; **66**:273–277.

135. Heesen BJ, Wolfenbuttel BHR, Leurs PB, Sels JPJ, Menheere PPCA, Jacklebeckers SEC, Kruseman ACN. Lipoprotein (a) levels in relation to diabetic complications in patients with non-insulin-dependent diabetes. *Eur J Clin Invest* 1993; **23**:580–584.

136. O'Brien T, N'Guyen TT, Harrison JM, Bailey KR, Dyck PJ, Kottke BA. Lipids and Lp(a) lipoprotein levels and coronary artery disease in subjects with non-insulin-dependent diabetes mellitus. *Mayo Clin Proc* 1994; **69**:430–435.

137. Ruiz J, Thillet J, Huby T, James RW, Ehrlich D, Flandre P, *et al*. Association of elevated lipoprotein (a) levels and coronary heart disease in NIDDM patients. Relationship with apolipoprotein (a) phenotypes. *Diabetologia* 1994; **37**:585–591.

138. Haffner SM, Moss SE, Klein BEK, Klein R. Lack of association between lipoprotein (a) concentrations and coronary heart disease mortality in diabetes: the Wisconsin epidemiologic study of diabetic retinopathy. *Metabolism* 1992; **41**:194–197.

139. Mayne EE. Haemostatic disorders in diabetes mellitus. In *Diabetes and Atherosclerosis*, ed. RW Stout, pp. 219–35 Amsterdam: Kluwer 1992

140. Lee P, Jenkins A, Bourke C, Santamaria J, Paton C, Janus E, Best J. Prothrombotic and antithrombotic factors are elevated in patients with type 1 diabetes complicated by microalbuminuria. *Diabet Med* 1993; **10**:122–128.

141. Knobl P, Schernthaner G, Schnack C, Pietschmann P, Griesmacher A, Prager R, Muller M. Thrombogenic factors are related to urinary albumin excretion rate in Type 1 (insulin-dependent) and Type 2 (non-insulin-dependent) diabetic patients. *Diabetologia* 1993; **36**:1045–1050.

142. Gruden G, Cavallo-Perin P, Bazzan M, Stella S, Vuolo A, Pagano G. PAI-1 and Factor VII activity are higher in IDDM patients with microalbuminuria. *Diabetes* 1994; **43**:426–429.

143. Baba T, Kodama T, Yasuda TK, Ishizaki T. Comparison of platelet aggregability in Japanese type 2 diabetic patients with and without microalbuminuria. *Diabet Med* 1993; **10**:643–646.

144. O'Donnell MJ, Le Guen CA, Lawson N, Gyde OHB, Barnett AH. Platelet behaviour and haemostatic behaviour in type 1 (insulin-dependent) diabetic patients with and without albuminuria. *Diabet Med* 1991; **8**:624–628.

145. Collier A, Rumley A, Rumley AG, Paterson JR, Leach JP, Lowe GDO, Small M. Free radical activity and hemostatic measures in NIDDM patients with and without microalbuminuria. *Diabetes* 1992; **41**:909–913.

146. Donders SHJ, Lustermans FAT, van Wersch JWJ. The effect of microalbuminuria on glycaemic control, serum lipids and haemostasis parameters in non-insulin-dependent diabetes mellitus. *Ann Clin Biochem* 1993; **30**:439–444.

147. Bent-Hanson L, Deckert T. Metabolism of albumin and fibrinogen in type 1 (insulin-dependent) diabetes mellitus. *Diabetes Res* 1988; **7**:159–164.
148. Ibbotson SH, Rayner H, Stickland MH, Davies JA, Grant PJ. Thrombin generation and factor VIII:C levels in patients with type 1 diabetes complicated by nephropathy. *Diabet Med* 1993; **10**:336–340.
149. Van Wersch JW, Donders SH, Westerhuis LW, Venekamp WJ. Microalbuminuria in diabetic patients:relationship to lipid, glyco-metabolic, coagulation and fibrinolysis parameters. *Eur J Clin Chem Clin Biochem* 1991; **29**:493–498.
150. Yagame M, Eguchi K, Suzuki D, Machimura H, Takeda H, Inoue W, *et al.* Fibrinolysis in patients with diabetic nephropathy determined by plasmin-alpha 2 plasmin inhibitor complexes in plasma. *J Diabet Comp* 1990; **4**: 175–178.
151. Gough SCL, Rice PJS, McCormack L, Chapman C, Grant PJ. The relationship between plasminogen activator inhibitor-1 and insulin resistance in newly diagnosed type 2 diabetes mellitus. *Diabet Med* 1993; **10**:638–642.
152. Mahmoud R, Raccah D, Alessi MC, Aillaud MF, Juhan-Vague I, Vague P. Fibrinolysis in insulin dependent diabetic patients with or without nephropathy. *Fibrinolysis* 1992; **6**:105–109.
153. Hendra T, Yudkin JS. Spontaneous platelet aggregation in whole blood in diabetic subjects with and without microvascular disease. *Diabet Med* 1992; **9**:247–251.
154. Wolff SP, Jiang ZY, Hunt JV. Protein glycation and oxidative stress in diabetes mellitus. *Free Rad Biol Med* 1991; **10**:339–352.
155. Jennings PE, Jones AF, Florkowski C, Lunec J, Barnett AH. Increased diene conjugates in diabetic subjects with microangiopathy. *Diabet Med* 1987; **4**:452–456.
156. Dyer RG, Stewart MW, Mitcheson J, Alberti KGMM, Laker MF. 7-Ketocholesterol, a specific indicator of lipoprotein oxidation, and malondialdehyde in non-insulin dependent diabetes and peripheral vascular disease. *Clin Chem Acta* 1997; **260**:1–13.
157. Collier A, Jackson M, Dawkes RM, Bell D, Clarke BF. Reduced free radical actvity detected by decreased diene conjugates in insulin-dependent diabetic patients. *Diabet Med* 1988; **5**:747–749.
158. Jones AF, Jennings PE, Wakefield A, Winkles JW, Lunec J, Barnett AH. The fluorescence of serum proteins in diabetic patients with and without retinopathy. *Diabet Med* 1988; **5**:547–551.
159. MacRury SM, Gordon D, Wilson R, Bradley H, Gemmell CG, Paterson JR, *et al.* A comparison of different methods of assessing free radical activity in type 2 diabetes and peripheral vascular disease. *Diabet Med* 1993; **10**:331–335.
160. Velazquez E, Winocour PH, Laker MF, Kesteven P, Alberti KGMM. Lipid peroxides in non-insulin dependent diabetes with macrovascular disease. *Diabet Med* 1991; **8**:752–758.
161. Ardron M, Macfarlane IA, Martin P, Walton C, Day J, Robinson C, Calverly P. Urinary excretion of albumin, α-1-microglobulin, and N-acetyl-B-D-glucosaminosidase in relation to smoking habits in diabetic and non-diabetic subjects. *J Diabet Comp* 1989; **3**:154–157.
162. Ekberg G, Grefberg N, Larsson LO. Cigarette smoking and urinary albumin excretion in insulin-treated diabetics without manifest nephropathy. *J Intern Med* 1991; **230**:435–442.

163. Chase HP, Garg SK, Marshall G, Berg CL, Harris S, Jackson WE, Hamman RE. Cigarette smoking increases the risk of albuminuria among subjects with type 1 diabetes. *J Am Med Ass* 1991; **265**:614–617.

164. Mulhauser I, Sawicki P, Berger M. Cigarette smoking as a risk factor for macroproteinuria and proliferative retinopathy in type 1 diabetes. *Diabetologia* 1986; **29**:500–502.

165. Bodmer CW, Valentine DT, Masson EA, Savage MW, Lake D, Williams G. Smoking attenuates the vasoconstrictor response to noradrenaline in Type 1 diabetic patients and normal subjects: possible relevance to diabetic nephropathy. *Eur J Clin Invest* 1994; **24**:331–336.

166. Kuusisto J, Mykkanen L, Pyorala K, Laakso M. Hyperinsulinaemic microalbuminuria. A new risk indicator for coronary herat disease. *Circulation* 1995; **91**:831–837.

167. Bianchi S, Bigazzi R, Valtriani C, Chiapponi I, Sgherri G, Baldari G, *et al.* Elevated serum insulin levels in patients with essential hypertension and microalbuminuria. *Hypertension* 1994; **23**:681–687.

168. Yip J, Mattock MB, Morocutti A, Sethi M, Trevisan R, Viberti GC. Insulin resistance in insulin-dependent diabetic patients with microalbuminuria. *Lancet* 1993; **342**:883–887.

169. Niskanen L, Laakso M. Insulin resistance related to albuminuria in patients with Type II (non-insulin-dependent) diabetes mellitus. *Metabolism* 1993; **42**:1541–1545.

170. Nosadini R, Cipollina MR, Solini A, Sambataro M, Morocutti A, Doria A, *et al.* Close relationship between microalbuminuria and insulin resistance in essential hypertension and non-insulin dependent diabetes mellitus. *J Am Soc Nephrol* 1992; **3** suppl 1; S56–S63.

171. Groop L, Ekstrand A, Forsblom CM, Widen E, Groop P-H, Teppo A-M, Eriksson J. Insulin resistance, hypertension and microalbuminuria in patients with Type 2 (non-insulin-dependent) diabetes mellitus. *Diabetologia* 1993; **36**:642–647.

172. Forsblom CM, Eriksson JG, Ekstrand AV, Teppo A-M, Taskinen M-R, Groop LC. Insulin resistance and abnormal albumin excretion in non-diabetic first-degree relatives of patients with NIDDM. *Diabetologia* 1995; **38**:363–369.

173. Barnett AH, Mijovic C, Fletcher J, Chesner I, Kulkusa-Langlands BM, Holder R, Bradwell AR. Low plasma C4 concentrations: association with microangiopathy in insulin dependent diabetes. *Br Med J* 1984; **289**:943–945.

174. Seifert PS, Kaztchkine MD. The complement system in atherosclerosis. *Atherosclerosis* 1988; **73**:91–104.

175. Figueredo A, Molino AM, Ibarra JL, Fernandez-Cruz A, Bagazgoitia J, Patino R, Rodriguez A. Plasma C3d levels and ischaemic heart diseasc in type II diabetes. *Diabetes Care* 1993; **16**:445–449.

176. Witztum JL, Steinbrecher UP, Kesaniem A, Fisher M. Autoantibodies to glycosylated proteins in the plasma of patients with diabetes mellitus. *Proc Natl Acad Sci* 1983; **81**:3204–3208.

177. Carrie BJ, Hilberman M, Schroeder JS, Myers BD. Albuminuria and the permselective properties of the glomerulus in cardiac failure. *Kidney Int* 1980; **17**:507–514.

178. Ellekilde G, Holm J, Von Eyben F, Hemmingsen L. Above-normal urinary excretion of albumin and retinol-binding protein in chronic heart failure. *Clin Chem* 1992; **38**:593–594.

179. Molgaard H, Christensen PD, Sorensen KE, Christensen CK, Mogensen CE. Association of 24-h cardiac parasympathetic activity and degree of nephropathy in IDDM patients. *Diabetes* 1992; **41**:812–817.

180. Lilja B, Nosslin B, Bergstrom B, Sundkvist G. Glomerular filtration rate, autonomic nerve function, and orthostatic blood pressure in patients with diabetes melitus. *Diabetes Res* 1985; **2**:179–181.

181. Ewing DJ, Campbell IW, Clarke BF. The natural history of diabetic autonomic neuropathy. *Q J Med* 1980; **49**:95–108.

182. Fisher BM, Gillen G, Lindop GBM, Dargie HJ, Frier BM. Cardiac function and coronary arteriography in asymptomatic type 1 (insulin-dependent) diabetic patients:Evidence for a specific diabetic heart disease. *Diabetologia* 1986; **29**:706–712.

183. Sampson MJ, Chambers JB, Sprigings DC, Drury PL. Abnormal diastolic function in patients with type 1 diabetes and early nephropathy. *Br Heart J* 1990; **64**:266–271.

184. Sampson MJ, Chambers J, Sprigings D, Drury PL. Intraventricular septal hypertrophy in type 1 diabetic patients with microalbuminuria or early proteinuria. *Diabet Med* 1990; **7**:126–131.

185. Watschinger B, Brunner Ch, Wagner A, Schnack Ch, Prager R, Weissel M, Burghuber OC. Left ventricular impairment in type 1 diabetic patients with microalbuminuria. *Nephron* 1993; **63**:145–151.

186. Gosling P, Hughes EA, Reynolds Tm, Fox JP. Microalbuminuria is an early response following myocardial infarction. *Eur Heart J* 1991; **12**:508–513.

187. Rouleau JL, Moye LA, deChamplain J, Klein M, Bichet D, Packer M, *et al*. Activation of neurohormonal systems following acute myocardial infarction. *Am J Cardiol* 1991; **68**:80D–86D.

188. von Eyben FE, Holm J, Hemmingsen L, Ellekilde G. Albuminuria with or without streptokinase (letter). *Lancet* 1993; **342**:365–366.

189. Damsgaard EM, Fröland A, Jörgensen OD, Mogensen CE. Microalbuminuria as a predictor of increased mortality in elderly people. *Br Med J* 1990; **300**:297–300.

190. Hickey NC, Shearman CP, Gosling P, Simms MH. Assessment of intermittent claudication by quantitation of exercise-induced microalbuminuria. *Eur J Vasc Surg* 1990; **4**:603–606.

191. Schmitz A, Vaeth M. Microalbuminuria: a major risk factor in non-insulin-dependent diabetes. A 10-year follow-up study of 503 patients. *Diabet Med* 1988; **5**:126–134.

192. Mogensen CE. Microalbuminuria predicts clinical proteinuria and early mortality in maturity-onset diabetes. *N Engl J Med* 1984; **310**:356–360.

193. Jarrett RJ, Viberti GC, Argyropoulos A, Hill RD, Mahmud U, Murrells TJ. Microalbuminuria predicts mortality in non-insulin-dependent diabetes. *Diabet Med* 1984; **1**:17–20.

194. Penno G, Giampietro O, Nannipieri M, Rizzo L, Rapuano A, Miccoli R, *et al*. Increased urinary albumin excretion aggregates with atherosclerotic risk factors in type 2 (non-insulin-dependent) diabetes mellitus. *Acta Diabetol* 1992; **29**:250–257.

195. Neil A, Thorogood M, Hawkins M, Cohen D, Potok M, Mann J. A prospective population-based study of microalbuminuria as a predictor of mortality in NIDDM. *Diabetes Care* 1993; **7**:996–1003.

196. MacLeod JM, Lutale J, Marshall SM. Albumin excretion and vascular deaths in NIDDM. *Diabetologia* 1995; **38**:610–616.
197. Stehouwer CDA, Nauta JJP, Zeldenrust GC, Hackeng WHL, Donker AJM, den Ottolander GHJ. Urinary albumin excretion, cardiovascular disease, and endothelial dysfunction in non-insulin-dependent diabetes mellitus. *Lancet* 1992; **340**:319–323.
198. Orchard TJ, Dorman JS, Maser RE, Becker DJ, Drash AL, Ellis D, *et al.* Prevalence of complications in IDDM by sex and duration. Pittsburgh Epidemiology of Diabetes Complications Study II. *Diabetes* 1990; **39**: 116–1124.
199. Messent JWC, Elliot TG, Hill RD, Jarrett RJ, Keen H, Viberti GC. Prognostic significance of microalbuminuria in insulin-dependent diabetes mellitus: a twenty-three year follow-up study. *Kidney Int* 1992; **41**:836-839.
200. Deckert T, Yokoyama H, Mathiesen E, Ronn B, Jensen T, Feldt-Rasmussen B, *et al.* Cohort study of predictive value of urinary albumin excretion for atherosclerotic vascular disease in patients with insulin dependent diabetes. *Br Med J* 1996; **312**:871–874.
201. Rossing P, Hougaard P, Borch-Johnsen K, Parving HH. Predictors of mortality in insulin dependent diabetes: 10 year observational follow up study. *Br Med J* 1996; **313**:779–784.
202. Bulpitt CJ, Beilihn LJ, Clifton P, Coles EC, Dollery CT, Gear JSS, *et al.* Risk factors for death in treated hypertensive patients. Report from the DHSS hypertension care computing project. *Lancet* 1979; **2**:134–137.
203. Kannel WB, Stampfer MJ, Castelli WP, Verter J. The prognostic significance of proteinuria: the Framingham study. *Am Heart J* 1984; **108**:1347–1352.
204. Borch-Johnsen K, Kreiner S. Proteinuria: value as predictor of cardiovascular mortality in insulin-dependent diabetes mellitus. *Br Med J* 1987; **294**: 1651–1654.
205. Borch-Johnsen K, Andersen PK, Deckert T. The effect of proteinuria on relative mortality in type 1 (insulin dependent) diabetes mellitus. *Diabetologia* 1985; **28**:590–596.
206. Nelson RG, Pettitt DJ, Carraher MJ, Baird HR, Knowler WC. The effect of proteinuria on mortality in non-insulin-dependent diabetes mellitus. *Diabetes* 1988; **37**:1499–1504.
207. Krolewski AS, Kosinski EJ, Warram JH, Leland OS, Busick EJ, Asmal AC, *et al.* Magnitude and determinants of coronary artery disease in juvenile onset insulin dependent diabetes. *Am J Cardiol* 1987; **59**:570–575.
208. Mathiesen ER, Borch-Johnsen K, Jensen DJ, Deckert T. Improved survival in patients with diabetic nephropathy. *Diabetologia* 1989; **32**:884–886.
209. Parving HH, Hommel E. Prognosis in diabetic nephropathy. *Br Med J* 1989; **299**:230–233.
210. Kofoed-Enevoldsen A, Borch-Johnsen K, Kriener S, Nerup J, Deckert T. Declining incidence of persistent proteinuria in type 1 (insulin-dependent) diabetic patients in Denmark. *Diabetes* 1987; **36**:205–209.
211. Bilous RW, Marshall SM. Diabetic nephropathy: clinical aspects. In KGMM Alberti, H. Keen, RW de Fronzo (eds) *International Textbook of Diabetes.* John Wiley, London, 1997, pp. 1363–1412.

7

Microalbuminuria as a non-specific marker of disease

The pathophysiology of microalbuminuria has focused primarily on its relevance to diabetes, hypertension and cardiovascular disease, but there is increasing interest in the importance of urinary protein excretion in other conditions. Indeed, it is only by awareness of the multiplicity of clinical situations in which microalbuminuria is recorded, that its relatively non-specific nature is apparent. The present chapter identifies those conditions where microalbuminuria has been described and, where relevant, discusses the clinical value in its detection.

Renal disease

Although the presence of microalbuminuria might be thought fundamental to the investigation and monitoring of virtually all non-diabetic renal disease, there is remarkably little written on this subject. It could be anticipated that any structural damage to the glomerular or tubular components of the nephron, or the distal urinary tract, would all be accompanied by microalbuminuria in a large proportion of cases. The additional presence of low molecular weight proteinuria would infer predominantly tubular disease or dysfunction. Albuminuria will accompany any other cause of major overflow proteinuria such as Bence–Jones proteinuria (see later), myoglobinuria or haemoglobinuria[1]. Microalbuminuria as a feature of genito-urinary tract neoplasm has been alluded to earlier in Chapter 6, and has been demonstrated to be of prognostic value in this setting, in both diabetic and elderly subjects[2-5]. Genito-urinary infection and nephrolithiasis are recognised causes of proteinuria, and microalbuminuria can be expected sometime in the course of events, usually following active treatment, although on occasion as a marker of unexpected structural pathology[6,7].

Glomerulonephritis and focal tubulo-interstitial disease are the most common nephropathic disease processes other than diabetic glomerulosclerosis, likely to be associated with microalbuminuria. The association is most commonly described in the context of albuminuria in diabetic patients where there is a suspicion of non-diabetic renal disease, and histological evidence of glomerulonephritis or focal interstitial fibrosis. Milder degrees of microalbuminuria in the absence of diabetes have been reported in glomerulonephritis, most commonly of the membranous variety[8], but mesangioproliferative, amyloid, IgA and lupus nephropathy are also recognised causes[9-12], and it has been suggested that the presence of microalbuminuria following apparent remission may be the most sensitive method of detection of relapse of glomerulonephritis[13]. Other studies did not find the degree of microalbuminuria to be predictive of recurrence[8,14] and, although microalbuminuria may be a feature of minimal change glomerulonephritis, it has been suggested that basal albuminuria and the response to exercise in children in apparent remission for 1–4 years is no different than in healthy control subjects[14].

Urinary albumin and lower molecular weight protein excretion has also been monitored during steroid therapy of minimal change nephropathy and nephrotic syndrome, supporting the concept that the filtered albumin load may lead to tubular dysfunction under these circumstances[15]. The mechanism of microalbuminuria in glomerulonephritis is likely to be multifactorial, and the consequence of immune complex deposition, complement activation and release of vasoactive substances, which together would be expected to increase glomerular permeability.

Basal microalbuminuria may be present in more than 50 % of children with renal scarring some six years after correction of vesico-ureteric reflux, and this appears to be exaggerated if hyperfiltration is induced by amino acid infusion[16].

The detection of microalbuminuria has also been examined as a marker of early graft rejection following renal transplants[17,18]. However the measurement of other markers of renal function, for example tubular proteins and enzymes such as N-acetyl-glucosaminidase (NAG), are probably more sensitive markers of graft rejection than albuminuria. The positive predictive value of microalbuminuria may be as low as 33 %, although the negative predictive value can be as high as 95 %. Concurrent urinary infection is the major cause of the high prevalence of false-positive microalbuminuria in this setting.

By contrast, urinary albumin excretion as a marker of glomerular dysfunction appears to be more sensitive than urinary retinol binding protein excretion (a low molecular weight protein excreted with tubular dysfunction) in response to long-term lithium therapy[19,20]. This reflects both structural and functional changes, and it appears that lithium treatment may increase glomerular permeability, perhaps as a result of structural damage in the form of glomerular sclerosis. However the early suggestion of a close correlation between duration of lithium treatment and extent of microalbuminuria[19] was not supported by the later longitudinal study[20], which rather suggested that functional impairment was an early feature and a more likely explanation. Use of sustained-release lithium was associated with greater microalbuminuria than with standard lithium carbonate, raising the possibility that regeneration of glomerular function takes place. Other factors such as lithium-induced alterations in electrostatic properties of albumin could either increase glomerular permeability and/or attenuate proximal tubular reabsorption of the ultrafiltered albumin.

Renal involvement in leprosy was first described over 50 years ago, and recently microalbuminuria (> 20 mg/l) was reported in over 15 % of multibacillary and paucibacillary cases, often in association with tubular proteinuria and microscopic haematuria[21]. These findings were interpreted as evidence of both glomerular and tubular disease secondary to the leprosy. The contribution of amyloidosis to these findings was not ascertained.

Microalbuminuria and renal disease in pregnancy

Physiological increases in glomerular filtration and albuminuria are a feature of the third trimester of healthy pregnancies. This could potentially exert a cumulative effect on renal function amongst those with pre-existing renal disease, and perhaps also have a bearing on the development of pre-eclamptic toxaemia, which is currently thought to be immunologically mediated through alterations in placental function.

Deterioration in renal function through pregnancy is well recognised in patients with glomerular disease[22]. Whilst this is usually reversible it may on occasion be progressive and rarely in the context of diabetic nephropathy, life-threatening[23]. Increases in microalbuminuria in pregnancy where glomerular dysfunction pre-existed thus seem likely. The nature of the established renal disease seems to have more bearing on the outcome than the degree of albuminuria (see Chapter 4), apart from in diabetes mellitus, where the outcome for mother and foetus is poorer if the mother has proteinuria.

There is less agreement as to whether or not monitoring of urinary albumin excretion can help in the prediction of pre-eclampsia. Severe proteinuric pre-eclampsia can develop rapidly without time to detect clearly a preceding phase of microalbuminuria, and is more clearly heralded by a rise in serum urate and a decreased platelet count[24]. However, the development of mild pre-eclampsia (increased blood pressure and serum urate without clinical proteinuria) was associated with a modest exaggerated increase in albuminuria in this study, and the majority of other reports have suggested that microalbuminuria is a marker for risk of pre-eclampsia[25–28], particularly in diabetic pregnancies[29], and in non-diabetic primigravidaes after 28 weeks' gestation, when microalbuminuria persists long after blood pressure has returned to normal[27]. The predictive value of an albumin:creatinine ratio > 10 mg/mmol at 20 weeks' gestation may be as high as 95 %[25], and such an elevation can precede hypertension in pre- eclampsia by an average of nine weeks[27]; thus it has been suggested to be a reasonable screening test for those considered to be at risk of pre-eclampsia.

The important paper of Rodriguez and colleagues[26] examined the clinical utility of microalbuminuria as a predictor for pre-eclampsia in a prospective study of 78 normotensive women. They noted that albuminuria > 11 mg/l at 24–34 weeks' gestation was reasonably specific (83 %), but of low sensitivity (56 %). This meant that 17 women whose albumin excretion exceeded this value remained normotensive. However incorporation of the urinary calcium:creatinine ratio increased the specificity to 99 %, although the sensitivity remained poor (50 %). This suggests that, although detection of microalbuminuria and other abnormalities will make pre-eclampsia almost inevitable for that individual, almost half the cases of pre-eclampsia appear to arise precipitously without any prodromal period.

More recently microalbuminuria has also been suggested to be a marker for premature birth, with 25 % of those women in the top quartile of albumin:creatinine ratios at 16 weeks gestation delivering at 32 weeks or less. This association was independent of maternal age, ethnic origin, body mass, blood pressure, smoking or gestational age at booking, and it was hypothesised that if microalbuminuria was indicative of endothelial dysfunction, then this in turn could be implicated in the inflammatory and/or vasculitic placental features amongst premature births[30]. A subsequent report in 500 normotensive nulliparous women refuted this association and found no relationship between gestational age and urinary albumin, creatinine, calcium and either the albumin:creatinine or calcium:creatinine ratios[31].

Surgery and trauma

The concept that microalbuminuria is a marker of an acute phase response has been advanced most clearly by Gosling and colleagues[32,33], who have charted in detail the time course of albuminuria excretion in response to various forms of acute physical stress. Microalbuminuria accompanies surgical procedures, with a three-fold increment apparent 90 minutes after the start of most forms of peritoneal and vascular operative procedures, in some instances in patients with cancer. The degree of microalbuminuria was proportional to the severity of surgery (i.e. less under conditions of local anaesthesia), but apparently no different following induction of anaesthesia[34]. This contrasts with observations of an increase in albumin:creatinine ratios (from 2.7 to 4.7 mg/mmol) following induction of anaesthesia, with a further increase peri-operatively (to 13.0 mg/mmol), and sustained post-operative microalbuminuria on recovery[35]. It was suggested in both reports that microalbuminuria reflected increased vascular permeability.

The changes during induction of anaesthesia could be specific to the use of certain agents, although the process of induction by whatever means is associated with reduced glomerular filtration but increased filtration fraction, as a result of increased intracapillary glomerular pressure, secondary to pressor effects of angiotensin, catecholamines and prostaglandins. This would compound the increased glomerular permeability due to the trauma of the surgery, a situation analogous to that following non-surgical trauma or burns[32,33], where microalbuminuria is also described within 60 minutes of the event, proportional to the severity of the stress, and transient, settling within several hours. Persistent microalbuminuria under such circumstances would suggest underlying sepsis or respiratory complications (*vide infra*).

Acute systemic illness

Transient proteinuria in acute illness was first documented over 60 years ago[36], and microalbuminuria has now been recorded in a variety of acute medical situations. Presumably the microalbuminuria is a non-specific response to the consequent haemodynamic alterations, complement activation and the release of kinins, prostaglandins, interleukins and other granulocyte factors which increase vascular permeability. As mentioned in Chapter 6, microalbuminuria is present in cardiac failure and following myocardial infarction, and also accompanies febrile illnesses, seizures and pancreatitis.

Hemmingsen and Skaarup[37] examined a battery of serum proteins during febrile illnesses and noted that the proteinuria was due to both glomerular and tubular dysfunction, with transient albuminuria ranging from 2.8 to 634.7 µg/min. The degree of fever (> 38 °C) was proportional to the amount of tubular proteinuria, and independent of the actual infection. This suggested that a centrally mediated release of, for example interleukins, was implicated in impaired reabsorption, although the increased plasma concentrations of some proteins as part of the acute phase response also played a role. Tubular proteinuria tended to subside after a period of three days. The mechanism of glomerular proteinuria (i.e. microalbuminuria) was somewhat more complex and thought to reflect the release of vasoactive substances from organisms, and the capacity of certain microbes to induce a low-grade autoimmune glomerulonephritis following immune complex activation.

This could explain why albuminuria could persist for many days following resolution of the febrile illness, but short-lived microalbuminuria and tubular proteinuria is a feature of febrile conditions without associated infection such as familial Mediterranean fever[38,39]. This suggests that tubular dysfunction also plays a role in albumin excretion, although the earlier study suggested that subclinical renal amyloidosis compromised orthostatic glomerular function, thus explaining why only increases in day-time albumin excretion were observed.

The pattern of microalbuminuria following other acute illness is similar, although the mechanism may differ somewhat. Transient proteinuria (and microalbuminuria) following seizures is probably in the main due to myoglobinuria-induced tubular damage[40], whereas microalbuminuria following pancreatitis is accompanied by increased IgG excretion, suggesting glomerular dysfunction. Markers of tubular dysfunction have however also been noted in acute pancreatitis[41]. Increased excretion rates of albumin and IgG have been noted on admission in two-thirds of patients with acute pancreatitis[42], and it has been suggested that the level of protein excretion is proportional to the extent of inflammation, and thus an aid to assess the prognosis and intensity of management over the first 24 h following hospital admission. The albuminuria usually subsides to normal over seven days.

In addition to the mechanisms alluded to previously in other acute illnesses, pancreatic enzymes may additionally activate the complement system leading to granulocyte release of anaphylotoxin C5a, which in experimental systems increases vascular permeability.

Microalbuminuria in malignancy and AIDS

Microalbuminuria is an anticipated and prevalent feature of neoplasms of the genito-urinary tract, and appears to be a prognostic marker for subsequent mortality in this group[3]. It is less well appreciated that increased urinary protein excretion has been described in association with a variety of non-urothelial tumours, including epithelial cancers (e.g. lung, breast), lympho-

and myeloproliferative disorders (including multiple myeloma), adenocarcinoma (e.g. gastrointestinal and ovarian), and melanoma[37,43–45]. Increased albumin excretion is also of prognostic importance in these conditions.

There has been extensive investigation into the clinical utility of so-called tumour markers, primarily as an aid to assess response to treatment, and thereafter to enable early detection of relapse. In practice the measurement of urinary excretion of albumin and other plasma proteins is not a standard procedure, apart from the measurement of low molecular weight tubular proteins in serum and urine in cases of myeloma and lymphoma. This is in part a reflection of the low specificity of microalbuminuria as a tumour marker, as well as a realisation that the majority of tumour markers are not sensitive enough to detect early relapse.

The mechanism of albuminuria or proteinuria in patients with malignant neoplasms is usually due to deposition of tumour products or antigens in glomerular basement membrane, or alternatively to deposition of immune complexes in glomeruli. Therafter activation of the complement system and release of vasoactive substances will alter glomerular albumin handling. Release of kinins and tumour necrosis factor from bulk tumour could also affect renal protein handling, and in the case of myeloma direct renal damage to tubules is the major determinant not only of low molecular weight proteinuria, but also of microalbuminuria.

Microalbuminuria in longitudinal studies in NIDDM and the elderly non-diabetic population is a marker of subsequent cancer-related mortality in 20 % of cases[3,4], and this complements findings in patients with a variety of malignancies, where the presence of Albustix-negative proteinuria (up to 100 mg/l) is associated with a 22 % survival rate over four years, in comparison with 36 % amongst those without detectable proteinuria[43]. In patients with myeloma, albuminuria is not necessarily related to excretion of light chain or other low molecular weight proteins, although a mixed pattern of glomerular (i.e. albuminuria) and tubular proteinuria (i.e. α_1-microglobulin and retinol binding protein) can be present in up to 10 % of cases of myelomatosis, prior to any reduction of glomerular filtration rate. Early detection of this type of proteinuria could mark those at risk for renal involvement of myeloma, and thereby affect management of such patients. Albuminuria is more evident however, when accompanying Bence–Jones proteinuria, and it is thought that this is mainly the consequence of increased permeability rather than impaired tubular reabsorption, since such increases are not evident following competitive inhibition in tubular protein absorption after intravenous administration of amino acids[45].

The relationship between microalbuminuria and infection with the human immunodeficiency virus (HIV) has been examined, in view of frequent renal involvement in acquired immunodeficiency syndrome (AIDS). This is usually manifest as acute renal failure or moderately severe proteinuria, but early detection of microalbuminuria could mark those at risk for progressive nephropathy, particularly in cases with AIDS-associated nephropathy (HIVAN), a syndrome characterised by normal renal filtration function, nephromegaly, focal and segmental histological glomerulosclerosis, and a rapid decline in renal function without any change in blood pressure.

The prevalence of microalbuminuria in non-hypertensive, non-azotaemic subjects without dip-stick proteinuria has been estimated at 10–30 % in ambulatory HIV-infected patients[46,47], with the majority exhibiting full blown AIDS or AIDS-related complex. Microalbuminuria was not correlated with race, gender, risk factors for AIDS (e.g. intravenous drug abuse), disease history, or concurrent drug therapy other than zidovudine which was associated with three-fold greater concentrations in one study[46] although not in another[47]. There was also no consensus as to whether greater microalbuminuria was a feature of more advanced disease, but urinary albumin concentrations were correlated with CD4 T-cell and white blood cell counts, tumour necrosis factor and serum α and β_2-microglobulin levels, and tended to be more common in patients with a history of *Pneumocystis carinii* pneumonia. The possibility that microalbuminuria could be associated with progression of AIDS would require confirmation in a longitudinal study, but these associations and the observation of raised urinary β_2-microglobulin excretion, suggest that both glomerular and tubular dysfunction are implicated in the microalbuminuria.

Drug and toxin-induced microalbuminuria

The variety of drugs known to induce proteinuria is legion. They essentially act either by immune complex formation, non-denatured DNA antibody or basement membrane antibody induction with subsequent glomerulonephritis, acute lupus erythematosus or Goodpasture syndrome, by interstitial nephritis, or by direct toxic effects or anaphylaxis acting on the renal tubules.

D-penicillamine is one of the drugs where screening for proteinuria is most commonly carried out, but antibiotics, anti-hypertensive agents, heavy metals, and anti-inflammatory drugs have all been implicated in proteinuria[1,48] (Table 7.1).

At present there are only anecdotal reports of microalbuminuria without clinical proteinuria as a result of drug therapy[1], but it is inevitable that lesser

Table 7.1 *Types of drug-induced proteinuria*

Glomerular albuminuria

Immune complex disease	*Lupus syndrome*	*Goodpasture syndrome*
D-penicillamine	Hydrallazine	D-penicillamine
Lithium	Procainamide	
Gold	Methyldopa	
Trimethadone	Griseofulvin	
Asparaginase	Sulphonamides	
Fenprofen	Chlorpromazine	
Probenecid	Nitrofurantoin	
Practolol	D-penicillamine	
	Isonicotinic acid	

Tubular proteinuria

Anaphylactic	*Directly toxic*	*Interstitial nephritis*
Foreign proteins	Gold, mercury,	Antibiotics
Antibiotics	lead, bismuth,	D-penicillamine
Analgesics	cadmium, copper,	Phenacetin
	chromium, oxalate	

degrees of protein excretion will be evident in a proportion of cases, although the clinical significance of such a finding is presently uncertain. In the majority of cases the evident renal damage is reversible within months of cessation of therapy.

Endocrine disease and microalbuminuria

Despite the knowledge that hormonal control of renal function plays an important role in glomerular protein handling, little is known of microalbuminuria in endocrine disease, other than in acromegaly, a condition which, like diabetes mellitus, is characterised by glomerular hyperfiltration. One study has in fact shown that microalbuminuria may be an inconsistent feature of untreated acromegaly, but that overnight albumin excretion is reduced by 22 % following treatment with the somatostatin analogue octreotide[49]. By contrast, recombinant human growth hormone therapy does not appear to increase microalbuminuria in children with short stature[50].

Table 7.2 *Microalbuminuria as a non-specific marker of disease*

Renal disease	*Malignant disease*
Glomerulonephritis	Epithelial (lung, breast)
Pyelonephritis	Adenocarcinoma (renal)
GU tract inflammatory disease	Melanoma
Pre-eclampsia	Lymphoreticular
Renal graft rejection	
Sickle cell disease	
Leprosy	
Refux nephropathy	
Nephrolithiasis	
Febrile illness	*Circulatory disease*
Familial Mediterannean fever	Myocardial infarction
HIV infection – AIDS	Cardiac failure
	Peripheral vascular disease
	Hypertension
Inflammatory disease	*Skin disease*
Pancreatitis	Psoriasis
Rheumatoid arthritis	Systemic sclerosis
SLE	
Trauma and surgery	*Respiratory disease*
Extensive Injury	COPD
Burns	Obstructive sleep apnoea
Abdominal and vascular surgery	Hypoia at high altitude
Induction of anaesthesia	
Drugs	*Endocrine disease*
Penicillamine	Acromegaly
Steroids	Diabetes mellitus

Microalbuminuria in connective tissue and skin disease

Most types of connective tissue disease may be associated with endothelial dysfunction and microvascular changes which theoretically could alter vascular permeability, and renal involvement is also known to complicate systemic lupus erythematosus (SLE) and progressive systemic sclerosis. In systemic sclerosis microalbuminuria was noted in 2 out of 26 cases without overt renal involvement, but the proportion increased to 25 % after a follow-up period of 12 months[51]. Interestingly, withdrawal of nifedipine therapy had no sustained consistent effect on microalbuminuria in these subjects. A high prevalence of microalbuminuria has been noted in SLE before the development of structural renal changes, and excretion appears to decrease following steroid therapy[12]. Microalbuminuria has also been associated with rheumatoid arthritis[1]. The mechanism of microalbuminuria in all these situations is most likely to be predominantly enhanced glomerular permeability.

Psoriasis is another disorder where microvascular pathology may be a feature, and where microalbuminuria has been recorded in as many as 40–50 % of normotensive subjects with diffuse psoriasis[52,53]. The degree of microalbuminuria is directly related to the extent of skin involvement[53]. There is thought to be an increased risk of cardiovascular risk factors (hypertension and diabetes mellitus) and coronary atherosclerosis in psoriasis; thus the interaction of microalbuminuria with blood pressure and hyperglycaemia is likely to be cumulative and of pathophysiological importance.

Microalbuminuria in respiratory disease

Microalbuminuria (> 10 mg albumin per mmol creatinine) has been noted in 50 % of patients with chronic obstructive pulmonary disease (COPD), although half had cor pulmonale[54]. The cardiac failure would of course have promoted albuminuria in its own right. The associated increase in excretion of N-acetyl-glucosaminidase suggests that tubular damage, perhaps as a result of tissue hypoxia, may have contributed to the microalbuminuria, although tissue hypoxia may also have increased glomerular permeability, and increased glomerular filtration would have been enhanced by the increases in glomerular size and ANP concentrations seen in COPD. A contribution from hypoxia is favoured by similar observations made in chronic sleep apnoea[55] and at high altitude[56]. The prognostic relevance of the microalbuminuria could not be elicited from these cross-sectional studies.

References

1. Shihabi ZK, Konen JC, O'Connor ML. Albuminuria as urinary total protein for detecting chronic renal disorders. *Clin Chem* 1991; **37**:621–624.
2. Yudkin JS, Forrest RD, Jackson CA. Microalbuminuria as predictor of vascular disease in non-diabetic subjects. Islington Diabetes Survey. *Lancet* 1988; **2**:530–533.
3. Damsgaard EM, Fröland A, Jörgensen OD, Mogensen CE. Microalbuminuria as a predictor of increased mortality in elderly people. *Br Med J* 1990; **300**:297–300.

4. Neil A, Thorogood M, Hawkins M, Cohen D, Potok M, Mann J. A prospective population-based study of microalbuminuria as a predictor of mortality in NIDDM. *Diabetes Care* 1993; 7:996–1003.
5. Stiegler H, Standl E, Schulz K, Roth R, Lehmacher W. Morbidity, mortality, and albuminuria in type 2 diabetic patients: a three-year prospective study of a random cohort in general practice. *Diabet Med* 1992; **9**:646–653.
6. Watts RWE. Urinary stone disease. In *Oxford Textbook of Medicine*, 2nd edn, ed. DJ Weatherall, JG Ledingham, DA Warrell. London, Oxford University Press, 1988; pp 18.87–18.95.
7. Winocour PH, Catalano C, Tapson JS. Nephrolithiasis and early onset microvascular disease in type 1 diabetes mellitus. *Nephron* 1994; 66:364–365.
8. Hong KS, Kim SY, Koo WS, Choi EJ, Cha BY, Chang YS, *et al.* The clinical utility of microalbuminuria in nephrotic syndrome with complete remission, isolated microscopic haematuria and renal transplantation donors. *Korean J Intern Med* 1988; **3**:117–121.
9. Tait JL, Billson VR, Nankervis A, Kincaid-Smith P, Martin FIR. A clinical–histological study of individuals with diabetes mellitus and proteinuria. *Diabet Med* 1990; 7:215–221.
10. Kasinath BS, Mujais SK, Spargo BH, Katz AI. Nondiabetic renal disease in patients with diabetes mellitus. *Am J Med* 1983; **75**:613–617.
11. Richards NT, Greaves I, Lee SJ, Howie AJ, Adu D, Michael J. Increased prevalence of renal biopsy findings other than diabetic glomerulopathy in type II diabetes mellitus. *Nephrol Dial Transplant* 1992; 7:397–399.
12. Terai C, Nojima Y, Takano K, Yamada F, Takaku F. Determination of urinary albumin by radioimmunoassay in patients with subclinical lupus nephritis. *Clin Nephrol* 1987; **27**:79–93.
13. Short CD, Winocour PH, Durrington PN, Mallick N. Microalbuminuria in patients in clinical remission from nephrotic syndrome. *10th International Congress of Nephrology*, London, 1987.
14. Berg U, Bohlin AB, Freyschuss U, Johansson BL, Lefvert AK. Renal function and albumin excretion during exercise in children during remission of the minimal change nephrotic syndrome. *Acta Paed Scand* 1988; **77**:287–293.
15. Beetham R, Newman D. Urinary albumin and low molecular weight excretion in the nephrotic syndrome – sequential studies during corticosteroid treatment. *Ann Clin Biochem* 1992; **29**:450–453.
16. Coppo R, Porcellini MG, Gianoglio B, Alessi D, Peruzzi L, Amore A, *et al.* Glomerular permselectivity to macromolecules in reflux nephropathy: microalbuminuria during acute hyperfiltration due to aminoacid infusion. *Clin Nephrol* 1993; **40**:299–307.
17. Hemmingsen L, Skaarup P. Urinary excretion of ten plasma proteins in patients with febrile diseases. *Acta Med Scand* 1977; **201**:359–364.
18. Morelet L, Legendre C, Kreis H, Lacour B. Sequential measurements of urinary albumin in recipients of renal allografts. *Clin Chem* 1991; **37**:472–473.
19. Jensen HV, Holm J, Hemmingsen L, Thiesen S, Andersen J. Urinary excretion of albumin and retinol-binding protein in lithium treated patients. *Acta Psychiat Scand* 1988; **78**:375–378.
20. Jensen HV, Hemmingsen L, Holm J, Christensen EM, Aggernaes H. Urinary excretion of albumin and retinol-binding protein in lithium-treated patients: a longitudinal study. *Acta Psychiat Scand* 1992; **85**:480–483.

21. Kirsztajn GM, Nishida SK, Silva MS, Ajzen H, Pereira AB. Renal abnormalities in leprosy. *Nephron* 1993; **65**:381–384.

22. Suriah M, Imbasciati E, Cosci P, Banfi G, di Belgiojoso GB, Brancaccio D, *et al.* Glomerular disease and pregnancy. A study of 123 pregnancies in patients with primary and secondary glomerular diseases. *Nephron* 1984; **36**:101–105.

23. Weinstock RS, Kopecky RT, Jones DB, Sunderji S. Rapid development of nephrotic syndrome, hypertension, and haemolytic anaemia early in pregnancy in patients with IDDM. *Diabetes Care* 1988; **11**:416–421.

24. Lopez-Esponoza I, Dhar H, Humphreys S, Redman WG. Urinary albumin excretion in pregnancy. *Br J Obstet Gynaecol* 1986; **93**:176–181.

25. Nakamura T, Ito M, Yoshimura T, Mabe K, Okamura H. Usefulness of the urinary microalbumin/creatinine ratio in prediciting pregnancy-induced hypertension. *Int J Gynaecol Obstet* 1992; **37**:99–103.

26. Rodriguez MH, Masaki DI, Mestman J, Kumar D, Rude R. Calcium / creatinine ratio and microalbuminuria in the prediction of pre-eclampsia. *Am J Obstet Gynaecol* 1988; **159**:1452–1455.

27. Misiani R, Marchesi D, Tiraboschi G, Gualandris L, Goglio A, Amuso G, *et al.* Urinary albumin excretion in normal pregnancy and pregnancy induced hypertension. *Nephron* 1991; **59**:416–422.

28. Konstantin-Hansen KF, Hesseldahl II, Pedersen SM. Microalbuminuria as a predictor of pre-eclampsia. *Acta Obstet Gynecol Scand* 1992; **71**:343–346.

29. Winocour PH, Taylor R. Possible predictive factors for the development of pre-eclampsia in insulin-dependent diabetic pregnancies. *Diabetes Res* 1989; **10**:159–164.

30. Perry IJ, Gosling P, Sanghera K, Churchill D, Luesley DM, Beevers DG. Urinary microalbumin excretion in early pregnancy and gestational age at delivery. *Br Med J* 1993; **307**:420–421.

31. Baker PN, Hackett GA. Urinary microalbumin excretion and preterm birth (letter). *Br Med J* 1993; **307**:802.

32. Gosling P, Sutcliffe AJ. Proteinuria following trauma. *Ann Clin Biochem* 1986; **23**:681–685.

33. Gosling P, Sutcliffe AJ, Cooper MACS, Jones AF. Burn and trauma associated proteinuria: the role of lipid peroxidation. *Ann Clin Biochem* 1988; **25**:53–59.

34. Gosling P, Shearman CP, Gwynn BR, Simms MH, Bainbridge ET. Microproteinuria: response to operation. *Br Med J* 1988; **296**:338–339.

35. Mercatello A, Hadj-Aissa A, Chery C, Sagnard P, Pozet N, Tissot E, *et al.* Microalbuminuria is acutely increased during anaesthesia and surgery. *Nephron* 1991; **58**:161–163.

36. Welty JW. Febrile albuminuria. *Am J Med Sci* 1937; **194**:70–74.

37. Hemmingsen L, Skaarup P. Urinary excretion of ten plasma proteins in patients with extrarenal epithelial carcinoma. *Acta Chir Scand* 1977; **143**: 177–183.

38. Oren S, Viskoper JR, Ilan S, Schlesinger M. Urinary albumin excretion in patients with familial Mediterranean fever: a pilot study. *Am J Med Sci* 1991; **301**:375–378.

39. Saatci U, Ozdemir S, Ozen S, Bakkaloglu A. Serum concentration and urinary excretion of β_2-microglobulin and microalbuminuria in familial Mediterranean fever. *Arch Dis Child* 1994; **70**:27–29.

40. Reuben DB, Wachtel TJ, Brown PC, Driscoll JL. Transient proteinuria in emergency medical admissions. *N Engl J Med* 1982; **306**:1031–1033.

41. Karlsson FA, Jacobson G. Renal handling of beta-2-microgloblin, amylase and albumin in acute pancreatitis. *Acta Chir Scand* 1979; **145**:59–63.
42. Shearman CP, Gosling P, Walker KJ. Is low proteinuria an early predictor of severity of acute pancreatitis? *J Clin Pathol* 1989; **42**:1132–1135.
43. Sawyer N, Wadsworth J, Wijnen M, Gabriel R. Prevalence, concentration and prognostic importance of proteinuria in patients with malignancies. *Br Med J* 1988; **296**:1295–1298.
44. Cooper EH, Forbes MA, Crockson RA, MacLennan IC. Proximal renal tubular function in myelomatosis. *J Clin Pathol* 1984; **37**:852–858.
45. Scarpioni L, Ballochi S, Bergonzi G, Cecchetin M, Dall'Aglio P, Fontana F, *et al*. Glomerular and tubular proteinuria in myeloma. Relationship with Bence Jones proteinuria. *Contrib Nephrol* 1981; **26**:89–102.
46. Luke DR, Sarnoski TP, Dennis S. Incidence of microalbuminuria in ambulatory patients with acquired immunodeficiency syndrome. *Clin Nephrol* 1992; **38**:69–74.
47. Kimmel PL, Umana WO, Bosch JP. Abnormal urinary protein excretion in HIV-infected patients. *Clin Nephrol* 1993; **39**:17–21.
48. Matthes KJ. Drug induced proteinuria. *Contrib Nephrol* 1981; **24**:109–114.
49. Dullaart RPF, Meijer S, Marbach P, Sluiter WJ. Effect of a somatostatin analogue, octreotide, on renal haemodynamics and albuminuria in acromegalic patients. *Eur J Clin Invest* 1992; **22**:494–502.
50. Levine D, Kreitzer P, Freedman S, Trachtmann H. Recombinant human growth hormone therapy does not increase microalbuminuria in children with short stature. *Clin Endocrinol* 1993; **39**:677–679.
51. Dawnay A, Wilson AG, Lamb E, Kirby JDT, Cattell WR. Microalbuminuria in systemic sclerosis. *Ann Rheum Dis* 1992; **51**:384–388.
52. Maddedu P, Ena P, Glorioso N, Cerimele D, Rappelli A. High prevalence of microproteinuria, an early index of renal impairment in patients with diffuse psoriasis. *Nephron* 1988; **48**:222–225.
53. Cecchi R, Seghieri G, Gironi A, Tuci F, Giomi A. Relation between urinary albumin excretion and skin involvement in patients with psoriasis. *Dermatology* 1992; **185**:93–95.
54. Wilkinson R, Milledge JS, Landon MJ. Microalbuminuria in chronic obstructive lung disease. *Br Med J* 1993; **307**:239.
55. Sklar AH, Chaudhery BA. Reversible proteinuria in obstructive sleep apnoea syndrome. *Arch Intern Med* 1988; **148**:87–89.
56. Winterborn MH, Bradwell AR, Chessner IM, Jones GT. The origin of proteinuria at high altitude. *Postgrad Med J* 1987; **63**:179–181.

8

The management of microalbuminuria in diabetes mellitus and essential hypertension

DIABETES MELLITUS

Introduction

As discussed in previous chapters, the presence of persistent microalbuminuria in insulin-dependent diabetic patients identifies a subgroup who will eventually progress to end-stage renal failure and who are at high risk of vascular disease. In non-insulin-dependent diabetes, the majority of patients with microalbuminuria will succumb prematurely to vascular disease, the minority who survive for long enough being at risk of progression to end-stage renal disease or cancer-related deaths. Thus microalbuminuria encompasses a spectrum of risk, the balance in insulin-dependent diabetes being towards renal disease and in non-insulin-dependent diabetes, as in the general population, to large vessel disease. The management of diabetic patients with microalbuminuria therefore has two main aspects: the reduction in the risk of nephropathy, which is of major importance in insulin-dependent diabetes, and the reduction in cardiovascular risk, which has predominance in non-insulin-dependent diabetes. In practice, both aspects are obviously interconnected, as measures to reduce renal risk may also reduce the risk of large vessel disease and vice versa.

Consideration of the features associated with microalbuminuria, as described in Chapter 4, and of the pathophysiological changes in diabetic nephropathy leads to a number of obvious therapeutic avenues worthy of exploration (Table 8.1). In dealing with the cardiovascular risk, in the absence of controlled trials specifically in diabetes, the assumption is made that measures which reduce the risk in the non-diabetic population will also be effective in people with diabetes.

Table 8.1 *Possible therapeutic avenues in reducing renal risk in microalbuminuria in diabetes mellitus*

Functional aspects	Structural aspects
Blood glucose	Glycation
Systemic blood pressure	Filtration surface area, charge and pore size
Intraglomerular pressure	Basement membrane thickness
Growth factors	Mesangial cell contraction
Angiotensins	
Kallekrins	
Prostaglandins	

Monitoring the effects of intervention

Current knowledge of the natural history of microalbuminuria suggests that in IDDM, the albumin excretion rate rises at approximately 20 % per year. Thus, on average it will take 12–13 years for the AER to rise from 20 µg/min to over 200 µg/min. Previous work suggests that, untreated, the average time for progression from persistent proteinuria to end-stage renal disease is 8–10 years[1]. Thus, a total of 20–25 years might elapse between the first appearance of microalbuminuria to the requirement for renal replacement therapy. Obviously, it becomes exceedingly difficult to carry out studies using the hard end-points of requirement for renal support, so that a variety of intermediate or surrogate renal end-points have been used in almost all studies to date. Little attention has been given as yet to cardiovascular morbidity or mortality, again because of the time constraints.

Most observers would accept a decline in glomerular filtration rate (GFR) as a good indicator of developing renal failure. Once persistent proteinuria is present, the GFR inevitably declines, so that at this advanced stage of diabetic nephropathy it is possible to use changes in GFR as a study end-point. However, patients with low levels of microalbuminuria may have a normal or even high GFR. Only as the albumin excretion approaches the proteinuric range does the GFR begin to fall. Thus, changes in GFR cannot be used as an end-point in monitoring intervention in microalbuminuria, unless the study continues for 5–10 years.

Serum creatinine concentrations are a less sensitive, albeit more readily measured, indicator of renal function than GFR. Serum creatinine levels are well within the normal range in microalbuminuria and in early proteinuria, only rising to pathological levels when persistent proteinuria has been present for some time. Thus, absolute levels of serum creatinine may not be useful until late in the course of diabetic nephropathy.

However, it is well recognised that there is an individual linear relationship between the inverse of the serum creatinine and time[2] and the slope of the line is used clinically to predict the time when renal replacement therapy will be required, and to monitor changes in renal function with treatment after the appearance of proteinuria. The regression slope of the line is only of prognostic value when the serum creatinine is > 200 μmol/l[2] and not in the microalbuminuric range when serum creatinine is within the normal range[3].

Other end-points, such as structural changes, are as yet relatively unresearched. Because of perceived risks in performing renal biopsies, particularly in patients with microalbuminuria, there is currently little cross-sectional or longitudinal information on the structural correlates of microalbuminuria.

Thus, most studies in microalbuminuria to date have used changes in albumin excretion as their major end-point, expressing the outcome either as absolute or fractional changes in albumin excretion rate or the number of patients developing persistent proteinuria. The strength and consistency of the association of persistent microalbuminuria to the later development of end-stage renal disease supports this approach, although it remains possible that alterations in albumin excretion do not reflect changes in glomerular filtration accurately.

Management possibilities

Blood glucose control

Acute effects in long-term diabetes

The effects of changes in glycaemia at diagnosis of diabetes and in short-term disease have been discussed in some detail in Chapter 4. Several studies have demonstrated that acute changes in blood glucose control are associated with short-term changes in albumin excretion in IDDM patients with relatively long duration of diabetes. Viberti and colleagues[4] studied seven patients with insulin-dependent diabetes, selected because of elevated albumin excretion rates, during ordinary metabolic control on subcutaneous injection therapy and after 48–72 h of improved blood glucose control using continuous subcutaneous insulin infusion (CSII). Mean 24-h blood glucose was around 11.5 mmol/l on injection therapy and 5.6 mmol/l on CSII. Urinary albumin excretion fell from 38.3 μg/min (range 18.3–70.8) on injection therapy to 17.4 μg/min (range 5.5–37.1) on CSII (Fig. 8.1).

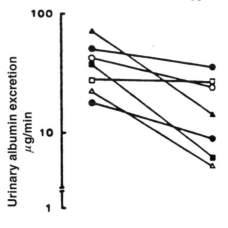

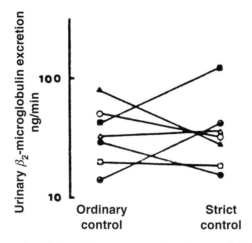

Fig. 8.1. Urinary excretion (log scale) of albumin and β_2-microglobulin during ordinary and strict glycaemic control in seven initially microalbuminuric IDDM patients who underwent continuous subcutaneous insulin infusion for one to three days. Reproduced from reference 4 with permission (copyright 1979 Massachusetts Medical Society; all rights reserved).

The same group also studied eight insulin-dependent diabetic patients whose 24-h urinary albumin excretion was normal under ordinary conditions of life[5]. However, the peak albumin excretion rate after standardised exercise on a bicycle ergometer was significantly higher in these patients than in matched non-diabetic control subjects (approximately 30 versus 6 µg/min). After a three-week period of improved glucose control using CSII, mean HbA_1 was reduced from 12.1 to 10.0 % and pre-exercise blood glucose from 13.1 to 7.6 mmol/l. Peak albumin excretion rate on CSII was also significantly reduced so that it was not different from that in the control subjects.

Mathiesen and colleagues[6] studied nine insulin-dependent diabetic patients with microalbuminuria (AER 30–300 mg/24 h) and ten matched normoalbuminuric diabetic subjects, before and after seven days of improved glucose control. Median blood glucose values were 15 mmol/l during poor control (induced by reduction in insulin dose in some cases) and 7 mmol/l during good control. Basal urinary albumin excretion was 60 (37–247) mg/24 h in the microalbuminuric group and 7 (4–30) mg/24 h in the normoalbuminuric patients. Urinary albumin excretion, fractional excretion of albumin, glomerular filtration rate, transcapillary escape rate of albumin and extracellular fluid volume did not change in either group during poor or good metabolic control.

Thus in established IDDM patients, the effect of acute changes in metabolic control seems controversial. In the studies cited above, patient age, duration of diabetes and blood glucose concentrations during 'good' and 'poor' control all appear similar. Albumin excretion rates, however were probably higher in the work by Mathiesen and colleagues[6]. Thus it may be that only lower levels of 'microalbuminuria' are reduced by short-term improvements in glycaemic control in long-duration diabetes.

Longer-term effects

Primary prevention The large scale Diabetes Control and Complications Trial (DCCT) was designed primarily to examine the effect of improved metabolic control on the development and progression of retinopathy, but details on albumin excretion during a 4-h day-time collection period were also gathered[7,8]. Seven hundred and twenty six insulin dependent diabetic patients, aged 13–39 years, duration of diabetes 1–5 years, with no retinopathy and with albumin excretion < 40 mg/24 h, entered the primary prevention cohort, and 715 with diabetes duration 1–15 years, with minimal retinopathy and albumin excretion < 200 mg/24 h entered the secondary prevention cohort. Randomisation with stratification by cohort was to conventional or intensive care. The entire cohort was followed for a mean of 6.5 years (range 3–9). A statistically significant difference in HbA_{1c} was maintained between the groups for the duration of the study, the mean in the intensively managed group being 7.2 % and in the conventionally treated group 9.1 % (upper limit of reference range 6.05 %). In the primary prevention cohort, the cumulative incidence of developing microalbuminuria was 16 % after nine years in the intensively treated group and 27 % in the conventionally treated group ($p = 0.04$, Fig. 8.2). The relative risk, adjusted for baseline AER, was 1.51 (95 % confidence limits 1.02–2.25) and the mean adjusted risk reduction by intensive therapy 34 % (95 % CI 2–56). In the secondary cohort, considering only those patients whose initial AER was < 40 mg/24 h (the vast majority), the cumulative incidence of microalbuminuria was 26 % after nine years in the intensively treated group and 42 % in the conventionally managed group ($p < 0.001$). The adjusted relative risk was 1.74 (95 % CI 1.26–2.39), giving a risk reduction on intensive therapy of 43 % (95 % CI 21–58). The cumulative incidence of more advanced microalbuminuria (AER > 100 mg/24 h) in the primary prevention cohort was 3.3 % after nine years in the intensively treated cohort and 7.0 % in the conventionally managed group (ns). In the secondary cohort, the equivalent cumulative incidences were 10.0 % and 20.2 %($p = 0.002$). The adjusted relative risk in the secondary cohort was 2.28 (95 % CI 1.35–3.85), with a mean reduction in absolute risk of 56 % (95 % CI 26–74). Only nine subjects in the primary cohort developed proteinuria, too few for statistical analysis. In the secondary cohort, the cumulative incidence of proteinuria was 5.2 % in the intensively treated group and 11.3 % with conventional care ($p < 0.01$). The adjusted relative risk was 2.27 (95 % CI 1.21–4.23), giving a mean reduction in absolute risk of 56 % (95 % CI 18–76).

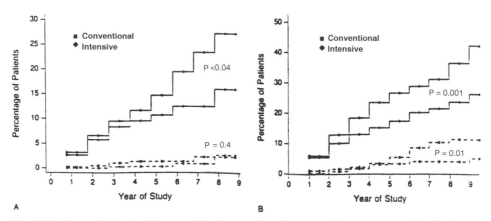

Fig. 8.2. Cumulative incidence of urinary albumin excretion > 300 mg/24 h (dashed line) and > 40 mg/24 h (solid line) in IDDM patients receiving intensive or conventional therapy in the DCCT: (A) primary prevention cohort; (B) patients with urinary albumin excretion < 40 mg/24 h in the secondary cohort. Reproduced from reference 7 with permission (copyright 1993 Massachusetts Medical Society; all rights reserved).

It is noteworthy, however, that despite apparently much improved glycaemic control, some DCCT patients in the intensively managed group did develop microalbuminuria and proteinuria. We await further analysis to determine if these were patients with relatively poor control within the intensively treated group: the 25th and 75th centile HbA_{1c} values within the group were approximately 6.5 % and 7.8 % , and less than 5 % of patients maintained HbA_{1c} within the reference range (< 6.05 %) for the duration of the study. Alternatively, other confounding factors, such as blood pressure, may be as or more important than glycaemic control. Data from the UK Microalbuminuria Study Group suggests that both glycaemic control and blood pressure are important driving factors in the transition from normo- to microalbuminuria[9].

There are no other primary prevention studies exactly equivalent to the DCCT, but in several smaller European studies the vast majority of patients have had normal albumin excretion or very low levels of microalbuminuria at entry (Table 8.2). These studies and a large amount of animal evidence would support the findings of the DCCT that improved glycaemic control is effective in reducing the risk of nephropathy when the albumin excretion rate is normal or only minimally elevated. One such study has also suggested that improved glycaemic control may also have a beneficial effect on renal structure in insulin-dependent diabetic patients[12]. In this study, 18 patients with initial overnight AER 15-200 µg/min were randomised to CSII or conventional therapy. Renal biopsies were performed at baseline and after 2–3 years. HbA_{1c} declined from 10.1 to 8.6 % in the CSII group but was unchanged at 10.1% in the conventionally managed group. Of the structural parameters measured, only basement membrane thickness increased significantly during the follow-up in the CSII group, whereas basement membrane thickness, matrix or mesangial volume fraction and matrix star volume all increased in the conventionally treated group. The increases in basement membrane thickness and matrix or mesangial volume fraction were significantly greater in the conventional group compared to the CSII group. Interestingly, the albumin excretion rates were stable throughout the study and similar in the two groups (CSII: 27 (10–75) versus 34 (12–98) µg/min; conventional group: 28 (12–67) versus 32 (12–83) µg/min), with albumin excretion actually being within the normal range in the majority of patients at baseline.

It is not clear whether the risk of progression of normoalbuminuria and low-level microalbuminuria is continuous with increasing glycated haemoglobin or whether there is a threshold, a level of glycated haemoglobin below which the risk is only marginally increased. One retrospective study from the Joslin clinic has suggested that there may be such a threshold[14]. In 1613

Table 8.2 *The effect of improved glycaemic control on the primary prevention of nephropathy in insulin-dependent diabetes*

Study	Patients with micro-albuminuria (%)	Duration of study (years)	Outcome	Achieved HbA$_{1c}$ CIT	Achieved HbA$_{1c}$ IIT	Non-diabetic reference HbA$_{1c}$
DCCT 1993[7]	0	9	Positive	9.1	7.1	<6.05
Reichard 1993[10]	28	7.5	Positive	8.5	7.1	<5.7
Dahl-Jorgensen 1988[11]	25	2 4	Negative Positive	10.5	9.0	<7.6*
Bangstad 1994[12]	33	2–3	Negative	9.7	8.6	<6.1
Kroc 1984[13]	33	0.75	Negative at normal AER Positive if AER >12 μg/min	10.3	8.0	<7.6*

*HbA$_1$.
CIT: conventional insulin therapy; IIT: intensified insulin therapy.
Reproduced from reference 146 with permission.

IDDM patients, the mean albumin:creatinine ratio and HbA_1 over three years were calculated and the risk of having microalbuminuria (albumin: creatinine ratio 17 μg/mg (1.87 mg/mmol) in men, 25 μg/mg (2.75 mg/mmol) in women) calculated at each level of HbA_1. A steep increase in risk of microalbuminuria was seen around a total HbA_1 of 10.1 % or HbA_{1c} of 8.1 % and further statistical analysis supported the concept of a threshold or breakpoint rather than a continuous relationship (Fig. 8.3). However, the Diabetes Control and Complications Trial Research Group have been unable to find such a threshold for nephropathy or retinopathy and suggest that there is no level of HbA_{1c} below which there is no risk of progression of complications[15]. In addition, the proportional rate of reduction of the risk of nephropathy was similar with proportional reductions in HbA_{1c} above and below 8.0 %. Although the concept of a threshold may be important in terms of the aetiology of nephropathy and also in terms of the risk–benefit ratio of improving glycaemic control, it is important to remember that all studies demonstrate that any improvement in glycaemic control, even though normoglycaemia is not achieved, is worthwhile in the primary prevention of nephropathy.

Only one study, in relatively young (mean age 49 years), non-obese, insulin-treated Japanese patients, has examined the effect of intensive insulin

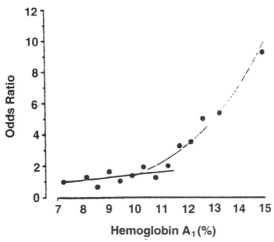

Fig. 8.3. Relationship between mean haemoglobin A_1 values and the risk of microalbuminuria in IDDM patients. Reproduced from reference 14 with permission (copyright 1995 Massachusetts Medical Society; all rights reserved).

therapy on the development of microvascular complications in NIDDM[16]. Fifty one patients with no retinopathy and AER < 30 mg/24 h at baseline were randomised to intensive or conventional insulin treatment. Mean HbA_{1c} over the six-year study was 7.1 % in the intensively treated group and 9.4 % in the conventionally managed group (upper limit of non-diabetic range 6.4 %). The cumulative percentage incidence of the development of microalbuminuria or proteinuria was significantly lower in the intensive group (7.7 versus 28.0 %, $p < 0.032$). This study would appear to support the results of the DCCT, although generalisation to obese, Caucasian NIDDM patients may not be appropriate.

Secondary prevention Only two studies have been designed specifically to examine the effect of improved blood glucose control on progression from microalbuminuria to proteinuria[17–19]. In addition, a sub-analysis of the 73 patients in the Diabetes Control and Complications Trial who were microalbuminuric at entry has also been published[8]. In the Steno study, 36 insulin dependent diabetic patients with microalbuminuria (AER 30–300 mg/24 h) were matched in pairs for AER, HbA_{1c} and gender and randomised to CSII or conventional insulin treatment[17]. Over 12 months there was a significant reduction in mean HbA_{1c} from 9.5 to 7.3 % (upper limit of reference range 6.3 %) in the CSII group, but unchanged control in the conventionally treated group. No significant changes in AER or GFR were seen over 12 months in either group, mean AER remaining around 62 (range 31–300) mg/24 h[17]. Results were also reported at two years[18]. Sustained improvement in metabolic control was seen in the CSII group (median HbA_{1c} 7.2 %) with unchanged control in the conventionally treated group (median HbA_{1c} 8.6 %). Proteinuria (AER > 300 mg/24 h) developed in five patients in the conventionally treated group but in none of the group on CSII. Absolute data on AER were not reported, albumin excretion being expressed as either fractional clearance of albumin or yearly percent change in AER from baseline. Fractional albumin clearance was unchanged over 24 months in the CSII group, at around 170 $x10^7$ but increased, apparently non-significantly, in the conventionally treated group from 160 to 360×10^7. Although there was no significant difference in these absolute values between the two groups, the change from baseline in fractional albumin clearance was significantly greater in the conventionally managed group. In addition, the mean percentage change per year in AER was significantly greater in the conventionally treated group, although the range of values in both groups was large (conventional: +7(–65 to +88) % per year, CSII: –9(–53 to

+43) % per year). In the discussion, the authors state that progression was most likely in patients with initial AER > 60 mg/24 h, the median increase in albumin excretion above this level being 45 % per year in the conventionally treated group. However, the effect of improved blood glucose control was apparently similar above and below this level. Glomerular filtration rate fell on CSII from 109 ± 4 to 99 ± 5 ml/min/m^2 and was unchanged on conventional therapy (116 ± 5 versus 114 ± 6 ml/min/1.73 m^2). The change in albumin excretion correlated with the mean HbA$_{1c}$ and with the change in mean blood pressure.

Although this study was formally terminated at the end of two years, and patients allowed to change treatment modality, an open follow-up over five years has been reported[20], in which data from these patients has been combined with results from similar patients in an earlier study. Although blood glucose control was improved in the conventionally treated groups over the entire study period, the fall in HbA$_{1c}$ was significantly greater in the intensively treated groups. However, in the last three years of follow-up, there was no significant difference in metabolic control. The change in albumin excretion correlated to the mean HbA$_{1c}$ over the entire follow-up period. No change in albumin excretion rate was observed in the 32 patients whose initial AER was 30–99 mg/24 h. In the 19 patients whose initial AER was 100–300 mg/24 h, clinical nephropathy developed in all ten of those originally on conventional therapy but in only two of the nine on intensive therapy. Arterial hypertension (> 160/95 mmHg) occurred in seven of the ten on conventional therapy and one of nine receiving intensive care. Glomerular filtration rate declined significantly by 23 ml/min/1.73 m^2 on conventional treatment and non-significantly by 13 ml/min/1.73 m^2 on intensive therapy. The authors speculated that the beneficial effects on renal function of improved glycaemic control may persist for longer than the actual period of improved control, suggesting perhaps that the mechanism of improvement is structural rather than haemodynamic.

The UK Microalbuminuria Collaborative Study Group have reported a similar trial over five years[19]. Seventy insulin-dependent diabetic patients with microalbuminuria (overnight AER 20–200 µg/min) were randomised to intensive or conventional treatment. Blood glucose control was significantly better in the intensively treated group for three years only, HbA$_1$ in the conventionally managed group being around 9.8 % and in the intensively treated group 8.9 % (upper limit of reference range 7.5 %). Six patients in each group developed proteinuria (AER > 200 µg/min), 16 in the conventionally treated group and 17 in the intensively treated group remained microalbuminuric, and 12 and 13 respectively became normoalbuminuric,

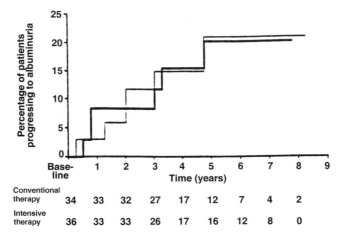

Fig. 8.4. Cumulative incidence of proteinuria in microalbuminuric IDDM
patients receiving intensive therapy (thick solid line) or conventional therapy (thin solid line). Reproduced with permission from
reference 19.

with no significant difference between the groups (Figure 8.4). At the end of
the study, the mean AER was 48.2 μg/min in the conventionally treated
group and 47.6 μg/min in the intensively managed group.

In the DCCT, perhaps as a result of the selection criteria, only 73 patients
had microalbuminuria (AER 40–200 mg/24 h) at entry[8]. Fortuitously, 35
were randomised to conventional and 38 to intensive care. In each treatment
group, eight developed proteinuria, with AER > 200 mg/24 h, and the rate
of change of albumin excretion was similar. Unfortunately, no details of
achieved glycaemic control or confounding variables such as blood pressure,
have been published.

A number of other studies, primarily designed to examine the effect of
improved glycaemic control on the progression of retinopathy, have also
reported on albumin excretion[10,11,13,21,22]. All have purported to show that
improved blood glucose control slows or prevents the progression of microalbuminuria to protcinuria. However, all of these studies included patients
with both normo- and microalbuminuria at entry, and in most, the majority
of patients had albumin excretion within the normal range at baseline (Table
8.2). A meta-analysis has concluded that intensive therapy apparently
reduces the risk of progression of nephropathy, with an odds ratio of 0.34
(95 % confidence limits 0.20-0.58)[23]. Again, however, almost all of the studies
analysed included patients with normoalbuminuria and microalbuminuria or
exclusively normal albumin excretion.

In 51 lean, relatively young, Japanese patients with microalbuminuria (AER 30–300 mg/24 h), intensive insulin therapy reduced the risk of proteinuria from 44.0 to 19.2 % ($p < 0.049$)[16]. The cumulative percentage incidences of proteinuria were 11.5 and 32.0 % in the intensive and conventional groups respectively ($p < 0.044$).

Thus, there is no doubt that improved glycaemic control is important in the primary prevention of diabetic nephropathy. The benefits of intensive management once microalbuminuria has developed are less apparent. The small size of the available studies suggests that a type 1[18] or type 2[8,19] statistical error is possible. However, if the DCCT and MCS patient groups[8,19] are combined, the sample size is large enough to detect a 33 % reduction in the risk of progression to proteinuria, a reduction of similar magnitude to that observed in many studies examining the effect of antihypertensive therapy (*vide infra*). Blood glucose control in the UK Microalbuminuria Collaborative Study[19] was not ideal, and no information on achieved glycated haemoglobin levels has been given for the microalbuminuric patients included in the DCCT[8]. It is thus possible that tighter glycaemic control, perhaps approaching normoglycaemia, may have an impact. However, such strict control has its inherent risks, particularly of hypoglycaemia[7]. Overall, there is currently no good evidence to suggest that improving glycaemic control affects progression of microalbuminuria to clinical proteinuria. Good glycaemic control is nonetheless an important factor in the management of the other microvascular complications which often co-exist.

These longer-term results must also be reconciled with the acute studies, where there is reasonable agreement that improving glycaemic control does reduce albumin excretion. Part of the explanation may be that in the acute studies, initial blood glucose levels were higher than in the later, longer-term studies. In the presence of glycosuria, the normal glomerular vasoconstrictive response to increased distal tubular flow is blunted, resulting in relative hyperfiltration[24]. In hyperfiltering normoglycaemic insulin dependent diabetic patients, during hyperglycaemia (blood glucose 12.5 mmol/l), both the filtration fraction and renal plasma flow are raised, whereas in normoglycaemia (blood glucose around 5 mmol/l), only the renal plasma flow is elevated[25]. The precise level of glycaemia at which the haemodynamic responses change is unknown, but it may be that when control is improved in patients in particularly poor glycaemic control, the initial fall in blood glucose, perhaps to levels under the renal threshold, leads to an acute reduction in filtration fraction with a consequent reduction in albumin excretion. However, if the basal blood glucose concentration is already under the renal threshold, then further lowering of the level will not reduce the filtration fraction and thus not affect albumin excretion. Such an argument might suggest that changes in albumin excretion immediately following acute reductions in blood glucose are secondary to acute haemodynamic effects and only occur when the blood glucose is reduced from a level above the renal threshold. In the primary prevention of nephropathy by good glycaemic control, these haemodynamic mechanisms may not be relevant. Instead, the prevention of structural damage, such as glycation, loss of the anionic charge on the basement membrane or retention of the normal pore size, may be of greater importance.

Antihypertensive agents

As discussed in Chapter 4, cross-sectional studies have shown that blood pressure is higher in microalbuminuric diabetic patients compared with matched normoalbuminuric patients. In addition, the progressive rise in albumin excretion from normo- to micro- to macroproteinuria is very closely linked to steadily increasing blood pressure. It is thus not surprising that much attention has been given to the effects of antihypertensive agents on the progression of all stages of diabetic nephropathy.

It is now widely accepted that when persistent proteinuria is present, reduction in systemic blood pressure reduces proteinuria but more importantly also slows the rate of decline in glomerular filtration. In general, blood pressure has been reduced to $< 140/90$ mmHg and the rate of fall of GFR from around 10 ml/min/year untreated to < 5 ml/min/year. Beneficial effects have been demonstrated with a variety of ACE inhibitors[26–30], diltiazem[26] and β-blockers[27–29,31,32], all with or without the addition of a loop or thiazide diuretic. There is some evidence to suggest that treatment with ACE inhibitors may be more beneficial than other agents in terms of greater slowing in the fall of GFR[28,29,33] and in reduction in the combined end-point of death, dialysis or transplantation[32], and that at least part of their effect may be independent of any lowering of blood pressure. But what of the earlier stage of microalbuminuria?

Acute and short-term effects of reduction of systemic blood pressure on microalbuminuria

Intravenous injection of antihypertensive agents appears to reduce resting albumin excretion immediately. In 12 insulin-dependent microalbuminuric diabetic patients, intravenous injection of clonidine 225 μg reduced systemic blood pressure from $125/79 \pm 13/8$ to $104/68 \pm 9/7$ mmHg and albumin excretion rate from 68 (31–369) to 46 (6–200) μg/min[34]. Fractional clearance of albumin fell in all patients whilst glomerular filtration rate was unchanged, at around 111 ± 11 ml/min/1.73 m². In IDDM patients with clinical proteinuria (AER 368–2979 µg/min), acute reduction of systemic blood pressure with intravenous clonidine also reduces the transcapillary escape rate of labelled albumin[35].

The short-term effect of antihypertensive medication on exercise-induced increases in albumin excretion is unclear. Two very small studies in normoalbuminuric and microalbuminuric IDDM patients have suggested that metoprolol has no effect on albumin excretion, despite significantly reducing the exercise-induced rise in systemic blood pressure[36,37]. However, captopril does reduce exercise-induced increases in albumin excretion in normoalbuminuric and microalbuminuric IDDM and NIDDM patients but not in non-diabetic control subjects[38]. The effect of captopril on albumin excretion appears to be greater than the effect of placebo and nifedipine, despite unchanged systemic blood pressure with captopril[39] (Fig. 8.5).

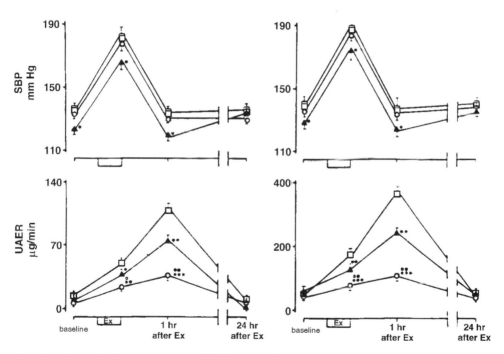

Fig. 8.5. Systolic blood pressure (SBP) and albumin excretion rate (UAER) ar rest, at end of standard exercise and 1 and 24 h after exercise performed after placebo (□), captopril (○) and nifedipine (▲) in normotensive, normoalbuminuric (left) and microalbuminuric (right) IDDM patients.
 * $p < 0.05$, ** $p < 0.01$, *** $p < 0.001$ versus placebo; ° $p < 0.05$, °° $p < 0.01$ versus nifedipine. Reprinted from reference 39 with permission.

Several studies have examined changes in albumin excretion over 4–6 weeks using a variety of antihypertensive agents. Entry criteria vary greatly, measures of albumin excretion are not standardised and systemic blood pressure quoted in different forms, making it difficult to compare studies. However, in general all conclude that reduction in systemic blood pressure over a few weeks leads to a significant reduction in albumin excretion in both insulin dependent and non-insulin dependent diabetes. In hypertensive, microalbuminuric NIDDM patients treated with enalapril or nicardipine for 4 weeks, the reduction in systemic blood pressure (from 167/100 to 140/88 mmHg) and albumin excretion (from 33 to 20 μg/min in a 2 h clearance study) was similar with the two agents[40]. A small group of 'normotensive' microalbuminuric IDDM patients were randomly assigned to six weeks' treatment with nifedipine slow release, captopril or placebo in fixed dose[41,42]. In the placebo group, systemic blood pressure and albumin excretion were unchanged. Blood pressure was reduced to a similar extent in the groups receiving active agents, from around 136/80 to 129/76 mmHg, but albumin excretion was unchanged in the group taking placebo, rose in those on nifedipine from 86 to 122 μg/min, and fell in those on captopril from 86 to 51 μg/min.

Although these studies are of some interest, it is obviously difficult to draw firm conclusions from such small studies conducted over a short time span.

Longer-term effects of lowering systemic blood pressure on microalbuminuria

No studies have reported on the primary prevention of microalbuminuria using antihypertensive agents. Four relatively large, randomised studies have examined the effect of antihypertensive medication on the progression of microalbuminuria to proteinuria over 2–5 years[43–48]. The European Microalbuminuria Captopril Study[43] and the work from the North American Microalbuminuria Study Group[44] were essentially similar. In both, microalbuminuric (AER 20-200 μg/min), normotensive (BP < 140/90 mmHg) IDDM patients were enrolled to a two year study comparing the effects of captopril 50 mg or placebo twice daily. Blood pressure at baseline was similar in both studies, 124/77 mmHg or mean arterial pressure around 92 mmHg. Mean arterial pressure was unchanged[43] or rose by 2.8 mmHg[44] over two years in the placebo-treated groups and fell by 3–7 mmHg in the groups taking captopril, a significant drop. AER rose in the placebo groups but fell in the captopril groups, the difference between the groups being significant. Significantly more patients taking placebo progressed to persistent proteinuria in both studies. In the American study, creatinine clearance was stable in those taking captopril but fell in the placebo-treated group, the difference between the groups again reaching significance.

The results from these two studies have been combined and analysed together, a procedure which seems valid given the close similarities between protocols[45] (Fig 8.6). The risk of progression to proteinuria over 24 months was reduced by 69.2 % (95 % CI 31.7–86.1; $p < 0.004$). The degree of risk reduction was essentially unchanged (62.9 %, CI 16.1–83.6) when adjusted for changes in mean arterial pressure with time, suggesting that the beneficial effects of captopril were at least in part independent of its blood-pressure-lowering effects.

In a similar study in non-insulin-dependent diabetes, 94 patients aged less than 50 years, with normotension (BP $< 140/90$ mmHg) and microalbuminuria (AER 30–300 mg/24 h) were randomised to enalapril 10 mg daily or

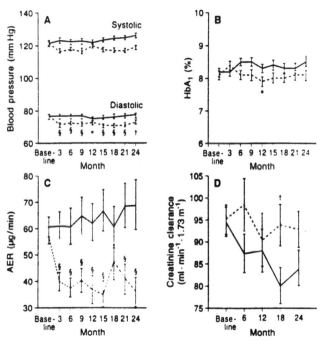

Fig. 8.6. Blood pressure (BP), HbA$_1$, albumin excretion rate (AER) and creatinine clearance (CrCl) in microalbuminuric IDDM patients receiving captopril (broken line) or placebo (solid line). Values are mean (AER geometric mean) ± SEM. * $p < 0.05$, $p < 0.01$, $p < 0.008$ for captopril versus placebo at a particular time point. Reproduced from reference 45 with permission (copyright Springer-Verlag).

placebo[46,47]. Follow-up was every 3–4 months for five years, nifedipine being added if blood pressure was consistently > 145/95 mmHg. In the enalapril treated group, a fall in AER was seen in the first year, from 143 to 122 mg/24 h. Thereafter, AER rose progressively, to a mean of 140 mg/24 h at the end of the study. In contrast, in the placebo group, AER rose throughout the study to a mean of 310 mg/24 h by the fifth year. Six patients in the enalapril group and 19 in the placebo group had final AER > 300 mg/24 h. Renal function, expressed as the reciprocal of the baseline serum creatinine, was stable in the enalapril group but declined by 13 % in the placebo group, this difference being significant (Fig. 8.7). Mean blood pressure in both groups was around 98 mmHg at the beginning of the study, remained stable in those given enalapril but rose from 99 to 100 mmHg ($p = 0.082$) in the placebo group. However, three patients in the enalapril group and nine in the placebo group required the addition of nifedipine. Interestingly, the frequency of the development of any retinopathy was less in the group taking enalapril (18 versus 29 %, $p < 0.002$).

In a fourth study, Sano and colleagues[48,49] have reported a four-year study of treatment with enalapril in microalbuminuric, normotensive (BP < 150/90 mmHg) non-insulin-dependent patients. Enalapril 5 mg/day significantly reduced the albumin excretion rate after four years from 115 ± 80 to 75 ± 45 mg/24 h, whereas in those receiving placebo AER rose from 94 ± 70 to 150 ± 145 mg/24 h. Other parameters, including systemic blood

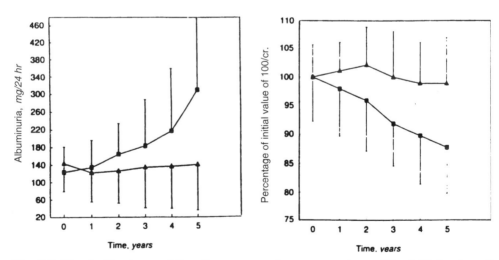

Fig. 8.7. The decline in renal function expressed as a percentage of the initial value of the reciprocal of the serum creatinine in microalbuminuric NIDDM patients treated with enalapril (▲) or placebo (●). Reproduced from reference 46 with permission.

pressure, creatinine clearance and glycated haemoglobin were similar in the treated and untreated groups and were unchanged for the duration of the study.

Thus, these four large studies demonstrate unequivocally that in both IDDM and NIDDM patients with microalbuminuria, treatment with anti-hypertensive medication will reduce albumin excretion and the risk of developing proteinuria. In addition, two of the studies have shown preservation of glomerular function with active treatment[44,46].

These reports consolidate and extend the findings of many previous, smaller and shorter studies demonstrating the effects of a variety of antihypertensive agents on albumin excretion. These are summarised in Table 8.3. In almost all of the studies, the use of antihypertensive medication reduced albumin excretion rate. The only exceptions were two small studies using the thiazide diuretic hydrochlorothiazide[52,55] and one using metoprolol[55]. Interestingly, in both these studies a positive effect of ACE inhibition was seen in parallel groups[52,55].

Effects of antihypertensive agents on albuminuria independent of systemic blood pressure – a specific intra-renal effect?

In several of the studies cited above, changes in albumin excretion have been observed with minimal or no change in systemic blood pressure, leading to the suggestion that antihypertensive agents and ACE inhibitors in particular may reduce albuminuria by a mechanism independent of changes in arterial pressure. An observational study of diabetic patients with end-stage nephropathy and gross proteinuria first suggested this[62] and work in microalbuminuric patients would support the concept.

Mathiesen and colleagues[53] followed 44 normotensive (mean blood pressure 127/78), microalbuminuric (AER 30–300 mg/24 h) IDDM patients for four years in an open, randomised controlled trial of captopril versus placebo. The initial dose of captopril of 25 mg daily was increased to a maximum of 100 mg daily in all treated patients, the aim being to prevent the expected rise in systemic blood pressure and, if possible, to lower diastolic blood pressure by 5 mmHg. Bendrofluazide 2.5 mg daily was added after 30 months. Perhaps surprisingly, clinic blood pressure was identical in the two groups throughout the study and remained remarkably constant over the four years; 24-h ambulatory blood pressure monitoring was performed only once, at 36 months. Diastolic blood pressure was significantly lower in those on active therapy at 0900 h and between 1900 and 2300 h, whilst systolic pressure was lower at 2100, 2300 and 0100 h. However, the mean 24-h

Table 8.3 *Studies examining the effects of antihypertensive agents on albumin excretion in microalbuminuric patients*

Study	Population	Duration (months)	Agent	Blood pressure		Result
				Initial	Final	
Marre[50]	IDDM and NIDDM	6	ACE	137/82	124/72	Pos
Marre[51]	IDDM and NIDDM	12	ACE	90[a]	86[a]	Pos
Hallab[52]	IDDM	12	ACE	94[a]	88[a]	Pos
			Thiazide	97[a]	90[a]	Neg
Mathiesen[52]	IDDM	48	ACE	127/78	127/78	Pos
MDNSG[54]	IDDM and NIDDM	12	ACE	102[a]	95[a]	Pos
			Ca	108[a]	99[a]	Pos
Lacourciere[55]	NIDDM	36	β-Blocker	159/95	152/80	Neg
			Thiazide	162/99	145/81	Neg
			ACE	158/95	146/81	Pos
Hermans[56]	IDDM	36	ACE	170/100	155/83	Pos
Slomowitz[57]	IDDM	4	ACE	130/77	123/72	Pos
Chan[58]	NIDDM	12	Ca	166/91	→	Pos
			ACE	174/92	→	Pos
Lebovitz[59]	NIDDM	36	ACE	101[a]	96[a]	Pos
Flack[60]	NIDDM	12	ACE	144/85	136/80	Pos
			Indapamide	144/85	135/77	Pos
Romero[61]	NIDDM	6	ACE	132/75	127/68	Pos

[a] mean arterial blood pressure, Pos: albumin excretion reduced, Neg: albumin excretion unchanged, ↓: blood pressure reduced by treatment.
ACE: angiotensin-converting enzyme inhibition; Ca: calcium channel blocking agent.

systolic (124 versus 127 mmHg) and diastolic (71 versus 75 mmHg) pressures were not statistically different (Fig. 8.8). Despite these very similar blood pressure levels over the four years, seven of the patients taking placebo but none of those taking captopril progressed to clinical proteinuria. Mean AER rose from 105 (77–153) to 166 (83–323) mg/24 h in the untreated group, but fell progressively from 82 (66–1060) to 57 (39–85) mg/24 h in those on captopril. GFR was unchanged in both groups throughout. Thus, this study would suggest that captopril may exert beneficial effects on renal function in diabetic nephropathy without changes in systemic blood pressure.

Wiegmann and colleagues[63] studied twelve normotensive, normoalbuminuric IDDM patients and eight patients with microalbuminuria (AER 20–200 µg/min) in a double-blind placebo-controlled study. Baseline casual systolic and diastolic blood pressure measurement were similar in the two groups, as were 24-h systolic (126 ± 2.7 versus 124 ± 2.4 mmHg) and diastolic (74 ± 1.9 versus 72 ± 1.9 mmHg) blood pressures after three months' treatment with captopril 25 mg three times a day or placebo. There was a substantial, although statistically non-significant, fall in 24-h AER on captopril, from 59 ± 29.8 to 27.7 ± 13.9 µg/min. Results were not given for the normoalbuminuric and microalbuminuric patients separately, although the change in AER was significantly correlated to the initial AER.

In the combined report of the Microalbuminuria Captopril Study Group[45], the magnitude of the reduction in the risk of progression from microalbuminuria to clinical proteinuria with ACE inhibitor treatment was similar before and after adjustment for differences in arterial blood pressure with time. This also supports the concept that the effect of ACE inhibition on progression is not simply a consequence of reduction in arterial blood pressure. These studies are in keeping with the results of meta-analyses which have included studies at all stages of diabetic nephropathy[64,65].

Possible mechanisms for an intra-renal effect of antihypertensive agents

In experimental diabetic glomerulosclerosis, single nephron glomerular filtration is raised, as a result of concomitant increases in glomerular plasma flow rate and mean glomerular capillary hydraulic pressure[66]. These early haemodynamic changes are thought by some to be primarily responsible for the subsequent development of diabetic glomerulopathy[67]. Afferent, efferent and total arteriolar resistance are all decreased in experimental diabetes, but the decrease is most marked in the afferent arteriole (Fig. 8.9). There is thus relative afferent arteriolar dilation, or efferent arteriolar constriction, so that mean glomerular capillary hydraulic pressure and the glomerular trans-

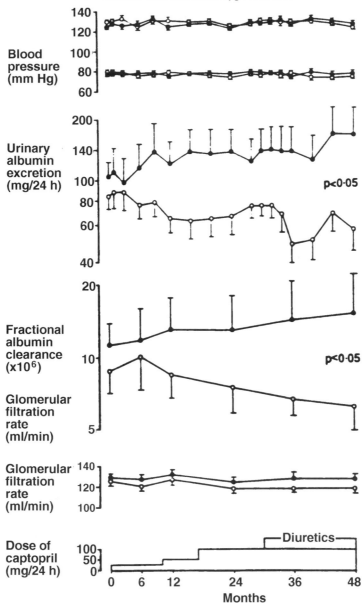

Fig. 8.8. Time course of mean arterial pressure, urinary albumin excretion, fractional albumin clearance and glomerular filtration rate in normotensive insulin-dependent diabetic patients with microalbuminuria. Twenty one patients received captopril (○) and 23 served as untreated control subjects (●). Mean ± SEM. Reproduced from reference 53 with permission.

A

Afferent
arteriole

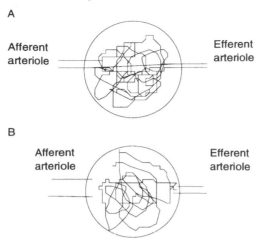

Efferent
arteriole

B

Afferent
arteriole

Efferent
arteriole

Fig. 8.9. Glomerular haemodynamics in normal (A) and diabetic animals
(B). In diabetes, afferent, efferent and total vascular resistance are
decreased, but the decrease is most marked in the afferent arteriole.
Thus, glomerular capillary hydraulic pressure and the glomerular
transcapillary pressure difference are increased.

capillary hydraulic pressure difference are increased[67]. After four weeks'
treatment with the ACE inhibitor enalapril, whole kidney glomerular filtration rate and single nephron glomerular filtration rate were similar in enalapril-treated diabetic and control diabetic animals[67]. However, because of a
significant fall in systemic blood pressure and in efferent arteriolar resistance,
the glomerular transcapillary hydraulic pressure difference was significantly
reduced in the enalapril-treated diabetic animals, to a level equivalent to that
in non-diabetic control animals. Animals given enalapril did not develop the
albuminuria or histological features seen in untreated diabetic animals
despite similar glycaemic control. This study has been interpreted as showing
that altered intra-renal haemodynamics are the cause of diabetic glomerulopathy, and that ACE inhibition can normalise the intrarenal hypertension
and prevent glomerulopathy even in the face of continuing glomerular hyperfiltration and hyperfusion.

Support for the above has come from several other studies. After 70 weeks
of therapy with either captopril or triple therapy (reserpine, hydralazine and
hydrochlorothiazide), efferent arteriolar resistance and mean glomerular
capillary hydraulic pressure were controlled in those animals receiving captopril but not in those on triple therapy[68]. Albumin excretion and the number
of sclerosed glomeruli were significantly greater in the animals on triple
therapy compared to those on captopril.

streptozotocin-diabetic rats after 10–15 days of diabetes before and during intravenous infusion of glycine[77]. In non-diabetic rats, glycine increased single nephron plasma flow and glomerular filtration rate. Basal single nephron plasma flow (SNPF) and SNGFR were similar in diabetic and non-diabetic animals, but infusion of glycine had no effect in the diabetic rats, suggesting loss of renal functional reserve. In animals given the ACE inhibitor enalapril, SNPF, SNGFR and ultrafiltration coefficient increased with glycine, whereas in animals given an angiotensin II receptor antagonist SNPF was unchanged and SNGFR slightly but significantly decreased. Thus, the restoration of renal functional reserve seen after administration of enalapril may not be due to ACE inhibition and the fall in angiotensin II but to other mechanisms such as an increase in bradykinin. Bradykinin is known to stimulate endothelium-derived relaxing factor, which in non-diabetic rats plays a major role in the renal response to amino acid infusion.

The effect of calcium channel blockers on intra-renal haemodynamics is controversial, some studies suggesting a relaxation of the afferent glomerular arteriole leading to increased intraglomerular pressure[78] whilst others suggest a relaxation of the efferent arteriole[79]. The class of calcium channel blocker used may be important: in animal models of hyperfiltration, verapamil and ACE inhibitors affect glomerular size and charge selectivity in a similar fashion[80] and in diabetic beagle dogs ACE inhibition and a diltiazem-like compound both decrease proteinuria to a similar extent through a comparable reduction of intracapillary pressure and mesangial matrix expansion[81]. Thus, calcium channel blockers other than nifedipine may be of use in diabetic nephropathy.

Trials comparing different classes of antihypertensive agents in humans

Few long-term human studies have compared the effects of different antihypertensive agents. These studies are difficult to carry out, as they require a precisely similar effect of the agents on systemic blood pressure. The largest study so far has been in 407 IDDM patients with advanced nephropathy[33], in which the addition of captopril to other antihypertensive therapy was associated with significant reductions in the risk of doubling of the serum creatinine, the rate of decline of creatinine clearance and in the risk of the combined end-point of death, dialysis or transplantation, compared with the addition of placebo. A smaller study in patients at a similar stage of nephropathy compared the effects of enalapril and metoprolol for a mean follow-up of 2.2 years[29]. The rate of decline in GFR was significantly less in those patients taking enalapril (2.0 versus 5.6 ml/min/year) and urinary albumin excretion was reduced by approximately 60 %. However, a small, two-year study comparing captopril and atenolol in IDDM patients with early clinical nephropathy found a similar effect on blood pressure, albuminuria and total proteinuria[82]. The rate of decline of GFR was also similar, around 4 ml/min/year.

In microalbuminuria, the largest comparative study included both normotensive and hypertensive insulin–dependent and non-insulin–dependent patients followed for one year[54]. Perindopril and nifedipine had similar effects on systemic blood pressure and albumin excretion. In another study, 21 microalbuminuric, normotensive (< 160/95 mmHg) IDDM patients were randomised to one year's treatment with enalapril 20 mg or hydrochlorothiazide 25 mg once daily[52]. Mean arterial pressure was similar before (around 98 mmHg) and after one year's treatment (88 mmHg) in the two groups. Mean urinary excretion of albumin fell from 59 (37–260) to 38 (14–146) mg/24 h with enalapril and from 111 (33–282) to 109 (33–262) mg/24 h with hydrochlorothiazide. In the last three months of the study, in the enalapril group five patients were persistently normoalbuminuric, 5 had low-level microalbuminuria and 1 high level microalbuminuria, whilst in the group taking hydrochlorothiazide the figures were one, three and six respectively.

A mixed population of hypertensive Chinese NIDDM patients with normal albumin excretion ($n = 44$), microalbuminuria ($n = 36$) and macroproteinuria ($n = 22$), were randomised to one year's treatment with enalapril or nifedipine, the doses being adjusted to lower the systolic blood pressure to < 140 mmHg[58]. Indapamide or frusemide were added if required to meet this target. Significantly more patients in the enalapril group required the addition of a diuretic. At one year, mean arterial blood pressure was similar in the two groups, whereas albuminuria decreased by 54 % in the enalapril group and by 11 % in the nifedipine group. Creatinine clearance fell similarly in the groups but serum creatinine rose by 20 % in the enalapril group compared with 8 % in the nifedipine group, a significant difference. This rather concerning rise in serum creatinine may have been related to acute haemodynamic changes and seems to be reversible.

One study in NIDDM patients, the majority of whom had normal albumin excretion or very low-level microalbuminuria[55], confirmed the beneficial effects of ACE inhibition with or without a diuretic on albumin excretion but, interestingly, failed to show any effect of metoprolol on albuminuria despite a significant fall in systemic blood pressure.

Two other very short and small studies showed contrasting results, one showing equivalent effects on microalbuminuria of enalapril and nicardipine[40] whilst the other showed a reduction in AER with captopril but an increase with nifedipine[41,42].

In a small study of hypertensive (> 170/105 mmHg), microalbuminuric NIDDM patients, subjects received either nitrendipine or enalapril for eight months[83]. There was a non-significant fall in systolic pressure but a significant fall in diastolic pressure with nitrendipine, and a significant fall in systolic pressure and a non-significant fall in diastolic pressure with enalapril. Excretion of albumin fell and excretion of epidermal growth factor rose significantly with enalapril treatment, whilst both parameters were unchanged with nitrendipine.

Thus, overall there is relatively strong evidence that ACE inhibition in the late stages of diabetic nephropathy has effects which are independent of a reduction in arterial pressure and are more efficacious than other classes of antihypertensive agents in terms of renal and patient survival. However, in microalbuminuria and early proteinuria, these superior benefits of ACE inhibition, compared with other classes of antihypertensive agents, have not been demonstrated clearly in controlled trials.

Possible deleterious effects of antihypertensive medication

Given that microalbuminuric diabetic patients already are more insulin resistant and have more extreme dyslipidaemias than their normoalbuminuric peers, the metabolic effects of antihypertensive drugs must be considered carefully. Thiazide diuretics may worsen glucose tolerance and dyslipidaemias, but the antihypertensive effect of a low dose is equivalent to higher doses and the metabolic effects may not be seen[84].

The Hypertension in Diabetes Study Group[85] reported the metabolic effects of two years' treatment with captopril or atenolol in a large group of hypertensive NIDDM subjects. Blood pressure reduction and rates of hypoglycaemia were similar, but weight increase was higher (2.3 versus 0.7 kg) and serum triglyceride levels non-significantly higher on atenolol. In addition, β-blockade may mask the warning signs of hypoglycaemia and worsen peripheral vascular disease.

ACE inhibitors and calcium channel blockers are generally regarded as being metabolically 'neutral' or even having a beneficial effect on glucose sensitivity. In a 12-week study of Chinese NIDDM patients, circulating levels of HbA_1 and apoB were reduced more by enalapril than nifedipine, whilst blood pressure reduction was significantly greater with enalapril[86]. In a similar study, 30 hypertensive NIDDM patients were treated for three months with either captopril, nifedipine or doxazocin[87]. A similar reduction in blood pressure was achieved with all three agents. Captopril and nifedipine were considered to be metabolically 'neutral', fasting plasma glucose and HbA_{1c} levels, and glucose, insulin and NEFA levels during an oral glucose tolerance test all being similar to untreated levels. Insulin-mediated glucose uptake, glucose oxidation and non-oxidative glucose disposal during a euglycaemic insulin clamp were also all unchanged from baseline and similar in these two treatment groups. However, after treatment with doxazocin, glucose and NEFA concentrations during the oral glucose tolerance test were lower, and glucose uptake and glucose oxidation during the clamp higher than in the untreated state, suggesting that the α-blocker had a beneficial effect on glucose and fat metabolism[87]. In IDDM, despite comparable hypotensive effects, atenolol and doxazosin had different metabolic effects: fructosamine and the total cholesterol:HDL cholesterol ratio rose with atenolol but not doxazocin[88].

An increase in serum creatinine may be observed soon after the introduction of an ACE inhibitor, particularly in NIDDM patients[58]. This may be due to immediate alteration in intrarenal haemodynamics but also to unmasking of atheromatous renal artery stenosis. The presence of peripheral vascular disease might identify patients at particular risk of a significant decline in renal function on commencement of an ACE inhibitor. Hyperkalaemia may also be a problem, perhaps relating to autonomic neuropathy and low serum renin and aldosterone levels.

Thus, when choosing an antihypertensive agent, the metabolic effects of the agents and potential interactions with other concomitant diseases should be considered (Table 8.4). Therapy should begin with a small dose which can be titrated upwards gradually, with frequent monitoring of renal function in the first few months.

Target blood pressure

Almost all of the studies described above have used a blood pressure level of < 140/90 mmHg as an entry criterion or as a target level of treatment. Justification for this cut-off comes from several studies showing that the rate of decline in GFR is greater above this level[89–91]. However, in many of the studies of microalbuminuric patients, it is clear that arterial pressure was reduced much below this level (Table 8.3). Thus it may be that introduction of antihypertensive medication when arterial blood pressure is < 140/90 mmHg may be beneficial, especially in younger patients. Use of age and gender-related centile charts may be worthwhile[92], beginning antihypertensive medication when the arterial pressure is above the 75th centile for age

Table 8.4. *Summary of the effects of different classes of antihypertensive agents*

Agent	Advantages	Possible disadvantages
ACEI	Reduce albumin excretion Preserve renal function No or +ve effect on insulin sensitivity No effect on NEFA ?Reduce serum lipids	Precipitous decline in renal function Hyperkalaemia
Ca channel blockers	Reduce albumin excretion[a] No effect on insulin sensitivity No effect on NEFA	No evidence on effect on renal function Peripheral oedema*
α-blockers	Reduce albumin excretion +ve effect on insulin sensitivity +ve effect on NEFA	No evidence on effect on renal function
β-blockers	Reduce albumin excretion Preserve renal function	Raise serum lipids Reduce insulin sensitivity
Thiazide diuretics		No effect on albumin excretion or renal function[b] Deleterious effect on lipids[b] Deleterious effect on insulin sensitivity[b]

ACEI: Angiotensin converting enzyme inhibitors.
*Dihydropyridine derivatives.
[a]Except nifedipine, [b]Except bendrofluazide 2.5 mg daily. +ve: Beneficial effect.

and sex, and aiming to lower it to < 50th centile. Alternative approaches are to reduce blood pressure to around 130/80 mmHg or indeed to commence ACE inhibitor therapy regardless of the level of blood pressure. Our current pragmatic approach is to begin therapy if systemic blood pressure is > 130/80 mmHg in younger patients and > 140/90 mmHg in older subjects. In younger subjects, angiotensin-converting enzyme inhibitors are the first line choice unless there are contraindications to their use. In older patients, ACE inhibitors should be used cautiously, commencing with a small dose and titrating upwards gradually to the maximum tolerated dose, with frequent checks on serum creatinine and potassium. If ACE inhibitors are not tolerated or are contraindicated, calcium channel-blocking drugs or alpha-blocking agents should be considered.

In the primary prevention of nephropathy, treatment of normotensive, normoalbuminuric patients with ACE inhibitors is of interest because of their effects on renal haemodynamics. Indeed, a three month study has shown that treatment with ACE inhibitors reduces fractional albumin excretion and filtration fraction in such patients[93]. Currently however it is not realistic to treat all IDDM patients from diagnosis with ACE inhibitors in the hope of preventing or delaying nephropathy in only a minority.

Dietary manipulations

Low protein diet

Experimental evidence suggests that dietary protein contributes to the rise in intraglomerular pressure and the increase in glomerular filtration rate observed in diabetes and which is thought to be implicated in the development of glomerular sclerosis[94,95]. Manipulation of dietary intake has therefore been tried therapeutically. In clinical proteinuria, a reduction of protein intake by approximately half has been shown to reduce proteinuria in the short term[96,97] and the rate of decline of GFR in the longer term[98–100]. Few studies have included microalbuminuric patients.

In a small study of 12 IDDM patients, with either normal albumin excretion or microalbuminuria, dietary change from their usual protein diet (about 103 g protein/day) to a low protein diet (about 45 g/day, half from animal and half from vegetable sources) lowered AER, GFR and filtration fraction whilst renal plasma flow and renal vascular resistance were similar after three weeks[101]. In eight microalbuminuric IDDM patients, a reduction in protein intake of approximately half to 47 g protein/day for three weeks significantly lowered AER, glomerular filtration rate and fractional excretion of albumin[102]. The effects of reducing protein intake may be most marked on patients who are initially hyperfiltering[103].

In a two-year study, 30 IDDM patients with initial overnight AER 10–200 µg/min were randomised to continue their usual protein diet (1.05 ± 0.32 g protein/kg body weight/day) or to a low protein diet[104]. The diets were isocaloric, with a similar amount of vegetable protein, but more car-bohydrate in the low protein diet. The target of the low protein diet was an intake of 0.6 mg/kg/day; however, the actual mean intake was 0.79 ± 0.16 mg/kg/day, significantly less than on the usual protein diet. Only 7 out of 14 patients consistently achieved an intake < 0.8 mg/kg/day. Baseline AER was around 36 µg/min in the low protein diet and 31 µg/min in the group continuing on their usual diet. There was a small but apparently significant drop in AER to 30 µg/min over the two years in those patients on the lower protein diet, whilst AER was unchanged in the group on the usual diet. However, AER, expressed as absolute values or as a percentage of baseline, was not statistically different in the two groups at any time point over the two years (Fig. 8.10). In the subgroup of patients with baseline AER > 20 µg/min, AER in those on the low protein diet fell from 91 to 70 µg/min, but was steady at 49 µg/min in those consuming their usual diet. Systolic and diastolic blood pressure in the two groups were similar at baseline (130/ 80 mmHg) but mean arterial pressure tended to be higher in the group on reduced protein intake, the overall difference in mean arterial pressure between the two groups being 3.5 mmHg ($p < 0.09$). In multiple regression analysis, the prevailing mean arterial pressure and duration of diabetes independently contributed to the progression of microalbuminuria, whereas the decrease in dietary protein intake reduced microalbuminuria ($p < 0.005$). When the change in AER was adjusted for mean arterial pressure and duration of diabetes, the mean fall in AER in the low protein group was 26 %, compared with a 5 % increase in the usual diet group (difference between the groups $p < 0.005$). The low protein diet led to a fall in effective renal plasma flow and GFR (indirectly via the effects on ERPF) at one year, with only minor changes in renal haemodynamics occurring in the second year.

Thus, there is a limited amount of evidence to suggest that reducing the total amount of dietary protein intake reduces microalbuminuria in the short and long term. The strength of the evidence and the difficulties with com-pliance perhaps suggest that moderating protein intake perhaps to around 1 g/kg body weight/day, rather than true restriction, is appropriate.

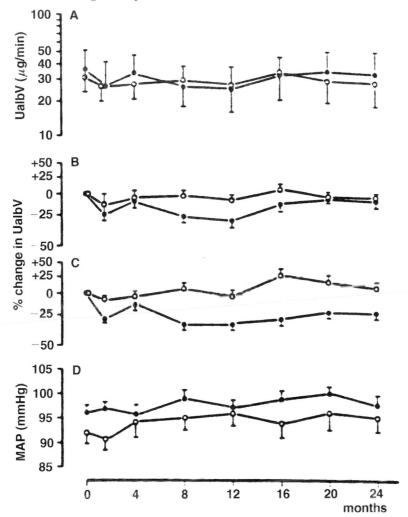

Fig. 8.10. The effects of reduction of dietary protein intake in IDDM patients from 1.05 (○) to 0.79 (●) g/kg body weight/day. (A) Urinary albumin excretion rate (UalbV). (B) Percentage change in urinary albumin excretion rate, unadjusted. (C) Percentage change in urinary albumin excretion rate adjusted for mean arterial pressure and diabetes duration. (D) Mean arterial blood pressure throughout the study. Mean ± SEM. Reproduced form reference 104 with permission.

Type of dietary protein

The source of dietary protein, in addition to the total amount, may also be important. In a short study in small numbers of insulin-dependent patients with microalbuminuria or proteinuria, albumin excretion fell after eight weeks on a diet where the major source of protein was predominantly vegetable rather than animal[105]. The fall in albumin excretion was not accompanied by changes in glycaemic control or blood pressure, although the total dietary protein intake was slightly but significantly lower on the vegetable diet.

In another study, a group of normoalbuminuric insulin-dependent diabetic patients followed three diets each for three weeks: usual protein diet (1.4 g protein/kg body weight/day); test diet (chicken and fish substituted for red meat at 1.4 g/kg body weight/day); low protein diet (0.5 g/kg/day)[106]. In the group as a whole, isotopically measured GFR fell significantly on the test and the low protein diets, and to a similar extent. On subgroup analysis, it was apparent that the change in GFR was confined to those patients who were hyperfiltering at baseline, GFR falling from around 160 to 130 ml/min/1.73 m^2. Albuminuria was unaffected by the dietary changes.

Fatty acids

Because of the increased cardiovascular mortality and the disadvantageous lipid and lipoprotein profiles in patients with microalbuminuria, it would seem appropriate to recommend a diet low in saturated and high in polyunsaturated fats such as linoleic acid. However, the renal effects of linoleic acid are controversial. In normal subjects, a high dietary intake of linoleic acid has been reported to stimulate creatinine clearance, perhaps by increasing the synthesis of vasodilatory prostaglandins[107]. A two-year study has been performed in 38 insulin-dependent diabetic patients with overnight AER 10–200 μg/min[108]. Patients were randomised to a diet with increased polyunsaturated:saturated fatty acid ratio of 1.0 by replacement of saturated fat with linoleic acid products or to continue their usual diet (polyunsaturated:saturated ratio 0.6). In the group consuming their usual diet, albumin excretion increased non-significantly by 16 % during the second year, whereas in the group taking a modified diet, albumin excretion rose 58 % in the first year and 55 % in the second year. Glomerular filtration rate, mean arterial blood pressure and glycated haemoglobin were similar in the two groups.

A three-week study in ten microalbuminuric NIDDM patients of a diet rich in monounsaturated fat found no effect on 24-h blood pressure, albumin excretion rate, glycaemic control, and serum lipid levels, although the LDL:HDL rato was reduced[109]. Thus increasing the ratio of dietary polyunsaturated:saturated fat intake does not have a beneficial effect on renal function and may even be deleterious.

In a double-blind crossover study in IDDM patients with high microalbuminuria or proteinuria, the effects of eight weeks' supplementation with cod-liver oil or olive oil on endothelial permeability, blood pressure and plasma lipids were compared[110]. Significant reductions in blood pressure and transcapillary escape rate of albumin were seen with cod-liver oil but not olive oil. Plasma HDL concentrations increased and VLDL-cholesterol and triglycerides decreased with cod-liver oil whilst LDL-cholesterol concentrations were unchanged. In contrast, with olive oil, LDL-cholesterol decreased, VLDL cholesterol and triglycerides increased and HDL-cholesterol was unchanged. GFR and albumin excretion were unaffected by supplementation with either oil. Thus the overall value of such dietary manipulation is uncertain.

Antiprostaglandins

It has been suggested that hyperfiltration and raised intraglomerular pressure are at least partly dependent on high concentrations of vasodilatory prostaglandins. In two small studies of IDDM patients with nephropathy (AER 200–972 µg/min and GFR 94–155 ml/min/1.73 m^2)[111] and microalbuminuria[112], urinary excretion of prostaglandin E_2 was significantly elevated compared with normoalbuminuric IDDM patients. Following three days' treatment with indomethacin 150 mg/day, urinary prostaglandin E_2 excretion, AER and fractional clearance of albumin were all significantly reduced. GFR was reduced in proteinuric but not microalbuminuric patients.

In another small study of young insulin-dependent diabetic patients with microalbuminuria, indomethacin (1 mg/kg) given orally 2 h before a standard exercise test significantly reduced the rise in AER with exercise, without an effect on systemic blood pressure[37].

It is obviously difficult to draw long-term conclusions from these very short studies.

Aldose reductase inhibitors

An increase in aldose reductase mRNA and activity and increased glomerular accumulation of sorbitol[113] has been reported in experimental diabetes. Albumin excretion is reduced, but not to normal, by two structurally different aldose reductase inhibitors, ponalrestat and sorbinil, given from the time of induction of streptozotocin diabetes[114]. Both inhibitors also reduced the glomerular production of prostaglandins, but again not to normal, and without an effect on glomerular filtration rate. This suggests that the effect of aldose reductase inhibitors on albumin excretion is not mediated by changes in glomerular filtration brought about by reduction in glomerular production of prostaglandins.

Other investigators have examined the effects of the aldose reductase inhibitor tolrestat begun two months after the induction of streptozotocin diabetes in animals with low (0.2–1.0 mg/24 h) and high (1.9–5.9 mg/24 h) rates of albumin excretion[115]. After six months, albumin excretion was reduced only in the group with initially low rates. However, total proteinuria was reduced in both groups. In another study, using male Sprague–Dawley streptozotocin diabetic rats, sorbinil 20 and 50 mg/kg for three months, had no effect on albuminuria, kidney weight or glomerular filtration rate, despite completely preventing renal cortical accumulation of sorbinil[116].

In a six-month, placebo-controlled study of the effects of tolrestat 200 mg/day in 20 IDDM patients with microalbuminuria (AER < 300 µg/day), GFR fell from 158 to 124 ml/min/1.73 m^2 on active treatment whilst renal plasma flow was unchanged; thus filtration fraction fell[117]. This was accompanied by a significant fall in AER from 219 ± 32.5 to 159 ± 19 mg/24 h, with a significant correlation between GFR and AER in the group taking tolrestat only. All parameters remained constant on placebo treatment.

Thus the effects of aldose reductase inhibitors are unclear and their clinical use is limited because of side-effects. We await trials of a new generation of agents with interest.

Inhibition of advanced glycation end-product formation

The formation of advanced glycation end-products can be measured by collagen-related fluorescence at specific wavelengths. In streptozotocin diabetes in the rat, fluorescence is increased in aorta and kidney[118]. Treatment with aminoguanidine prevents the increase in fluorescence in aorta, isolated glomeruli and renal tubules, and also prevents the rise in albuminuria and expansion of mesangium without affecting basement membrane thickness.

In chronically hypertensive, diabetic rats, aminoguanidine decreases the urinary albumin excretion rate by 75 %, without an effect on blood pressure[119]. Work from another group has suggested that eight weeks' treatment with aminoguanidine has no effect on urinary albumin excretion in the streptozotocin diabetic rat, but does reduce the clearance of radiolabelled iodine in various organs, including the eye, muscle and skin, but not lung[120].

Aminoguanidine also prevents the formation of interleukin-1-induced nitrite formation and cGMP accumulation, suggesting that aminoguanidine inhibits the formation of nitric oxide and may therefore be useful in preventing the vascular complications of diabetes[121,122].

Work with inhibitors of cross-linking is currently in progress in proteinuric diabetic patients.

Heparin and glycosaminoglycans

Heparin treatment has been shown to ameliorate proteinuria and histological changes in several experimental models of mesangioproliferative disease, including streptozotocin diabetes[123,124]. The mechanism of action of heparin is unclear, but heparin is known to stimulate the synthesis and sulphation of heparan sulphate proteoglycans in endothelial cells *in vitro* and to inhibit glomerular epithelial and mesangial cell proliferation, possibly via interactions with a variety of growth factors[125–128].

One human study has been reported of microalbuminuric IDDM patients[129]. Both unfractioned and whole heparin significantly reduced albumin excretion in a three-month treatment period. However, in a six-month study in streptozotocin diabetic rats, although heparin treatment prevented the increase in basement membrane thickness and mesangial volume classically seen in diabetes, albumin excretion was increased ten-fold with heparin[130]. Thus the value of heparin treatment remains unclear.

The use of the naturally occurring glycosaminoglycan sulodexide, which is extracted from porcine intestinal mucosa and which contains a fast-moving heparan-like fraction, has also been explored. Twelve hypertensive, insulin-treated NIDDM patients with either micro- or macroalbuminuria participated in a double-blind placebo-controlled study with four months active treatment[131]. Plasma fibrinogen levels were reduced significantly with active treatment, whilst a non-significant reduction in systolic blood pressure was observed. Albumin excretion decreased significantly on active treatment, and in the group given sulodexide first, AER remained reduced during the subsequent four month treatment with placebo. However, these results may have been influenced by two patients in whom very large changes in AER occurred. Further work with these compounds is obviously required.

Lipid lowering agents

Dyslipidaemias are common in diabetic patients with proteinuria and may contribute to the high cardiovascular mortality in patients with nephropathy. The presence of lipid abnormalities in diabetic patients with microalbuminuria suggests that the dyslipidaemia may not simply occur secondary to the renal disease but is an integral part of the process. Several studies[132,133,134], including several in diabetes[49,135,136] suggest that the hyperlipidaemia may contribute to the development and progression of renal disease. One three-month study has examined the effects of simvastatin in proteinuric IDDM patients[137]. There was a significant reduction in serum total- and LDL-cholesterol on active treatment, but no change in albuminuria or glomerular filtration rate. In a two-year, placebo-controlled study of proteinuric NIDDM patients, lovastatin was given in a dose sufficient to reduce total serum cholesterol to < 5.2 mmol/l[138]. Total serum cholesterol was reduced from a mean of 6.6 to 4.9 mmol/l, LDL cholesterol from 4.3 to 3.0 mmol/l, HDL cholesterol was unchanged at 1.1 mmol/l and triglycerides unchanged at 2.2 mmol/l. GFR was unchanged in patients receiving lovastatin but fell significantly in those taking placebo (Fig. 8.11).

Zhang and colleagues[139] performed a double-blind, randomised, cross-over study of 12 weeks' treatment with pravastatin 20 mg or placebo in 20 microalbuminuric IDDM patients. Plasma total cholesterol (5.4 versus 4.8 mmol/l) and LDL-cholesterol (3.2 versus 2.6 mmol/l) were significantly reduced on active treatment, but albumin excretion remained unchanged at around 65 μg/min. It is perhaps optimistic to expect changes in albumin excretion in such a short time, and over much longer periods, in both IDDM and NIDDM patients, the total serum cholesterol concentration is significantly related to percent changes in albumin excretion rate[49,140]. Intriguingly, in addition, in two studies in NIDDM patients with microalbuminuria or proteinuria, treatment with ACE inhibitors has apparently led to a significant reduction in serum total cholesterol levels[140,141], along with a beneficial effect on albumin excretion and renal function. The mechanism of action, and whether this is a direct effect or simply secondary to beneficial effects on renal function, remains unknown[142]. However, the data adds weight to the argument that ACE inhibitors have beneficial metabolic effects. Further work is obviously needed.

Growth factor antagonists

A role for many growth factors has been suggested in the development of diabetic nephropathy, in particular for growth hormone and insulin-like growth factor 1 (for review see Flyvbjerg and colleagues[143]). However, little work has been done in human diabetic nephropathy. In one study, the synthetic analogue of somatostatin, octreotide, was infused acutely in normotensive, normoalbuminuric insulin-dependent diabetic patients. GFR and renal plasma flow were reduced, whilst filtration fraction and total renal resistance rose[144]. Urinary albumin excretion, blood pressure and blood glucose levels were unchanged and plasma growth hormone and glucagon levels were suppressed. The reductions in GFR and renal plasma flow corre-

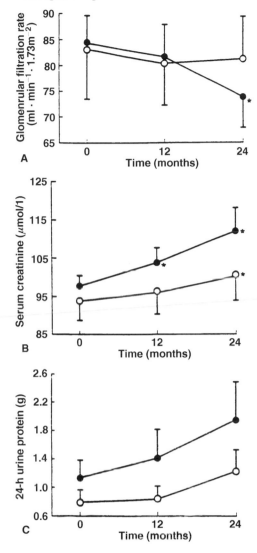

Fig. 8.11. Changes in glomerular filtration rate (A), serum creatinine (B) and 24-h urine protein excretion (C) in proteinuric NIDDM patients taking lovastatin (○) or placebo (●). $*p < 0.025$ versus pre-treatment. Reproduced from reference 138 with permission (copyright Springer-Verlag).

lated to the fall in circulating glucagon levels. An antidiuretic effect of the drug was also observed, with no change in arginine vasopressin, atrial natriuretic peptide, angiotensin II or aldosterone. In a nine month study of the long-acting somatostatin analogue somatulin, in hyperfiltering IDDM patients, GFR and RPF were significantly reduced after three months' active treatment compared to placebo[145]. However, after nine months, no significant differences in GFR, RPF or AER were seen between the treatment groups.

It is likely that major advances will arise in this field of work in the future.

Other management factors

Patients with microalbuminuria are more likely to have evidence of other microvascular complications of diabetes and are at higher risk of cardiovascular disease. Screening for and management of retinopathy, neuropathy and peripheral vascular disease should thus be undertaken with special care, and efforts made to reduce cardiovascular risk factors, particularly smoking and dyslipidaemias. As discussed above, this may also reduce the rate of progression of the renal disease. Because of the very high risk of large vessel disease, an argument could be made for prophylaxis with aspirin[146].

Overall conclusions and practical management of diabetic patients with microalbuminuria

For both IDDM and NIDDM patients, there is now good evidence that active treatment, particularly with antihypertensive agents, will reduce the rate of progression to proteinuria, and some evidence that the rate of decline of GFR is also slowed. The effect of improving blood glucose control is currently uncertain and a reduced protein intake has been shown to be beneficial only in the relatively short term. The use of all other agents is currently limited to trials. It should be remembered that no trial has yet shown any cardiovascular benefit. This is particularly important for patients with non-insulin-dependent diabetes, where the risk of large vessel disease vastly outweighs the risk of end-stage renal disease. However, there is no *a priori* reason why we should not aim for a reduction in classical cardiovascular risk factors. Plans of management for microalbuminuric diabetic patients are shown in Tables 8.5 and 8.6. In the choice of therapeutic agents, it is important that deleterious metabolic effects, particulary on insulin sensitivity and lipid levels, are avoided if possible.

ESSENTIAL HYPERTENSION

It is perhaps surprising that, since Parving and colleagues observed increased albumin excretion in insufficiently treated benign essential hypertension[147], there has been relatively little research into the impact of treatment of microalbuminuria on the clinical outcome of essential hypertension.

Table 8.5. *Management of microalbuminuria in IDDM*

Objective

Reduce risk of end-stage renal disease
Reduce risk of cardiovascular disease
Reduce impact of other complications

Aims
Normal albumin excretion

Targets
?HbA_{1c} less than 7.5%
Blood pressure <75th centile for age and sex
  (maximum 140/90 mmHg; ACE inhibitors first line)
Moderate dietary protein intake
  (1 g/kg body weight/day)
Non-smoking
Serum total cholesterol <5.2 mmol/l; LDL-cholesterol <3.9 mmol/l
?Aspirin

Table 8.6. *Management of microalbuminuria in NIDDM*

Objective
Reduce risk of premature vascular death
Reduce risk of end-stage renal disease

Aims
?Normal albumin excretion rate

Targets
Blood pressure <140/90 mmHg (ACE inhibitors with caution)
Serum total cholesterol <5.2 mmol/l; LDL-cholesterol <3.9 mmol/l
Non-smoking
Aspirin
?HbA_{1a} <7.5%

Pedersen and Mogensen[148] examined the impact of two months' treatment with the beta blocker alprenolol in 20 patients with moderate to severe hypertension. Left ventricular hypertrophy was present in over 50 % of cases, and a similar proportion required the addition of hydrallazine to achieve adequate blood pressure control. Blood pressure reduction was accompanied by falls in albumin excretion, although those whose diastolic pressure fell below 100 mmHg achieved lower albumin excretion rates. The improvements were not accompanied by changes in renal plasma flow (RPF) or glomerular filtration rates (GFR), and neither renal haemodynamic measure was correlated with albumin excretion. A later study from the same group[149] suggested that long-term propranolol treatment does not abolish exercise-induced albuminuria but is associated with a modest reduction in β_2-microglobulin secretion, and an exaggerated fall in GFR and RPF.

This in part can be interpreted as a demonstration that the mechanism of exercise-induced protein excretion is complex, and the consequence not only of systemic and renal haemodynamic changes, but also of changes in capillary permeability and tubular function, in part mediated by prostaglandin and the renin–angiotensin–aldosterone systems. This is supported by the lack of change in albuminuria despite altered GFR and RPF, and other reports of reductions in AER in response to non-steroidal anti-inflammatory drugs in salt-replete healthy subjects basally and following submaximal exercise, without accompanying changes in blood pressure and renal haemodynamics[150,151]. Notwithstanding these findings, effective antihypertensive treatment in general seems to reduce microalbuminuria in mild to moderate essential hypertension.

More recent reports have attempted to examine whether the type of hypotensive agent is important in determining the change in albumin excretion. At present β-adrenergic blockers have been studied in most detail. Although the pharmacological properties of these agents can vary according to their degree of water or lipid solubility, cardioselectivity, and intrinsic sympathomimetic activity (ISA), they do not modify albuminuria in normotensive normoalbuminuric healthy subjects, regardless of variation in the aforementioned properties. The overall impression is that β-blockers do reduce microalbuminuria when they lower blood pressure, although not in normoalbuminuric hypertensive subjects and perhaps less with atenolol than with other less hydrophilic agents such as metoprolol and the specifically cardioselective agent bisoprolol[152–156].

The role of metoprolol in reducing microalbuminuria (from 18.6 to 10.2 µg/min) has been demonstrated over a seven-year period, in association with good blood pressure control and restoration of echocardiographic left ventricular hypertrophy to normal[156]. GFR fell at the same rate as an untreated age-matched control group. Although the addition of thiazide diuretics and hydrallazine was required in several cases, this is to date the only long-term demonstration of the beneficial impact of any antihypertensive treatment on both cardiac and renal function.

The effect of the dihydropyridine group of calcium channel blockers has only been studied for periods of up to three months. Nifedipine, nitrendipine and nicardipine appear not to influence albumin excretion[154,157,158], whereas reductions in microalbuminuria have been noted with isradipine and felodipine[159,160]. The pharmacological characteristics of these latter two agents is not dramatically different, although it is feasible that less reduction in myocardial contractility could explain why they reduced albuminuria.

As in diabetes, short-term studies of up to three months have raised the possibility of a specific effect of ACE inhibitors in reducing albuminuria because of preferential reductions in efferent arteriolar tone. Enalapril, captopril, lisinopril and ramipril have all been demonstrated to reduce blood pressure and albuminuria[152–154,157,160], with two studies suggesting that this was a specific class effect independent of changes in blood pressure[153,154]. However, at least two short-term studies found that ACE inhibition in essential hypertension reduced blood pressure without affecting albuminuria[161,162], and the differential benefit in albuminuria over ß-blockers may be no longer evident after 12 months' treatment[152].

One study has shown that α-adrenergic blockade with doxazosin reduces both blood pressure and albuminuria over three months[160], whereas no such effect was noted with thiazide diuretics[154].

Thus, at present there is no definitive proof that ACE inhibitors exert specific long-term effects on renal function in essential hypertension which offer any advantage over virtually all other antihypertensive agents. Long-term studies addressing this and the more important question of the relationship between reduced albuminuria and cardiovascular outcome in essential hypertension are clearly necessary.

References

1. Watkins PJ, Blainey JD, Brewer DB, Fitzgerald MG, Malins JM, O'Sullivan DJ, Pinto JA. The natural history of diabetic renal disease. *Q J Med* 1972; **164**:437–456.
2. Jones RH, Hayakawa H, MacKay JD, Parsons V, Watkins PJ. Progression of diabetic nephropathy. *Lancet* 1979; **1**:1105–1106.
3. Mackin P, MacLeod JM, Jones SC, Marshall SM. Serum creatinine is not a reliable predictor of renal function in patients with long duration IDDM and microalbuminuria. *Diabet Med* 1995; **12** suppl 2:S40–S41.
4. Viberti GC, Pickup JC, Jarrett RJ, Keen H. Effect of control of blood glucose on urinary excretion of albumin and β_2-microglobulin in insulin-dependent diabetes. *N Engl J Med* 1979; **300**:638–641.
5. Viberti GC, Pickup JC, Bilous RW, Keen H, MacKintosh D. Correction of exercise-induced microalbuminuria in insulin-dependent diabetics after 3 weeks of subcutaneous insulin infusion. *Diabetes* 1981; **30**:818–823.

6. Mathiesen ER, Gall M-A, Hommel E, Skott P, Parving HH. Effects of short-term strict metabolic control on kidney function and extracellular fluid volume in incipient diabetic nephropathy. *Diabet Med 1989;* **6**:595–600.

7. The Diabetes Control and Complications Trial Research Group. The effect of intensive treatment of diabetes on the development and progression of long-term complications in insulin-dependent diabetes mellitus. *N Engl J Med* 1993; **329**:977–986.

8. The Diabetes Control and Complications Trial Research Group. Effect of intensive therapy on the development and progression of diabetic nephropathy in the Diabetes Control and Complications Trial. *Kidney Int* 1995; **47**:1703–1720.

9. Microalbuminuria Collaborative Study Group, UK. Risk factors for development of microalbuminuria in insulin-dependent diabetic patients: a cohort study. *Br Med J* 1993; **306**:1235–1239.

10. Reichard P, Nilsson B-Y, Rosenqvist U. The effect of long-term intensified insulin treatment on the development of microvascular complications of diabetes mellitus. *N Engl J Med* 1993; **329**:304–309.

11. Dahl-Jorgensen K, Hanssen KF, Kierulf P, Bjoro T, Sandvik L, Aagenaes O. Reduction of urinary albumin excretion after 4 years of continuous subcutaneous insulin infusion in insulin-dependent diabetes mellitus. The Oslo Study. *Acta Endocrinol (Copenh)* 1988; **117**:19–25.

12. Bangstad H-J, Osterby R, Dahl-Jorgensen K, Berg KJ, Hartmann A, Hanssen KF. Improvement of blood glucose control in IDDM patients retards the progression of morphological changes in early diabetic nephropathy. *Diabetologia* 1994; **37**:483–490.

13. The Kroc Collaborative Study Group. Blood glucose control and the evolution of diabetic retinopathy and albuminuria. A preliminary multicenter trial. *N Engl J Med* 1984; **311**:365–372.

14. Krolewski AS, Laffel LMB, Krolewski M, Quinn M, Warram JH. Glycosylated haemoglobin and the risk of microalbuminuria in patients with insulin-dependent diabetes mellitus. *N Engl J Med* 1995; **332**:1251–1255.

15. The Diabetes Control and Complications Trial Research Group. The absence of a glycemic threshold for the development of long-term complications: the perspective of the Diabetes Control and Complications Trial. *Diabetes* 1996; **45**:1289–1298.

16. Ohkubo Y, Kishikawa H, Araki E, Miyata T, Isami S, Motoyoshi S, *et al.* Intensive insulin therapy prevents the progression of diabetic microvascular complications in Japanese patients with non-insulin-dependent diabetes mellitus: a randomised prospective 6-year study. *Diabetes Res Clin Pract* 1995; **28**:103–117.

17. Feldt-Rasmussen B, Mathiesen ER, Hegedus L, Deckert T. Kidney function during 12 months of strict metabolic control in insulin-dependent diabetic patients with incipient nephropathy. *N Engl J Med* 1986; **314**:665–670.

18. Feldt-Rasmussen B, Mathiesen ER, Deckert T. Effect of two years of strict metabolic control on progression of incipient nephropathy in insulin-dependent diabetes. *Lancet* 1986; **2**:1300–1304.

19. Microalbuminuria Collaborative Study Group. Intensive therapy and progression to clinical albuminuria in patients with insulin-dependent diabetes and microalbuminuria. *Br Med J* 1995; **311**:973–977.

20. Feldt-Rasmussen B, Mathiesen ER, Jensen T, Lauritzen T, Deckert T. Effect of improved metabolic control on loss of kidney function in Type 1 (insulin-dependent diabetic patients: an update of the Steno studies. *Diabetologia* 1991; **34**:164–170.

21. Deckert T, Lauritzen T, Parving HH, Sandhl Christiansen J and the Steno Study Group. Effect of two years of strict metabolic control on kidney function in long-term insulin-dependent diabetics. *Diabet Nephropathy* 1984; **3**:6–10.

22. Steno Study Group. Effect of 6 months of strict metabolic control on eye and kidney function in insulin-dependent diabetics with background retinopathy. *Lancet* 1982; **1**:121–124.

23. Wang PH, Lau J, Chalmers TC. Meta-analysis of effects of intensive blood-glucose control on late complications of insulin-dependent diabetes. *Lancet* 1993; **341**:1306–1309.

24. Blantz RC, Petersen OW, Gushwa L, Tucker BJ. Effect of modest hyperglycaemia on tubuloglomerular feedback activity. *Kidney Int* 1982; **22** suppl 12:S206–S212.

25. Wiseman MJ, Mangilli R, Alberetto M, Keen H, Viberti GC. Glomerular response mechanisms to glycaemic changes in insulin-dependent diabetics. *Kidney Int* 1987; **31**:1012–1018.

26. Bakris GL. Effects of diltiazem or lisinopril on massive proteinuria associated with diabetes mellitus. *Ann Intern Med* 1990; **112**:707–708.

27. Stornello M, Valvo EV, Scapellato L. Comparative effects of enalapril, atenolol and chlorthalidone on blood pressure and kidney function of diabetic patients affected by arterial hypertension and persistent proteinuria. *Nephron* 1991; **58**:52–57.

28. Bjork S, Mulec H, Johnsen SA, Nyberg G, Aurell M. Contrasting effects of enalapril and metoprolol in diabetic nephropathy. *Br Med J* 1990; **300**:904–907.

29. Bjork S, Mulec H, Johnsen SA, Norden G, Aurell M. Renal protective effect of enalapril in diabetic nephropathy. *Br Med J* 1992; **304**:339–343.

30. Parving HH, Hommel E, Smidt UM. Protection of kidney function and decrease in albuminuria by captopril in insulin-dependent diabetics with nephropathy. *Br Med J* 1988; **297**:1086–1091.

31. Mogensen CE. Long-term antihypertensive treatment inhibiting progression of diabetic nephropathy. *Br Med J* 1982; **285**:685–688.

32. Parving H-H, Andersen AR, Smidt UM, Svendsen PA. Early aggressive antihypertensive treatment reduces rate of decline in kidney function in diabetic nephropathy. *Lancet* 1983; **1**:1175–1179.

33. Lewis EJ, Hunsicker LG, Bain RP, Rohde RD for the Collaborative Study Group. The effect of angiotensin-converting-enzyme inhibition on diabetic nephropathy. *N Engl J Med* 1993; **329**:1456–1462.

34. Hommel E, Mathiesen ER, Edsberg B, Bahnsen M, Parving HH. Acute reduction of arterial blood pressure reduces urinary albumin excretion in Type 1 (insulin-dependent) diabetic patients with incipient nephropathy. *Diabetologia* 1986; **29**:211–215.

35. Parving HH, Kastrup J, Smidt UM. Reduced transcapillary escape of albumin during acute blood pressure-lowering in Type 1 (insulin-dependent) diabetic patients with nephropathy. *Diabetologia* 1985; **28**:797–801.

36. Christensen CK, Mogensen CE. Acute and long-term effect of antihypertensive treatment on exercise-induced albuminuria in incipient diabetic nephropathy. *Scand J Clin Lab Invest* 1986; **46**:553–559.

37. Rudberg S, Satterstrom G, Dahlqvist R, Dahlquist G. Indomethacin but not metoprolol reduced exercise-induced albumin excretion rate in Type 1 diabetic patients with microalbuminuria. *Diabet Med 1993;* **10**:460-464.

38. Romanelli G, Giustina A, Cimino A, Valentini U, Agabiti-Rosei E, Muiesan G, Giustina G. Short-term effect of captopril on microalbuminuria induced by exercise in normotensive diabetics. *Br Med J* 1989; **298**:284–288.

39. Romanelli G, Giustina A, Bossoni S, Caldonazzo A, Cimino A, Cravarezza P, Giustina G. Short-term administration of captopril and nifedipine and exercise-induced albuminuria in normotensive diabetic patients with early-stage nephropathy. *Diabetes* 1990; **39**:1333–1338.

40. Baba T, Murabayashi S, Takebe K. Comparison of the renal effects of angiotensin converting enzyme inhibitor and calcium antagonist in hypertensive Type 2 (non-insulin-dependent) diabetic patients with microalbuminuria: a randomised controlled trial. *Diabetologia* 1989; **32**:40–44.

41. Insua A, Ribstein J, Mimran A. Comparative effect of captopril and nifedipine in normotensive patients with incipient diabetic nephropathy. *Postgrad Med J* 1988; **64** suppl 3:59–62.

42. Mimran A, Insua A, Ribstein J, Bringer J, Monnier L. Comparative effects of captopril and nifedipine in normotensive patients with incipient diabetic nephropathy. *Diabetes Care* 1988; **11**:850–853.

43. Viberti GC, Mogensen CE, Groop LC, Pauls JF for the European Microalbuminuria Captopril Study Group. Effect of captropril on progression to clinical proteinuria in patients with insulin-dependent diabetes and microalbuminuria. *J Am Med Ass* 1994; **271**:275–279.

44. Laffel LMB, McGill JB, Gans DJ on behalf of the North American Microalbuminuria Study Group. The beneficial effect of angiotensin-converting enzyme inhibition with captopril on diabetic nephropathy in normotensive IDDM patients with microalbuminuria. *Am J Med* 1995; **99**: 497–504.

45. The Microalbuminuria Captopril Study Group. Captopril reduces the risk of nephropathy in IDDM patients with microalbuminuria. *Diabetologia* 1996; **39**:587–593.

46. Ravid M, Savin H, Jutrin I, Bental T, Katz B, Lishner M. Long-term stabilising effect of angiotensin-converting enzyme inhibition on plasma creatinine and on proteinuria in normotensive Type 2 diabetic patients. *Ann Intern Med* 1993; **118**:577–581.

47. Ravid M, Savin H, Jutrin I, Bental T, Lang R, Lishner M. Long-term effect of ACE inhibition on development of nephropathy in diabetes mellitus Type 2. *Kidney Int* 1994; **45** suppl 45:S161–S164.

48. Sano T, Kawamura T, Matsumae H, Sasaki H, Nakayama M, Hara T, *et al.* Effects of long-term enalapril treatment on persistent microalbuminuria in well-controlled hypertensive and normotensive NIDDM patients. *Diabetes Care* 1994; **17**:420-424.

49. Sano T, Hotta N, Kawamura T, Matsumae H, Chaya S, Sasaki H, *et al.* Effects of long-term enalapril treatment on persistent microalbuminuria in normotensive Type 2 diabetic patients: results of a 4-year, prospective, randomised study. *Diabet Med* 1996; **13**:120–124.

50. Marre M, Leblanc H, Suarez L, Guyenne T-T, Menard J, Passa P. Converting enzyme inhibition and kidney function in normotensive diabetic patients with persistent microalbuminuria. *Br Med J* 1987; **294**:1448–1452.

51. Marre M, Chatellier G, Leblanc H, Guyenne T-T, Menard J, Passa P. Prevention of diabetic nephropathy with enalapril in normotensive diabetics with microalbuminuria. *Br Med J* 1988; **297**:1092–1095.

52. Hallab M, Gallois Y, Chatellier G, Rohmer V, Fressinaud P, Marre M. Comparison of reduction in microalbuminuria by enalapril and hydrochlorothiazide in normotensive patients with insulin-dependent diabetes. *Br Med J* 1993; **306**:175–182.

53. Mathiesen ER, Hommel E, Giese J, Parving HH. Efficacy of captopril in postponing nephropathy in normotensive insulin-dependent diabetic patients with microalbuminuria. *Br Med J* 1991; **303**:81-87.

54. Melbourne Diabetic Nephropathy Study Group. Comparison between perindopril and nifedipine in hypertensive and normotensive diabetic patients with microalbuminuria. *Br Med J* 1991; **302**:210–216.

55. Lacourciere Y, Nadeau A, Poirier L, Tancrede G. Comparative effects of converting enzyme inhibition and conventional therapy in hypertensive non-insulin-dependent diabetics with normal renal function. *Clin Invest Med* 1991; **14**:652–660.

56. Hermans MP, Brichard SM, Colin I, Borgies P. Long-term reduction of microalbuminuria after 3 years of angiotensin converting enzyme inhibition by perindopril in hypertensive insulin-treated diabetic patients. *Am J Med* 1992; **92** suppl 48: 102S–107S.

57. Slomowitz LA, Bergamo R, Grosvenor M, Kopple JD. Enalapril reduces albumin excretion in diabetic patients with low levels of microalbuminuria. *Am J Nephrol* 1990; **10**:457–462.

58. Chan JCN, Cockram CS, Nicholls MG, Cheung CK, Swaminathan R. Comparison of enalapril and nifedipine in treating non-insulin-dependent diabetes associated with hypertension: one year analysis. *Br Med J* 1992; **305**:981–985.

59. Lebovitz HE, Wiegmann TB, Cnaan A, Shahinfar S, Sica D, Broadstone V, *et al.* Renal protective effects of enalapril in hypertensive NIDDM: role of baseline albuminuria. *Kidney Int* 1994; **45**: suppl 45:S150–S155.

60. Flack JR, Molyneaux L, Willey K, Yue DK. Regression of microalbuminuria: results of a controlled study, indapamide versus captopril. *J Cardiovasc Pharmacol* 1993; **22**: suppl 6:S75–S77.

61. Romero R, Salinas I, Lucas A, Abad E, Reverter JL, Johnston S, Sanmarti A. Renal function changes in microalbuminuric normotensive Type 2 diabetic patients treated with angiotensin-converting enzyme inhibitors. *Diabetes Care* 1993; **16**:597–600.

62. Taguma Y, Kitamoto Y, Futaki G, Ueda H, Monma H, Ishizaki M, *et al.* Effect of captopril on heavy proteinuria in azotemic diabetics. *N Engl J Med* 1985; **313**:1617–1620.

63. Wiegmann TB, Gigh Herron K, Chonko AM, MacDougall ML, Moore WV. Effect of angiotensin-converting enzyme inhibition on renal function and albuminuria in normotensive Type 1 diabetic patients. *Diabetes* 1992; **41**:62–67.

64. Kasiske BL, Kalil RSN, Ma JZ, Liao M, Keane WF. Effect of antihypertensive therapy on the kidney in patients with diabetes: a meta-regression analysis. *Ann Intern Med* 1993; **118**:129–138.

65. Weidmann P, Boehlen LM, de Courten M, Ferrari P. Antihypertensive therapy in diabetic patients. *J Hum Hypertens* 1992; **6** suppl 2:S23–S36.

66. Hostetter TH, Troy JL, Brenner BM. Glomerular haemodynamics in experimental diabetes mellitus. *Kidney Int* 1981; **19**:410–415.
67. Zatz R, Dunn BR, Meyer TW, Anderson S, Rennke HG, Brenner BM. Prevention of diabetic glomerulopathy by pharmacological amelioration of glomerular capillary hypertension. *J Clin Invest* 1986; **77**:1925–1930.
68. Anderson S, Rennke HG, Garcia DL, Brenner BM. Short and long-term effects of antihypertensive therapy in the diabetic rat. *Kidney Int* 1989; **36**: 526–536.
69. Anderson S, Rennke HG, Brenner BM, Zayas MA, Lafferty HM, Troy JL, Sandstrom DJ. Nifedipine versus fosinopril in uninephrectomized diabetic rats. *Kidney Int* 1992; **41**:891–897.
70. Cooper ME, Allen TJ, MacMillan PA, Clarke BE, Jerums G, Doyle AE. Enalapril retards glomerular basement membrane thickening and albuminuria in the diabetic rat. *Diabetologia* 1989; **32**:326–328.
71. Cooper ME, Allen TJ, O'Brien RC, Papazoglou D, Clarke BE, Jerums G, Doyle AE. Nephropathy in model combining genetic hypertension with experimental diabetes: enalapril versus hydralazine and metoprolol therapy. *Diabetes* 1990; **39**:1575–1579.
72. Cooper ME, Rumble JR, Allen TJ, O'Brien RC, Jerums G, Doyle A. Antihypertensive therapy in a model combining spontaneous hypertension with diabetes. *Kidney Int* 1992; **41**:898–903.
73. O'Brien RC, Cooper ME, Jerums G, Doyle AE. The effects of perindopril and triple therapy in a normotensive model of diabetic nephropathy. *Diabetes* 1993; **42**:604–609.
74. Fujihara CK, Padilha RM, Zatz R. Glomerular abnormalities in long-term experimental diabetes. *Diabetes* 1992; **41**:286–293.
75. Morelli E, Loon N, Meyer T, Peters W, Myers BD. Effects of converting-enzyme inhibition on barrier function in diabetic rats. *Diabetes* 1990; **39**:76–82.
76. Reddi AS, Ramamurthi R, Miller M, Dhuper S, Lasker N. Enalapril improves albuminuria by preventing glomerular loss of heparan sulphate in diabetic rats. *Biochem Med Metab Biol* 1991; **45**:119–131.
77. de Nicola L, Blantz RC, Gabbai B. Renal functional reserve in the early stage of experimental diabetes. *Diabetes* 1992; **41**:267–273.
78. Loutzenhiser R, Epstein M. Effects of calcium antagonists on renal haemodynamics. *Am J Physiol* 1985; **249**:F619–629.
79. Ichikawa I, Miele JF, Brenner BM. Reversal of renal cortical actions of angiotensin II by verapamil and manganese. *Kidney Int* 1979; **16**:137–147.
80. Yoshioka T, Shiraga H, Yoshida T, Fogo A, Glick AD, Deen WM, *et al.* Intact nephrons as the primary origin of proteinuria in chronic renal disease. *J Clin Invest* 1988; **82**:1614–1623.
81. Brown S, Walton C, Crawford P, Bakris GL. Renal response to angiotensin converting enzyme inhibition of calcium channel blockade in diabetic beagles. *J Am Soc Nephrol* 1991; **2**:286 (abstract).
82. Elving LD, Wetzels JFM, van Lier HJJ, de Nobel E, Berden JHM. Captopril and atenolol are equally effective in retarding progression of diabetic nephropathy. *Diabetologia* 1994; **37**:604–609.
83. Josefsberg Z, Ross SA, Lev-Ran A, Hwang DL. Effects of enalapril and nitrendipine on the excretion of epidermal growth factor and albumin in hypertensive NIDDM patients. *Diabetes Care* 1995; **18**:690–693.

84. Harper R, Ennis CN, Heaney AP, Sheridan B, Gormley M, Atkinson AB, *et al.* A comparison of the effects of low- and conventional-dose thiazide diuretic on insulin action in hypertensive patients with NIDDM. *Diabetologia* 1995; **38**:853–859.

85. Hypertension in Diabetes Study Group. Hypertension in diabetes III. Prospective study of therapy of hypertension in Type 2 diabetic patients: efficacy of ACE inhibition and B-blockade. *Diabet Med* 1994; **11**:773–782.

86. Chan JCN, Yeung VTF, Leung DHY, Tomlinson B, Nicholls MG, Cockram CS. The effects of enalapril and nifedipine on carbohydrate and lipid metabolism in NIDDM. *Diabetes Care* 1994; **17**:859–862.

87. Giordano M, Matsuda M, Sanders L, Canessa ML, DeFronzo RA. Effects of angiotensin-converting enzyme inhibitors, Ca^{2+} channel antagonists, and α- and β-adrenergic blockers on glucose and lipid metabolism in NIDDM patients with hypertension. *Diabetes* 1995; **44**:665–671.

88. Winocour PH, Catalano C, New J, Alberti KGMM. Contrasting renal and metabolic effects of alpha- and beta-adrenergic blockade in mildly hypertensive type 1 (insulin-dependent diabetic subjects. *Nutr Metab Cardiovasc Dis* 1995; **5**:217–224.

89. Walker WG, Hermann J, Murphy RP, Russell RP. Prospective study of the impact of hypertension upon kidney function in diabetes mellitus. *Nephron* 1990; **55** suppl 1:21–26.

90. Mogensen CE. Progression of nephropathy in long-term diabetics with proteinuria and effect of initial anti-hypertensive treatment. *Scand J Clin Lab Invest* 1976; **36**:383–388.

91. Sampson MJ, Griffith VS, Drury PL. Blood pressure, diet and the progression of nephropathy in patients with Type 1 diabetes and hypertension. *Diabet Med* 1994; **11**:150–154.

92. Drury P, Tarn AC. Are the WHO criteria for hypertension appropriate in young insulin-dependent diabetics? *Diabet Med* 1985; **2**:79–82.

93. Mau Pedersen M, Schimtz A, Bjerregaard Pedersen E, Danielsen H, Sandahl Christiansen J. Acute and long-term renal effects of angiotensin converting enzyme inhibition in normotensive, normoalbuminuric insulin-dependent diabetic patients. *Diabet Med* 1988; **5**:562–569.

94. Brenner BM, Meyer TW, Hostetter TW. Dietary intake and the progressive nature of kidney disease: the role of haemodynamically mediated glomerular injury in the pathogenesis of progressive glomerular sclerosis in aging, renal ablation and intrinsic renal disease. *N Engl J Med* 1982; **307**:652–659.

95. Zatz R, Meyer TW, Rennke HG, Brenner BM. Predominance of hemodynamic rather than metabolic factors in the pathogenesis of diabetic glomerulopathy. *Proc Natl Acad Sci USA* 1985; **82**:5963–5967.

96. Ciavarella A, di Mizio GF, Stefoni S, Borgnino LC, Vannini P. Reduced albuminuria after dietary protein restriction in insulin-dependent diabetic patients with clinical nephropathy. *Diabetes Care* 1987; **10**:407–413.

97. Bending JJ, Dodds RA, Keen H, Viberti GC. Renal response to restricted protein intake in diabetic nephropathy. *Diabetes* 1988; **37**:1641–1646.

98. Zeller K, Whittaker E, Sullivan L, Raskin P, Jacobson HR. Effect of restricting dietary protein on the progression of renal failure in patients with insulin-dependent diabetes mellitus. *N Engl J Med* 1991; **324**:78–84.

99. Evanoff G, Thompson C, Brown J, Weinman E. Prolonged dietary protein restriction in diabetic nephropathy. *Arch Intern Med* 1989; **149**:1129–1133.

100. Walker JD, Dodds RA, Murrells TJ, Bending JJ, Mattock MB, Keen H. Restriction of dietary protein and progression of renal failure in diabetic nephropathy. *Lancet* 1989; **2**:1411–1415.
101. Wiseman MJ, Bognetti E, Dodds R, Keen H, Viberti GC. Changes in renal function in response to protein restricted diet in type I (insulin-dependent) diabetic patients. *Diabetologia* 1987; **30**:154–159.
102. Cohen D, Dodds R, Viberti GC. Effect of protein restriction in insulin-dependent diabetics at risk of nephropathy. *Br Med J* 1987; **294**:795–798.
103. Rudberg S, Dahlquist G, Aperia A, Persson B. Reduction of protein intake decreases glomerular filtration rate in young Type 1 (insulin-dependent) diabetic patients mainly in hyperfiltering patients. *Diabetologia* 1988; **31**: 878–883.
104. Dullaart RPF, Beusekamp BJ, Meijer S, van Doormaal JJ, Sluiter WJ. Long-term effects of protein-restricted diet on albuminuria and renal function in IDDM patients without clinical nephropathy and hypertension. *Diabetes Care* 1993; **16**:483–492.
105. Jibani MM, Bloodworth LL, Foden E, Griffiths KD, Galpin OP. Predominantly vegetarian diet in patients with incipient and early nephropathy: effects on albumin excretion rate and nutritional status. *Diabet Med* 1991; **8**:949–953.
106. Pecis M, de Azevedo M, Gross JL. Chicken and fish diet reduces glomerular hyperfiltration in IDDM patients. *Diabetes Care* 1994; **17**:665–672.
107. Adam O, Wolfram G. Effect of different linoleic acid intakes on prostaglandin biosynthesis and kidney function in man. *Am J Clin Nutr* 1984; **40**:763–770.
108. Dullaart RPF, Beusekamp BJ, Meijer S, Hoogenberg K, van Doormaal JJ, Sluiter WJ. Long-term effects of linoleic-acid-enriched diet on albuminuria and lipid levels in Type 1 (insulin-dependent) diabetic patients with elevated urinary albumin excretion. *Diabetologia* 1992; **35**:165–172.
109. Nielsen S, Hermansen K, Rasmussen OW, Thomsen C, Mogensen CE. Urinary albumin excretion rate and 24 h ambulatory blood pressure in NIDDM with microalbuminuria: effects of a monounsaturated-enriched diet. *Diabetologia* 1995; **38**:1069–1075.
110. Jensen T, Stender S, Goldstein K, Holmer G, Deckert T. Partial normalisation by dietary cod-liver oil of increased microvascular albumin leakage in patients with insulin-dependent diabetes and albuminuria. *N Engl J Med* 1989; **321**:1572–1577.
111. Hommel E, Mathiesen ER, Arnold-Larsen S, Edsberg B, Olsen UB, Parving HH. Effects of indomethacin on kidney function in Type 1 (insulin-dependent) diabetic patients with nephropathy. *Diabetologia* 1987; **30**:78–81.
112. Mathiesen ER, Hommel E, Olsen UB, Parving HH. Elevated urinary prostaglandin excretion and the effect of indomethacin on renal function in incipient diabetic nephropathy. *Diabet Med* 1988; **5**:145–149.
113. Beyer-Meyers A, Ku L, Cohen MP. Glomerular polyol accumulation in diabetes and its prevention by oral sorbinil. *Diabetes* 1984; **33**:604–607.
114. Chang WP, Dimitriadis E, Allen T, Dunlop ME, Cooper M, Larkins RG. The effect of aldose reductase inhibitors on glomerular prostaglandin production and urinary albumin excretion in experimental diabetes mellitus. *Diabetologia* 1991; **34**:225–231.

115. McCaleb ML, McKean ML, Hohman TC, Laver N, Robinson Jr WG. Intervention with the aldose reductase inhibitor, tolrestat, in renal and retinal lesions of streptozotocin-diabetic rats. *Diabetologia* 1991; **34**:695–701.

116. Korner A, Celsi G, Eklof A-C, Linne T, Persson B, Aperia A. Sorbinil does not prevent hyperfiltration, elevated ultrafiltration pressure and albuminuria in streptozotocin-diabetic rats. *Diabetologia* 1992; **35**:414–418.

117. Passariello N, Sepe J, Marrazzo G, De Cicco A, Peluso A, Pisano MCA, *et al.* Effect of aldose reductase inhibitor (tolrestat) on urinary albumin excretion rate and glomerular filtration rate in IDDM subjects with nephropathy. *Diabetes Care* 1993; **16**:789–795.

118. Soulis-Liparota T, Cooper M, Parazoglou D, Clarke B, Jerums G. Retardation by aminoguanidine of development of albuminuria, mesangial expansion and tissue fluorescence in streptozotocin-induced diabetic rat. *Diabetes* 1991; **40**:1328–1334.

119. Edelstien D, Brownlee M. Aminoguanidine ameliorates albuminuria in diabetic hypertensive rats. *Diabetologia* 1992; **35**:96–97.

120. Huijberts MSP, Wolffenbuttel BHR, Crijns FRL, Nieuwenhuijzen Kruseman AC, Bemelmans MHA, Struijker Boudier HAJ. Aminoguanidine reduces regional albumin clearance but not urinary albumin excretion in streptozotocin-diabetic rats. *Diabetologia* 1994; **37**:10–14.

121. Corbett JA, Tilton RG, Chang K, Hasan KS, Ido Y, Wang Jl, *et al.* Aminoguanidine, a novel inhibitor of nitric oxide formation, prevents diabetic vascular dysfunction. *Diabetes* 1992; **41**:552–556.

122. Tilton RG, Chang K, Hasan KS, Smith SR, Petrash JM, Misko TP, *et al.* Prevention of diabetic vascular disease by guanidines. Inhibition of nitric oxide synthesis versus advanced glycation end-product formation. *Diabetes* 1993; **42**:221–232.

123. Floege J, Eng E, Young BA, Couser GH, Johnson RJ. Heparin suppresses mesangial cell proliferation and matrix expansion in experimental mesangioproliferative glomerulonephritis. *Kidney Int* 1993; **43**:369–380.

124. Gambaro G, Cavazzana AO, Luzi P, Piccoli A, Borsatti A, Crepaldi G, *et al.* Glycosaminoglycans prevent morphological renal alterations and albuminuria in diabetic rats. *Kidney Int* 1993; **42**:285–291.

125. Nadar HB, Bounassisi V, Colburn P, Dietrich CP. Heparin stimulates the synthesis and modifies the sulfation pattern of heparan sulfate proteoglycan from endothelial cells. *J Cell Physiol* 1989; **140**:305–310.

126. Tan M-S, Tsai J-C, Lee Y-J, Chen H-C, Shin S-J, Lai Y-H, *et al.* Induction of heparin-binding epidermal growth factor-like growth factor mRNA by protein kinase C activators. *Kidney Int* 1994; **46**:690–695.

127. Groggel GC, Marinides GN, Hovingh P, Hammond E, Linker A. Inhibition of rat mesangial cell growth by heparan sulphate. *Am J Physiol* 1990; **258**:F259–F265.

128. Wolthuis A, Boes A, Berden JHM, Grond J. Heparins modulate extracellular matrix and protein synthesis of cultured rat mesangial cells. *Virchows Archiv B Cell Pathol* 1993; **63**:181–189.

129. Myrup B, Hansen PM, Jensen T, Kofoed-Enevoldsen A, Feldt-Rasmussen B, Gram J, *et al.* Effect of low-dose heparin on urinary albumin excretion in insulin-dependent diabetes mellitus. *Lancet* 1995; **345**:421–422.

130. Marshall SM, Hansen KW, Osterby R, Frystyk J, Orskov H, Flyvbjerg A. The effects of heparin on renal morphology and albuminuria in experimental diabetes. *Am J Physiol* 1996; **217** E326–E332.

131. Solini A, Vergnani L, Ricci F, Crepaldi G. Glycosaminoglycans delay the progression of nephropathy in NIDDM. *Diabetes Care* 1997; **20**:819–823.

132. Moorhead JF, El-Nahas M, Chan MK, Varghese Z. Lipid nephrotoxicity in chronic progressive glomerular and tubulo-intestital disease. *Lancet* 1982; **2**:1310–1311.

133. Diamond JR, Karnovsky MJ. Exacerbation of chronic aminonucleoside nephrosis by dietary cholesterol supplementation. *Kidney Int* 1987; **32**:671–677.

134. Kasiske BI, O'Donnell M, Cleary MP, Keane WF. Effects of reduced renal mass on tissue lipids and renal injury in hyperlipidaemic rats. *Kidney Int* 1989; **35**:40–47.

135. Mulec H, Johnson S-AA, Bjorck S. Relation between serum cholesterol and diabetic nephropathy. *Lancet* 1990; **335**:1537–1538.

136. Scanferla F, Landini S, Fracasso A, Morachiello P, Righetto F, Toffoletto P-P, *et al*. Risk factors for progression of diabetic nephropathy: role of hyperlipidaemia and its correction. *Acta Diabetol* 1992; **29**:268–272.

137. Hommel E, Andersen P, Gall M-A, Nielson F, Jensen B, Rossing P, *et al*. Plasma lipoproteins and renal function during simvastatin treatment in diabetic nephropathy. *Diabetologia* 1992; **35**:447–451.

138. Lam KSL, Cheng IKP, Janus ED, Pang RWC. Cholesterol-lowering therapy may retard the progression of diabetic nephropathy. *Diabetologia* 1995; **38**:604–609.

139. Zhang A, Vertommen J, Van Gaal L, De Leeuw I. Effects of pravastatin on lipid levels, in vitro oxidizability of non-HDL lipoproteins and microalbuminuria in IDDM patients. *Diabetes Res Clin Prac* 1995; **29**: 189–194.

140. Ravid M, Neumann L, Lishner M. Plasma lipids and the progression of nephropathy in diabetes mellitus type II: effect of ACE inhibitors. *Kidney Int* 1995; **47**:907–910.

141. Keilani T, Schlueter WA, Levin ML, Batlle DC. Improvement of lipid abnormalities associated with proteinuria using fosinopril, an angiotensin-converting enzyme inhibitor. *Ann Intern Med* 1993; **118**:246–254.

142. Owens D, Stinson J, Collins P, Johnson A, Tomkin GH. Improvement in the regulation of cellular cholesterologenesis in diabetes: the effect of reduction in serum cholesterol by simvastatin. *Diabet Med* 1991; **8**:151–156.

143. Flyvbjerg A, Frystyk Y, Sillesen IB, Orskov H. Growth hormone and insulin-like growth factor 1 in experimental and human diabetes. In: KGMM Alberti, LP Krall (eds). *The Diabetes Annual*, vol. 6. Elsevier Science Publishers, BV, Amsterdam, 1991, pp 562–590.

144. Mau Pedersen, Engkjaer Christensen S, Sandahl Christiansen J, Bjerregaard Pedersen E, Mogensen CE, Orskov H. Acute effects of a somatostatin analogue on kidney function in Type 1 diabetic patients. *Diabet Med* 1990; **7**:304–309.

145. Jacobs ML, Derkx FHM, Stijnen T, Lamberts SWJ, Weber RFA. Effect of long–acting somatostatin analogue (Somatulin) on renal hyperfiltration in patients with IDDM. *Diabetes Care* 1997; **20**:632–636.

146. Bilous RW, Marshall SM. Diabetic nephropathy: clinical aspects. In KGMM Alberti, H. Keen, RW de Fronzo (eds) *International Textbook of Diabetes.* John Wiley, London. 1997, pp 1363–1412.

147. Parving H-H, Jensen H, Mogensen CE, Evrin PE. Increased urinary albumin excretion rate in benign essential hypertension. *Lancet* 1974; **1**:1190–1192.

148. Pedersen EB, Mogensen CE. Effect of antihypertensive treatment on urinary albumin excretion, glomerular filtration rate, and renal plasma flow in patients with essential hypertension. *Scand J Clin Lab Invest* 1976; **36**:231–237.

149. Pedersen EB, Mogensen CE, Larsen JS. Effects of exercise on urinary excretion of albumin and ß$_2$-microglobulin in young patients with mild essential hypertension without treatment and during long-term propranolol treatment. *Scan J Clin Lab Invest* 1981; **41**:493–498.

150. Gosling P, Andrews DJ, Chesner IM. Effect of anti-inflammatory drugs on urinary microalbumin excretion. *Lancet* 1991; **337**:855.

151. Mittleman KD, Zambraski EJ. Exercise-induced proteinuria is attenuated by indomethacin. *Med Sci Sport Exercise* 1992; **24**:1069–1074.

152. De Venuto G, Andreotti C, Matterei M, Pegoretti G. Long term captopril therapy at low doses reduces albumin excretion in patients with essential hypertension and no signs of renal impairment. *J Hypertens* 1988; **6**:919–923.

153. Samuelsson O, Hedner T, Ljungman S, Herlitz H, Widgren B, Pennert K. A comparative study of lisinopril and atenolol on low degree urinary albumin excretion, renal function and haemodynamics in uncomplicated, primary hypertension. *Eur J Clin Pharmacol* 1992; **43**:469–475.

154. Bianchi S, Bigazzi R, Baldari G, Campese VM. Microalbuminuria in patients with essential hypertension: efects of several antihypertensive drugs. *Am J Med* 1992; **93**:525–528.

155. Laville M, Doche C, Fauvel JP, Pozet N, Hadj-Aissa A, Zech P. Effect of beta-blockade on albumin excretion rate in essential hypertension. *Nephron* 1990; **54**:183–184.

156. Hartford M, Wendelhag I, Berglund G, Wallentin I, Ljungman S, Wikstrand J. Cardiovascular and renal effects of long-term antihypertensive treatment. *J Am Med Ass* 1988; **259**:2553–2557.

157. Bianchi S, Bigazzi R, Baldari G, Campese VM. Microalbuminuria in patients with essential hypertension: effects of an angiotensin converting enzyme inhibitor and of a calcium channel blocker. *Am J Hypertens* 1991; **4**:291–296.

158. Reams GP, Hamory A, Lau A, Bauer JH. Effect of nifedipine on renal function in patients with essential hypertension. *Hypertension* 1988; **11**:452–456.

159. Persson B, Andersson OK, Wysocki M, Hedner T, Karlberg B. Calcium antagonism in essential hypertension: effect on renal haemodynamics and microalbuminuria. *J Intern Med* 1992; **231**:247–252.

160. Erley CM, Haefele U, Heyne N, Braun N, Risler T. Microalbuminuria in essential hypertension. Reduction by different antihypertensive drugs. *Hypertension* 1993; **21**:810–815.

161. Valvo E, Casagrande P, Bedogna V, Antiga L, Alberti D, Zamboni M, *et al.* Systemic and renal effects of a new angiotensin converting enzyme inhibitor, benazepril, in essential hypertension. *J Hypertens* 1990; **8**:991–995.

162. Ribstein J, Du Cailar G, Brouard R, Mimran A. Comparative renal and cardiac effects of tertatolol and enalapril in essential hypertension. *Cardiology* 1993; **83**, suppl 1,57–63.

Index

ACE inhibitors, 111, 204, 209–16, 221, 233
  comparative trials, 217–18
  lipid lowering effect, 228
  possible deleterious effects, 218–19
  see also individual drugs
acquired immunodeficiency syndrome (AIDS), 184
acromegaly, 185
acute phase response, 180–1, 182
adenocarcinoma, 183
age influences, 45, 46–7, 64
Albufast, 17
albumin, 7
  albumin:creatinine ratio, 22–7, 41–7
  excretion rate (AER)
    day-to-day variation, 21
    diurnal variation, 19–21
    influencing factors, 8–9
    microalbuminuria progression and, 84
    pregnancy and, in diabetes, 84–6
  structure and function of, 7
  transcapillary escape, 109
  urinary excretion mechanisms, 5–6
  see also microalbuminuria; urinary protein
    excretion
albuminuria *see* microalbuminuria; urinary protein
  excretion
Albuscreen, 15
Albusure kit, 15–16
alcohol intake, 45, 49, 133
aldose reductase inhibitors, 225–6
alpha-blocking agents, 221, 233
alpha-1-microglobulin, 7, 73
alprenolol, 230
aminoguanidine, 226
amylase, 71
anaesthesia, 181
angina, 154–5, 158
angiotensin converting enzyme (ACE), 100, 107,
  112
  see also ACE inhibitors
angiotensin II, 5, 100
  receptor antagonist, 216

antihypertensive agents, 204–21
  comparative trials, 216–18
  deleterious effects of, 218–19
  effects of blood pressure reduction
    acute and short-term effects, 204–6
    longer-term effects, 206–9
  specific intra-renal effect, 209–11
    mechanisms for, 211–16
  target blood pressure, 219–21
  see also blood pressure; hypertension; *individual*
    drugs
antioxidants, 147
antiprostaglandins, 225
antithrombin III, 143, 144, 145
apolipoproteins, 130, 137–9, 141 2
arachidonic acid, 101, 102
aspirin, 111, 230
atenolol, 216, 218, 219
atherosclerosis, 116, 163
  endothelium role in, 106–7
  free radical activity and, 147
  in diabetic subjects, 157–60
    insulin-dependent diabetes, 160
    non-insulin-dependent diabetes, 149, 157–60
  in non-diabetic subjects, 154–6
  see also cardiovascular disease
autoregulation, 3

basement membrane, 3, 105
Bence–Jones proteinuria, 177, 183
bendrofluazide, 209
beta blockers, 133, 204, 218, 232
  see also individual drugs
beta-2-microglobulin, 7
blood glucose *see* glycaemia; hyperglycaemia
blood glucose control, 193–204
  acute effects in long-term diabetes, 193–5
  primary prevention, 195–200
  secondary prevention, 200–4
blood pressure, 40
  definition of, 117
  microalbuminuria relationships, 45, 46, 47–8, 64